Springer
Tokyo
Berlin
Heidelberg
New York
Barcelona
Hong Kong
London
Milan
Paris
Singapore

S. Tanaka, C. Hamanishi (Eds.)

Advances in Osteoarthritis

With 127 Figures

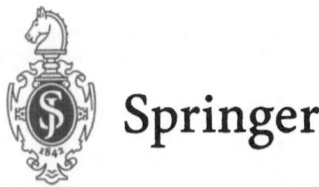

Springer

Seisuke Tanaka, M.D.
Dean
Kinki University School of Medicine
377-2 Ohno-Higashi, Osaka-Sayama
Osaka 589-8511, Japan

Chiaki Hamanishi, M.D.
Professor
Department of Orthopedic Surgery
Kinki University School of Medicine
377-2 Ohno-Higashi, Osaka-Sayama
Osaka 589-8511, Japan

ISBN-13: 978-4-431-68499-2   e-ISBN-13: 978-4-431-68497-8
DOI: 10.1007/978-4-431-68497-8

Library of Congress Cataloging-in-Publication Data

Advances in osteoarthritis / S. Tanaka, C. Hamanishi (eds.)
    p. cm.
    Includes bibliographical references and indexes.

    1. Osteoarthritis—Congresses.   I. Tanaka, S. (Seisuke). 1930–   II.
Hamanishi, C. (Chiaki), 1946–
    RO931.067   A38   1999
    616.7′223—dc21   98-46286
                                                       CIP

Printed on acid-free paper

© Springer-Verlag Tokyo 1999
Softcover reprint of the hardcover 1st edition 1999

Typesetting: Best-set Typesetter Ltd., Hong Kong

SPIN: 10694225

Preface

Basic research on osteoarthritis has been carried out mainly from the histological and biochemical aspects of the degenerating chondrocytes, collagen fibers, and matrix proteoglycans. Undue mechanical stress has been shown to be the principal factor in the initiation of osteoarthritis. Although the exact process by which mechanical stress leads to the total destruction of cartilage tissue remains unclear, several new research methods have enabled us to gain a deeper understanding of the process of degeneration.

In October 1997, we organized an international symposium titled "Advances in Osteoarthritis" in Kobe, with the main topics being updated research, diagnosis, and treatment of osteoarthritis. The proceedings of the symposium are presented here in five sections: (1) Mechanical stress and reactions of chondrocytes, such as intracellular ion changes, changes in the cytoskeleton, intracellular messenger systems, release of gas mediators, and changes in electromechanical properties of cartilage; (2) Functional diagnosis of osteoarthritis by MR imaging, and using calpain and collagenase III as new cartilage markers; (3) Treatment with a promising simple washout technique and IL-1RA and MMP antagonists; (4) Cartilage repair by new grafting techniques; and (5) Problems following total joint replacement.

We sincerely hope that the advanced knowledge provided in this volume of proceedings will be valuable to our readers.

SEISUKE TANAKA
CHIAKI HAMANISHI

Table of Contents

F. Problems Following Total Joint Replacement

List of Contributors

A. Mechanical Stress and Chondrocyte Reactions

Extracellular Ions and Hydrostatic Pressure: Their Influence on Chondrocyte Intracellular Ionic Composition

JILL P.G. URBAN and ROBERT J. WILKINS

Summary. The maintenance of a constant intracellular ionic environment is vital for cell viability and its proper function. To this end, cells possess an elaborate set of membrane proteins that transport ions across the plasma membrane. Intracellular ionic composition is determined by the activity of these transporters and by the extracellular ionic environment. The matrix in which chondrocytes are embedded is highly unusual when compared with the surroundings of other mammalian cells. In addition, the physical environment of the chondrocytes is routinely altered by load. By altering ionic gradients and transporter activity, load-induced changes to the matrix have knock-on effects on intracellular composition. This has important consequences for intracellular reactions such as macromolecule synthesis and hence matrix integrity. The carrier proteins present in chondrocytes to regulate cell composition therefore have a vital role to play in maintaining matrix integrity. We consider the specific challenges presented by the physical environment of chondrocytes and the ways in which these cells respond to them.

Key Words. Membrane transport, pH, Cell volume, Osmotic pressure, Matrix synthesis

Introduction

Chondrocytes of cartilage are embedded in a dense extracellular matrix, and interactions between cells and matrix govern cellular behavior in a variety of ways. This brief review focuses on an aspect of matrix–cell interactions that has perhaps been rather neglected: it discusses the effect of the extracellular matrix and of hydrostatic pressure on the intracellular ionic composition of the chondrocyte and how this has a role in regulating chondrocyte behaviour.

University Laboratory of Physiology, Parks Road, Oxford OX1 3PT, U.K.

The Intracellular Ionic Environment

Maintenance of Intracellular Ionic Composition

The maintenance of a constant intracellular ionic environment is vital for cell viability and its proper function. To this end, cells possess an elaborate set of membrane proteins that include ion pumps, carriers, and channels [1]. The keystone transporter in this homeostasis is the Na^+-K^+ ATPase, or sodium pump; this carrier extrudes sodium ions from the cell in exchange for potassium ions, energized by the hydrolysis of ATP. As a consequence of this active transport, an asymmetry of these two major cations is established across the plasma membrane: potassium is the major intracellular cation, while sodium is mostly extracellular [2].

There are several important explanations for this partition, all of which reflect the role of the sodium pump in keeping intracellular composition steady. First, the pump serves to maintain steady-state volume by ensuring that impermeant intracellular osmotic particles such as structural proteins are balanced by extracellular sodium. By effectively "trapping" sodium outside the cell (creating a double Donnan arrangement), extracellular and intracellular osmolarities are kept in balance and cell volume is fixed. In addition, the sodium pump is responsible for bioelectricity: the separation of cations underpins the establishment of the resting membrane potential and provides the ionic gradients by which the action potential can be evoked in excitable tissues. Third, many intracellular enzymes are highly dependent on potassium concentration, so that changes in cell salt composition can affect macromolecular structure, thereby altering rates of intracellular reactions. Finally, and most importantly in the present context, the inwardly directed sodium electrochemical gradient and the outwardly directed potassium gradient can be coupled to the movement of other ions and solutes. Symport, where the cation moves down its gradient in concert with the movement of a solute in the same direction, and antiport, in which the cation is exchanged for solute on the opposite side of the membrane, are both vital processes for cellular homeostasis. The energy contained within the sodium and potassium gradients (established by the primary hydrolysis of ATP) is used to move other solutes such as glucose or H^+ against their electrochemical gradients [1,3].

Cellular Homeostasis and Membrane Transport

Three key cellular parameters that must be regulated are cellular volume, pH, and calcium concentration [1,4]. All three are well established as regulators of cellular function, and as we shall see, this is especially true in the case of chondrocytes. Furthermore, the three variables are interlinked: changes in cell volume often produce changes in cellular calcium, while calcium concentration may be reciprocally related to intracellular pH [5]. Not surprisingly, therefore, some overlap in the manner of their regulation has been found.

As Fig. 1 shows, a variety of symporters and antiporters are expressed by mammalian cells to restore cell composition following any disturbance. When cells shrink, volume is restored by the sodium-driven influx of chloride ions, followed by osmotically obliged water movement (regulatory volume increase, RVI). The Na^+-Cl^- influx may be by symport (Na^+-K^+-$2Cl^-$ cotransport) or by the parallel operation of two antiporters ($Na^+ \times H^+$ exchange and $Cl^- \times HCO_3^-$ exchange) [1,6]. In contrast, cell swelling is countered by potassium-driven chloride efflux (K^+-Cl^- cotransport) [1,6], or by the loss of potassium ions and other intracellular osmotic particles (such as sorbitol, betaine, taurine) through a membrane channel (regulatory volume decrease, RVD) [7]. pH is regulated by a series of sodium-driven carriers that either extrude H^+ ions ($Na^+ \times H^+$ exchange, this time operating without the anion exchanger) or

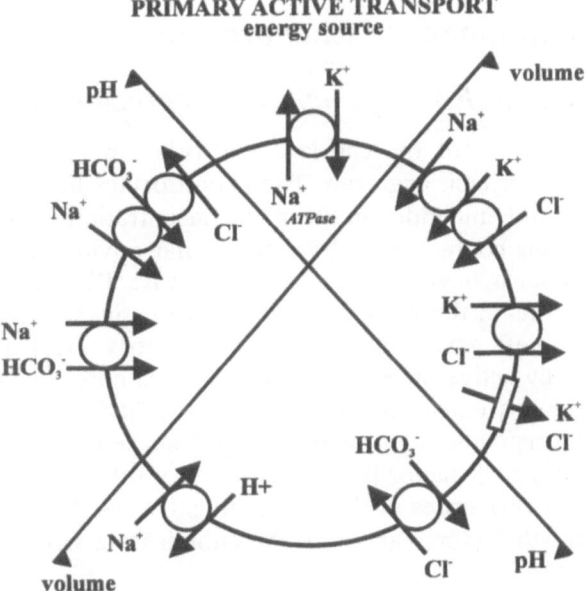

FIG. 1. Schematic of major transport proteins regulating cellular volume and pH in mammalian cells. Na^+ pumping in exchange for K^+, energized by the hydrolysis of ATP, establishes cation electrochemical gradients that can move other solutes. For volume regulation, recovery from shrinkage may be mediated by Na^+-K^+-$2Cl^-$ symport or the parallel operation of $Na^+ \times H^+$ and $Cl \times HCO_3^-$ antiport. Following swelling, the cell recovers using K^+-Cl^- symport or K^+ efflux via channels. For pH regulation, recovery from acidosis is mediated by the $Na^+ \times H^+$ antiport or by HCO_3^-, uptake either as Na^+-HCO_3^- antiport or by $Na^+ \times HCO_3^- \times Cl^-$ antiport. The Cl^- and HCO_3^- antiporter operates to restore pH following cellular alkalinization

import HCO_3^- ions, which buffer H^+ ($Na \times 2HCO_3^- \times Cl^-$ exchange or Na^+-HCO_3^- cotransport) [1]. Finally, disturbances of calcium concentration are countered by sodium-driven calcium ion extrusion ($Na^+ \times Ca^{2+}$ exchange) or primary active Ca^{2+} pumps (Ca^{2+}-ATPase) [8].

The matrix in which chondrocytes are embedded is highly unusual when compared with the surroundings of other mammalian cells, and the cells are subjected to marked variations in their extracellular environment. These changes have knock-on effects on intracellular composition, with important consequences for intracellular reactions such as macromolecule synthesis and hence matrix integrity. The carrier proteins present in chondrocytes to regulate parameters such as pH, cell volume, and calcium concentration therefore have a vital role to play in maintaining matrix integrity. We now consider the specific challenges presented by the physical environment of chondrocytes and the ways in which these cells respond to them.

Physical Environment of Chondrocytes

Regulation of the Environment by Aggrecan Content

The main components of the cartilage matrix are collagen and the large aggregating proteoglycan, aggrecan. The chondrocytes lie mainly separated from each other and embedded in this high concentration of aggrecan, which thus regulates their contact with the extracellular environment. The matrix may modify cellular behavior in many different ways. Binding of matrix components to integrins in the plasma membrane can trigger second-messenger responses and initiate gene expression [9]. The matrix affects the concentration of biologically active molecules around the chondrocyte by providing a selective permeability barrier that prevents large molecules from reaching the chondrocyte; matrix components may also bind and sequester molecules such as transforming growth factor-beta (TGF-β) or insulin-like growth factor-1 (IGF-1) [10]. The properties of the matrix thus govern the manner in which nutrients or growth factors can reach the chondrocyte from the circulation [11].

Aggrecan concentration also regulates extracellular ionic concentrations. The concentration of fixed negative charges on the glycosaminoglycan (GAG) side chains of these molecules regulates the ionic composition of the extracellular matrix through the Gibbs–Donnan equilibrium [11]. Both in vivo and in vitro, the concentration of free cations (including H^+) in the matrix is greater than in the surrounding serum or culture medium, whereas anion concentrations are depressed [12]. Ion concentrations and pH thus vary across the joint in relation to local gradients in aggrecan concentration and will change if aggrecan concentration falls (e.g., as a result of loss of proteoglycan in osteoarthritis or by dilution in vitro when cartilage swells) or if it increases (e.g., when water is expressed under compressive load). Because extracellular osmolality depends mostly on free diffusible species in the tissue, it is also influenced by ion concentrations and thus aggrecan content; the average osmolality in bovine metacarpophalangeal cartilage is about 400 mOsm, compared to 300 mOsm in serum [13].

In addition to the influence of GAG concentration, extracellular pH is regulated by cellular energy metabolism. Chondrocytes undergo aerobic glycolysis and thus produce lactic acid at a high rate [14]. Because cartilage is avascular, steep gradients in lactic acid develop through the depth of the tissue, with lactic acid concentrations being highest in regions furthest from synovial fluid or the blood supply. As extracellular pH is directly affected by lactic acid concentration, any change in energy production will also affect extracellular pH. The extent of changes has not been determined in articular cartilage, but concentrations greater than 12 mM lactic acid (compared to 1 mM lactic acid in serum) and pH levels below pH 6.5 have been measured in intervertebral disks [15].

Changes in the Physical Environment Induced by Load

Articular cartilage is routinely subjected to high external forces that arise from muscle contraction as well as from body weight, and thus vary with posture and movement [16]. Because joints are not congruent, some areas are loaded under most conditions while others are barely exposed to load. The degree of congruency varies from joint to joint, with the ankle, for example, being usually more congruent than the hip. Cartilage of the latter joint thus experiences higher peak stresses for the same applied load; peak pressures of 10–20 MPa have been measured in some regions of hip cartilage [17]. The loading pattern of cartilage from different joints is of interest because it is areas exposed to high load that initially develop osteoarthritic changes.

When cartilage is loaded, the matrix deforms, hydrostatic pressure rises, and the resulting pressure gradient leads to expression of fluid from the pressurized to less pressurized regions. During a normal walking cycle (about 1 Hz), fluid loss is minimal during the loading period of the cycle, recovery is virtually complete, and deformation is virtually at constant volume. However, if the period of cyclical loading is prolonged or long-term static loads occur, significant amounts of fluid can be lost from the tissue. Thus, the effect of load on the physical environment of cartilage depends on the duration and level of the load, and will depend on the material properties of the cartilage and vary from joint to joint. The same load will lead to a smaller rise of pressure in the ankle than the hip because of differences in congruity and will result in a greater degree of fluid loss and deformation in degenerate than normal cartilage [16].

Load and Cartilage Metabolism

It has long been known from in vivo and in vitro studies that mechanical load can influence chondrocyte metabolism and, despite the low cell density of these tissues, ultimately affect the composition of the cartilage matrix [18]. Studies on joints of animals subjected to strenuous exercise regimens have found that changes in customary loading pattern lead to alterations in cartilage composition and cell morphology [19]. In vitro studies have also found that production of different components of the extracellular matrix are affected by load, with response affected by loading pattern [20]. In general, loads that lead to net fluid expression depress matrix synthesis, whereas loads that lead to short applications of hydrostatic pressure or rapid pulses of fluid flow stimulate aggrecan production [21].

It is now apparent that chondrocytes do not respond to load as such but that their behavior is affected by load-induced changes in their extracellular environment [22]. Loading of the matrix induces both cell and matrix deformation and, in isolated chondrocytes at least, deformation of the cell affects membrane potential and second-messenger pathways [23]. The rise in hydrostatic pressure induced under load has been shown to affect rates of aggrecan expression and aggrecan synthesis, TGF-β1 and heat-shock protein expression, and matrix metalloproteinase production, with the respose depending on the duration and magnitude of pressure application [24,25]. Fluid shear has also been shown to increase aggrecan synthesis and also to influence expression of cytokines and growth factors, at least in isolated chondrocytes [26]. Expression of fluid under load, which leads to an increase in the concentration of cations and also a fall in extracellular pH, has been shown to suppress matrix synthesis [27]. These changes in ionic environment have been studied independently of changes in fluid content; response to these changes are similar to those seen after fluid expression [28].

The mechanisms by which such extracellular signals are translated into biochemical responses are not yet understood. However, it appears that strain and pressure at least can cause alterations in the chondrocyte cytoskeleton that may in turn affect signaling pathways or may even influence the nucleus directly [23,29]. Although these have not yet been fully investigated, it seems possible that stretch and pressure, for example, affect distinct second-messenger pathways and thus elicit specific responses. In this way the chondrocyte may regulate its response differentially in relation to changing aspects of load.

Load can also have a more direct effect on chondrocyte metabolism. Load-induced alterations in the extracellular matrix, particularly an increase in cation concentration and osmolality or a change in pressure, may affect transmembrane gradients of ions and transporter activity and thus alter intracellular ionic composition. The remainder of this chapter discusses the effects of changes in osmolality and pressure on matrix metabolism and show how these effects may be mediated in part at least by changes in intracellular ion concentrations.

Extracellular Ionic Environment

Effect of Extracellular Ions on Matrix Turnover

We have found that the rate of matrix synthesis in chondrocytes is strongly affected by changes in extracellular concentrations of Na^+, K^+, and H^+ and also by changes in osmolality. The change in synthesis rates induced by ions can be greater than that arising from growth factor or cytokine additions, and occurs much more rapidly, suggesting that the action of ions and that of growth factors occurs by different mechanisms.

Osmotic Pressure and Sodium

If bovine articular chondrocytes, isolated from the tissue by enzyme digestion, are incubated in tissue culture medium whose sodium concentration and osmotic pressure are increased by the addition of solid NaCl, aggrecan synthesis initially increases steeply and rapidly with rise in concentration from about 120–140 mM Na^+ (concentration in standard tissue culture medium) to about 200–220 mM Na^+ (in situ concentration in cartilaginous tissue). Synthesis rates can increase two- to threefold over this range of extracellular Na^+ concentration [30] (Fig. 2a). Similar results are seen with an increase in K^+, where the peak rate is at about 15 mM K^+ compared to 5 mM in serum or medium [13]. When Na^+ concentration or osmolality is increased further so that the medium becomes hyperosmotic relative to initial tissue osmolality, synthesis rates fall steeply in a dose-dependent manner. If cartilage slices rather than isolated cells are incubated in similar medium, synthesis rates decrease with increase in osmolality or Na^+ concentration [31,32]. The fall in synthesis is similar to that seen under static load, which also increases intratissue ion concentrations as fluid is expressed [32].

Extracellular pH and Ca^{2+}

Extracellular acidity is an important regulator of matrix metabolism: a complex bimodal relationship between matrix pH and synthesis has been described in rat mandibular condyles, bovine articular cartilage, and intervertebral disks where synthesis rates of aggrecan were about 40% higher at pH 6.9–7.1 than they were at pH 7.4; below pH 6.8, synthesis rates fall rapidly with the fall in pH [33,34]. Extremes of extracellular acidity are found to produce intracellular acidification in chondrocytes [34]; furthermore, we have found that direct imposition of intracellular acidosis can inhibit matrix metabolism [34]. In contrast to the effects of Na^+, H^+, and K^+, increases in extracellular Ca^{2+} over the physiological range (2–20 mM), although found to affect intracellular Ca^{2+} have little immediate effect on synthesis [13,32]. A rise in intracellular Ca^{2+} affects signal transduction, but the possible pathways involved in the response to this increase are as yet uncharacterized.

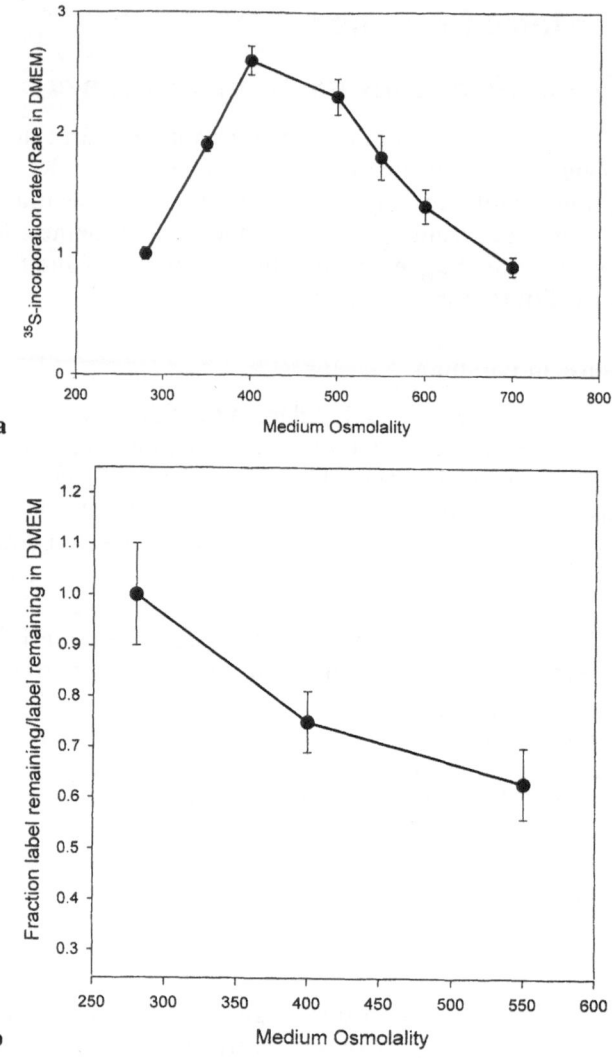

FIG. 2a,b. Effect of changes in osmolality of the medium (NaCl addition to Dulbecco's modified Eagle's medium [DMEM]) on matrix turnover. **a** Effect of medium osmolality on ^{35}S-sulfate incorporation rates in nucleus pulposus (adapted from [30, with permission]). **b** Effect of medium osmolality on loss of ^{35}S-sulfate-labeled GAG (glycosaminoglycan). Cartilage slices were labelled with ^{35}S-sulfate for 24h in DMEM and incubated in tracer-free medium of increasing osmolality for 7 days; the proportion of label remaining was then measured

Adaptation

We have found that there is a difference between the immediate (0–12 h) and long-term (>18 h) response of chondrocytes to an increase in external osmotic pressure. Initially, if chondrocytes are exposed to a hyperosmotic stress, matrix synthesis decreases in a dose-dependent manner as discussed earlier. However, if chondrocytes or cartilage are cultured for >18 h in hyperosmotic medium, synthesis rates return to or even exceed those measured in isoosmotic medium [13]. Similar effects have been seen for cartilage maintained under static load in vitro for >24 h; initially, sulfate incorporation rates fell relative to control rates but synthesis rates had recovered by the end of the experiment [28]. Chondrocytes are thus able to adapt to changes in their extracellular ionic and osmotic environment.

We and others have also found that increases in osmolality or ion concentration alter not only synthesis but also tissue breakdown. Chondrocytes incubated in alginate beads accumulate less matrix when incubated at high osmolalities [35]. Similarly, the rate of proteoglycan loss from cartilage explants increases as extracellular ion concentrations and osmolality rise (Fig. 2b). Matrix metalloproteinase production also increases. It therefore appears the rate of turnover is accelerated as extracellular osmolality rises because the rate of matrix loss as well as synthesis is increased.

Effect of Extracellular Ions on Cell Volume

Chondrocytes in the matrix, as well as those isolated from it, change their volume in response to changes in extracellular osmolality. After a fall in osmolality, chondrocytes swell and then exhibit RVD [36] (Fig. 3). If extracellular osmolality is increased by fluid expression under load, chondrocytes shrink, but do not show RVI [36]; although activity of the regulatory Na^+-K^+-$2Cl^-$ cotransporter is activated by cell shrinkage in these cells [37], they do not show RVI in the matrix because Cl^- gradients are unfavorable. Chondrocytes in situ can thus recover their initial volume when incubated in hypoosmotic medium, but remain shrunken while fluid is expressed under load. Microscopic examination of chondrocytes in statically loaded cartilage, where fluid expression has increased aggrecan and hence Na^+ concentration, has demonstrated their decrease in volume [38].

Effect on Intracellular Ionic Composition: Short-Term Responses

Osmolality and Na^+, K^+

Changes in extracellular ion concentrations lead to alterations in the intracellular ionic composition of chondrocytes. We have found that as extracellular osmolality increases, intracellular concentrations of Na^+ and K^+ rise in re-

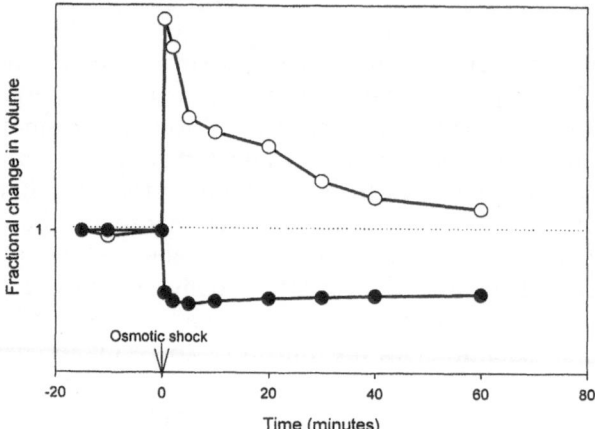

FIG. 3. Time course of volume change of isolated articular chondrocytes after 120mOsm hypoosmotic (*open circles*) and hyperosmotic (*closed circles*) shock. (Adapted from [36], with permission)

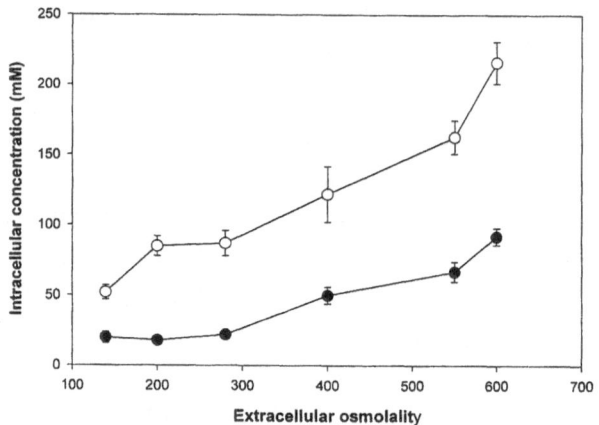

FIG. 4. Effect of change in extracellular osmolality (NaCl addition to DMEM) on intracellular concentrations of K^+ (*open circles*) and Na^+ (*closed circles*) in isolated bovine articular chondrocytes

sponse (Fig. 4). This increase arises partly from cell shrinkage, which concentrates intracellular solutes. It also arises because sodium fluxes into the cell rise as a result of steep inwardly directed transmembrane sodium gradients. The level of increase is however also regulated by the activity of the membrane transporters for these ions. Sodium pump activity increases with rises in intracellular $[Na^+]$ [39], thus the passive increase in Na^+ flux into the cell is balanced in part by increased rate of loss through the pump. The net effect of an increase in extracellular sodium or potassium concentration depends on the density of the various transport proteins per cell, the level of the transmembrane gradient, and activity of the transporters. After these have responded to the changed condition, the intracellular ion concentrations adjust to a new level.

Apart from the direct effect of an increase in extracellular $[Na^+]$ on intracellular $[Na^+]$, cell shrinkage can affect intracellular composition indirectly. For instance, shrinkage increases acid extrusion [40,41]. It is likely that this increased activity ensures that the acid challenges that follow fluid expression on joint loading can be effectively met.

pH and Ca^{2+}

Using the pH-sensitive fluorescent dye BCECF in articular chondrocytes to study pH-regulating properties of these cells, we have shown that chondrocytes have a resting pH of about 7.1 and possess powerful buffering and proton transport systems with which to counter any changes [42]. The intracellular buffering capacity is high in comparison with many cells but is consistent with the acidic environment and the H^+ sensitivity of the metabolism of these cells. Inhibitor and ion substitution studies have shown that imposition of intracellular acidification leads to a rapid sodium-dependent recovery not augmented in HCO_3^-/CO_2-buffered media [42]. These findings implicate the Na^+-H^+ antiporter as the sole regulator of intracellular pH following acidosis. Although these findings are unusual, they are consistent with the extracellular environment of the articular chondrocyte and with the observation that a modified anion exchanger operates to mediate the uptake of sulfate, an essential matrix precursor [42]. However, in avian growth plate chondrocytes HCO_3^--dependent carriers have been found to regulate pH [43], suggesting that development and environment both play an important role in determining expression of transport proteins in chondrocytes. Less is known about the regulation of Ca^{2+} in chondrocytes. Nevertheless, it seems that rises in intracellular Ca^{2+}, induced by agonists or resulting from raised extracellular Ca^{2+} or from other extracellular perturbations, can be rapidly countered by $Na^+ \times Ca^{2+}$ exchange [44].

Long-Term Effects on Intracellular Composition

Apart from the direct effects on changes in intracellular salts on synthesis, increased ion concentrations can also initiate gene expression of membrane transport proteins [45]. In other cell types, a rise in intracellular salts upregulates expression of membrane transporters such as the sodium pump; we have found that sodium pump density per chondrocyte increases with increase in extracellular sodium [46]. High intracellular salt also initiates expression of membrane transporters, which allow exchange of intracellular Na^+ and K^+ with neutral solutes such as betaine and choline [47], and also enhance metabolic production of osmotically active solutes such as glycerophosphocholine. Thus, intracellular osmolality is maintained as intracellular salt concentration falls. We have found that adaptation of chondrocytes to high extracellular osmolality occurs in part through such a mechanism [48]. After 24-h incubation in hyperosmotic medium, intracellular Na^+ and K^+ have returned to near initial values and intracellular betaine, choline, and myoinositol have risen 5- to 14 fold. These changes are necessary to restore matrix synthesis rates to their initial values. The time course of changes involved are shown schematically in Fig. 5.

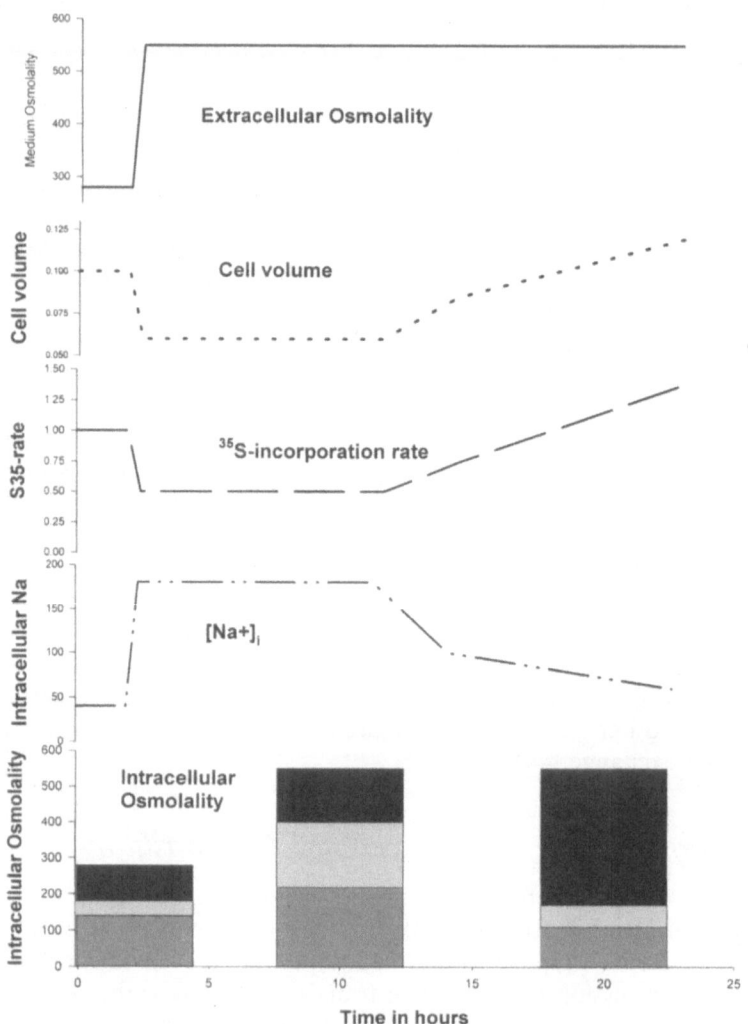

FIG. 5. Schematic of change in chondrocyte volume, ^{35}S-incorporation rates, intracellular Na^+, and intracellular solute concentrations with time after a step increase in extracellular osmolality. *Black bars*, neutral solutes; *light gray bars*, $[Na^+]_i$; *dark gray bars*, $[K^+]_i$)

Hydrostatic Pressure

Effect of Hydrostatic Pressure on Matrix Synthesis

Hydrostatic pressure has been shown to affect many aspects of cellular behavior. Because loading invariably induces an increase in hydrostatic pressure in cartilage, there have been several studies on the effect of pressure application on chondrocytes. An increase in hydrostatic pressure above a threshold level has been found to affect matrix synthesis rates and also expression of other macromolecules by chondrocytes [24,25,49,50], with the response very sensitive to the duration and magnitude of the applied pressure. In general, short applications of physiological pressures stimulate aggrecan production, whereas longer applications of high pressure inhibit it. The actual levels of pressure that elicit a particular response vary with the source of cartilage. A pressure of 7.5 MPa will stimulate aggrecan synthesis in articular chondrocytes but inhibit it in the intevertebral disk nucleus. Epiphyseal chondrocytes respond to pressures less than 1 MPa, but such pressures have no effect on articular chondrocytes [51]. Chondrocytes thus appear to adapt and respond to the pressures they routinely experience.

Hydrostatic Pressure and Membrane Transport

There has been some interest in elucidating the pressure-sensitive transport mechanism in chondrocytes. Early work in this area found pressure application led to a rise in cAMP, but nothing further is known about the effect of pressure on second-messenger systems in chondrocytes. More recently, pressure has been found to influence the cytoskeleton of chondrocytes, and the effects of high sustained pressure might be exerted in part through this mechanism.

There have also been some investigations of the effect of pressure on membrane transporters in chondrocytes. Pressure has been shown to inhibit Na^+-K^+ ATPase activity in chondrocytes with the extent of pump inhibition increasing with time at pressure and with pressure level [52] (Fig. 6a). Pressure has also been shown to stimulate the activity of $Na^+ \times H^+$ exchange [40] (Fig. 6b). The effect of pressure on $Na^+ \times H^+$ exchange can be inhibited by staurosporine and okadaic acid, indicating that a pressure-sensitive kinase is involved in the pressure response of this transporter. Pressure thus influences at least two membrane transporters, slowing Na^+ efflux from chondrocytes by inhibiting the sodium pump and increasing Na^+ influx by increasing $Na^+ \times H^+$ exchange activity. This mechanism could explain the rise in intracellular Na^+ seen with pressure and also explain the time- and level-dependent effects on synthesis in part. Short applications of low pressure only increase intracellular concentrations to a limited extent; these might actually increase synthesis rates, depending on the initial state of the chondrocyte.

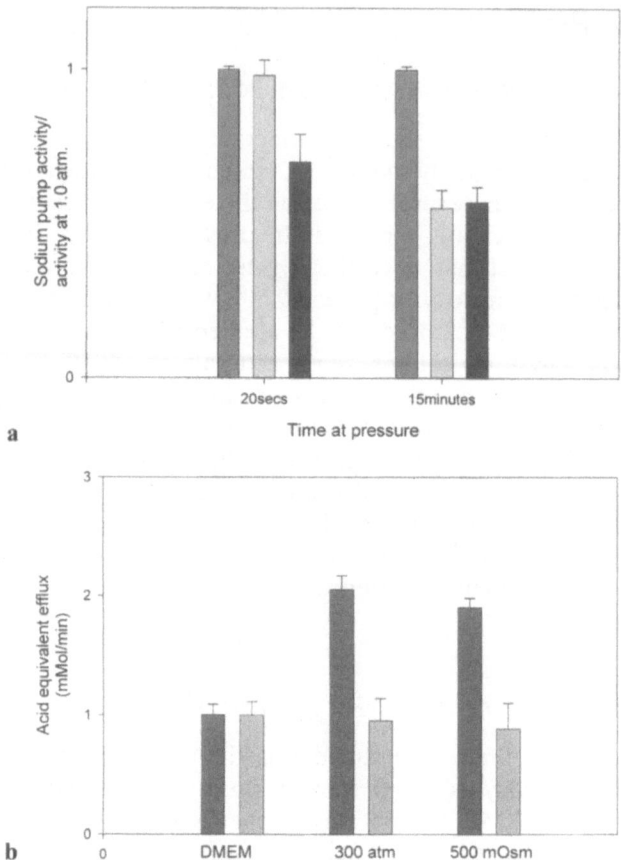

Fig. 6a,b. Effect of changes in the physical environment on membrane transporters. **a** Effect of pressure on $Na^+-K^+/ATPase$. *Darkly hatched bars (left)*, atmospheric pressure; *lightly hatched bars (middle)*, 2.5 atm; *black bars (right)*, ≥10 atm. (Adapted from [52], with permission). **b** Effect of pressure and hyperosmolality on $Na^+ \times H^+$ exchange. *Dark bars*, control; *light bars*, staurosporine added. (Adapted from [40], with permission)

Conclusions

We have shown that the extracellular ionic environment is a powerful regulator of matrix synthesis and breakdown in chondrocytes. In vivo, this ionic and osmotic environment is regulated by the aggrecan content of the matrix, and any change in aggrecan content is sensed by the chondrocyte as a change in ion concentration. We have seen that the chondrocyte can respond rapidly to such changes with short-term alterations in matrix synthesis rates. If the change is prolonged, indicating a long-term alteration in environment, the chondrocyte is able to adapt to this new condition. This response to the ionic environment is an important factor in allowing the chondrocyte to build and maintain a matrix that is appropriate for its customary mechanical and biochemical environment. There is currently a large interest in cartilage repair, but the potent effect of the ionic environment on tissue turnover is usually neglected. Understanding and utilizing its role in tissue turnover, however, is a necessary step for cartilage of the required composition and biomechanical properties to be produced by tissue engineering.

Acknowledgments. We thank the Arthritis Research Campaign (U0501, W0553), the Royal Society, and the Wellcome Trust for financial support.

References

1. Stein WD (1986) Transport and diffusion across cell membranes. Academic Press, London
2. Pedersen PI, Carafoli E (1987) Ion motive ATPases. 1. Ubiquity, properties, and significance to cell function. Trends Biol Sci 12:146–150
3. Hebert DN, Carruthers A (1991) Uniporters and anion antiporters. Curr Opin Cell Biol 3:702–709
4. Hoffman EK, Simonsen LO (1989) Membrane mechanisms in volume and pH regulation in vertebrate cells. Physiol Rev 69:315–382
5. McCarty NA, O'Neil RG (1992) Calcium signaling in cell volume regulation. Physiol Rev 72:1037–1061
6. Ellory JC, Hall AC (1988) Human red cell volume regulation in hypotonic media. Comp Biochem Physiol 90A:533–537
7. Jackson PS, Strange K (1993) Volume-sensitive anion channels mediate swelling-activated inositol and taurine efflux. Am J Physiol 265:C1489–C1500
8. Carafoli E (1987) Intracellular calcium homeostasis. Annu Rev Biochem 56:395–433
9. Yamada KM, Miyamoto S (1995) Integrin transmembrane signaling and cytoskeletal control. Curr Opm Cell Biol 7:681–689
10. Hildebrand A, Romaris M, Rasmussen LM, et al (1994) Interaction of small interstitial proteoglycans biglycan, decorin and fibromodulin with transforming growth factors beta. Biochem J 302:527–534
11. Maroudas A (1979) Physico-chemical properties of articular cartilage. In: Freeman M (ed) Adult articular cartilage. Pitman, London, pp 215–290
12. Maroudas A, Evans H (1974) A study of ionic equilibria in cartilage. Connect Tissue Res 1:69–79
13. Urban JPG, Hall AC, Gehl KA (1993) Regulation of matrix synthesis rates by the ionic and osmotic environment of articular chondrocytes. J Cell Physiol 154:262–270
14. Lee RB, Urban JPG (1997) Evidence for a negative Pasteur effect in articular cartilage. Biochem J 321:95–102
15. Diamant B, Karlsson J, Nachemson A (1968) Correlation between lactate levels and pH in discs of patients with lumbar rhizopathies. Experientia (Basel) 24:1195–1196

16. Weightman B, Kempson G (1979) Cartilage load carriage. In: Freeman MAR (ed) Adult articular cartilage. Pitman, London, pp 293–341
17. Hodge WA, Fuan RS, Carlson KL, Burgess RG, Harris WH, Mann RW (1986) Contact pressures in the human hip joint measured in vivo. Proc Natl Acad Sci USA 83:2879–2883
18. Helminen H, Jurvelin J, Kiviranta I, Paukkonen K, Saamanen A-M, Tammi M (1987) Joint loading effects on articular cartilage: a historical review. In: Helminen HJ, Kiviranta I, Tammi M, Saamanen A-M, Paukkonen K, Jurvelin J (eds) Joint loading: biology and health of articular structures. Wright, Bristol, pp 1–46
19. Arokoski J, Kiviranta I, Jurvelin J, Tammi M, Helminen HJ (1993) Long-distance running causes site-dependent decrease of cartilage glycosaminoglycan content in the knee joints of beagle dogs. Arthritis Rheum 36:1451–1459
20. Burton-Wurster N, Vernier-Singer M, Farquhar T, Lust G (1993) Effect of compressive loading and unloading on the synthesis of total protein, proteoglycan and fibronectin by canine cartilage explants. J Orthop Res 11:717–729
21. Sah R, Grodzinsky A, Plaas A, Sandy J (1992) Effects of static and dynamic compression on matrix metabolism in cartilage explants. In: Kuettner K, Shleyerbach R, Reyron J, Hascall V (eds) Articular cartilage and osteoarthritis. Raven Press, New York, pp 373–392
22. Kim Y-J, Bonasser LJ, Grodzinsky AJ (1995) The role of cartilage streaming potential, fluid flow and pressure in the stimulation of chondrocyte biosynthesis during dynamic compression. J Biomech 28:1055–1066
23. Wright M, Jobanputra P, Bavinton C, Salter DM, Nuki G (1996) Effects of intermittent pressure-induced strain on the electrophysiology of cultured human chondrocytes: evidence for the presence of stretch-activated membrane channels. Clin Sci (Colch) 90:61–71
24. Handa T, Ishihara H, Ohshima H, Osada R, Tsuji H, Obata K (1997) Effects of hydrostatic pressure on matrix synthesis and matrix metalloproteinase production in the human lumbar intervertebral disc. Spine 22:1085–1091
25. Takahashi K, Kubo T, Arai Y, et al (1997) High hydrostatic pressure induces Il-6 and tumor necrosis factor (TNF-α) mRNA in chondrocytes. Trans Orthop Res Soc 22:714
26. Smith RL, Donlon BS, Gupta MK, et al (1995) Effects of fluid-induced shear on articular chondrocyte morphology and metabolism in vitro. J Orthop Res 13:824–831
27. Jones IL, Klamfeldt A, Sandstrom T (1982) The effect of continuous mechanical pressure upon the turnover of articular cartilage proteoglycans in vitro. Clin Orthop 165:283–289
28. Boustany N, Gray ML, Black A, Chunziker EB (1995) Time-dependent changes in the response of cartilage to static compression suggest interstitial pH is not the only signaling mechanism. J Orthop Res 13:740–750
29. Guilak F, Donahue HJ, Zeil R, Grande DA, McLeod RJ, Rubin CT (1994) Deformation induced calcium signaling in articular chondrocytes. In: Mow VC, Guilak F, Transon-Tay R, Hochmuth RM (eds) Cell mechanics and cellular engineering. Berlin Heidelberg Springer, New York, pp 380–397
30. Ishihara H, Warensjo K, Roberts S, Urban JPG (1997) Proteoglycan synthesis in the intervertebral disk nucleus: the role of extracellular osmolality. Am J Physiol 272:C1499–C1506

31. Urban JPG, Bayliss MT (1989) Regulation of proteoglycan synthesis rate in cartilage in vitro: influence of extracellular ionic composition. Biochim Biophys Acta 992:59–65
32. Schneiderman R, Keret D, Maroudas A (1986) Effects of mechanical and osmotic pressure on the rate of glycosaminoglycan synthesis in the human adult femoral head. J Orthop Res 4:393–408
33. Ohshima H, Urban JPG (1992) The effect of lactate and pH on proteoglycan and protein synthesis rates in the intervertebral disc. Spine 17:1079–1082
34. Wilkins RJ, Hall AC (1995) Control of matrix synthesis in isolated bovine chondrocytes by extracellular and intracellular pH. J Cell Physiol 164:474–481
35. Aydelotte MB, Mok SS, Michai L, Schumacher BL (1993) Influence of changes in environmental osmotic pressure on synthesis and accumulation of proteoglycans in matrix assembled by cultured articular chondrocytes. Trans Am Orthop Res Soc 18:14
36. Urban JPG, Borghetti P, Hall AC, Deshayes C (1994) Volume regulatory behaviour of isolated and in situ chondrocytes in respone to changes in extracellular osmolarity. Trans Am Orthop Res Soc 19:490
37. Hall AC, Starks I, Shoults CL, Rashidbigi S (1996) Pathways for K^+ transport across the bovine articular chondrocyte membrane and their sensitivity to cell volume. Am J Physiol 270:C1300–C1310
38. Wong M, Wuethrich P, Buschmann MD, Eggli P, Hunziker E (1996) Chondrocyte biosynthesis correlates with local tissue strain in statically compressed adult articular cartilage. J Orthop Res 15:189–196
39. Horisberger J-D, Lemas V, Kraehenbuhl J-P, Rossier BC (1991) Structure-function relationship of Na,K-ATPase. Annu Rev Physiol 53:565–584
40. Wilkins RJ, Browning JA, Yamakazi N, Hall AC (1997) Hydrostatic pressure stimulates intracellular pH recovery from acidosis in bovine articular chondrocytes. Trans Orthop Res Soc 22:713
41. Descalu A, Korenstein R, Oron Y, Nevo Z (1996) A hyperosmotic stimulus regulates intracellular pH, calcium and S-100 protein levels in avian chondrocytes. Biochem Biophys Res Commun 227:368–373
42. Hall AC, Horowitz ER, Wilkins RJ (1996) The cellular physiology of articular cartilage. Exp Physiol 81:535–545
43. Descalu A, Nevo Z, Korenstein R (1993) The control of intracellular pH in cultured avian chondrocytes. J Physiol (Lond) 461:583–599
44. Ponte MR, Hall AC (1994) The effect of extracellular Ca^{2+} and Na^+ on $[Ca^{2+}]_i$ of porcine articular chondrocytes. J Physiol (Lond) 475P:105
45. Higgins C, Cairney J, Stirling D, Sutherland L, Booth I (1987) Osmotic regulation of gene expression: ionic strength as an intracellular signal? Trends Biol Sci 12:339–344
46. Mobasheri A, Hall AC, Urban JP, France SJ, Smith AL (1997) Immunologic and autoradiographic localisation of the Na^+, $K^{(+)}$-ATPase in articular cartilage: upregulation in response to changes in extracellular Na^+ concentration. Int J Biochem Cell Biol 29:649–657
47. Burg MB, Kwon ED, Kultz D (1996) Osmotic regulation of gene expression. FASEB J 10:1598–1606
48. Urban JPG, Hall AC (1993) Adaptive response of chondrocytes to changes in their physical environment. Trans Am Orthop Res Soc 18:650

49. Hall AC, Urban JPG, Gehl KA (1991) The effects of hydrostatic pressure on matrix synthesis in articular cartilage. J Orthop Res 9:1–10
50. Parkkinen JJ, Ikonen J, Lammi MJ, Laakonen J, Helminen HJ (1993) Effects of cyclic hydrostatic pressure on proteoglycan synthesis in cultured chondrocytes and articular cartilage explants. Arch Biochem Biophys 300:458–465
51. Lipiello L, Kaye C, Neumata T, Mankin HJ (1985) In vitro metabolic response of articular cartilage segments to low levels of hydrostatic pressure. Connect Tissue Res 13:99–107
52. Hall AC (1997) Hydrostatic pressure directly affects the activity of articular chondrocyte membrane transporters. Trans Orthop Res Soc 22:177

Cytoskeleton and Proteoglycan Synthesis in Chondrocytes Under Hydrostatic Pressure

Jyrki J. Parkkinen[1], Mikko J. Lammi[2], Matti O. Jortikka[2], Ritva I. Inkinen[2], Kai Kaarniranta[2], Heikki J. Helminen[2], and Markku I. Tammi[2]

Summary. Articular cartilage is normally subject to various magnitudes of pressures which control the content of matrix proteoglycans (PGs). Short-term cyclic hydrostatic pressurization (5 MPa, 1.5 h) stimulated PG synthesis in chondrocytes embedded in their natural environment in explants, but inhibited it when maintained in monolayer cultures. In long-term cyclic pressurization (5 MPa, 20 h), the inhibiting response of the cell cultures was reversed to stimulation. Continuous 30 MPa pressure reduced total PG synthesis and the steady-state mRNA level of aggrecan, while continuous 5 MPa pressure had no effect. Increased size of aggrecans, secreted under continuous 30 MPa pressure, was observed. Continuous 30 MPa hydrostatic pressure led to a reversible disorganization of microtubules, and the Golgi apparatus was packed into a perinuclear clump of vesicles. After depolymerization of the microtubules, pressurization did not influence the appearance of the Golgi apparatus or PG secretion. High hydrostatic pressure inhibited the organization of microfilaments and induced heat-shock protein 70 expression both at the mRNA and protein level. The results demonstrate that hydrostatic pressure controls the synthesis and structure of PGs in cultured chondrocytes. The simultaneous cytoskeletal changes may participate in the regulation of PG synthesis and secretion. The results further suggest that microtubules are important for PG metabolism. Hydrostatic pressure may control PG synthesis both at transcriptional and translational/posttranslational levels of biosynthesis.

Key Words: Hydrostatic pressure, Articular cartilage, Proteoglycans, Cytoskeleton, Golgi apparatus

Departments of [1] Pathology and [2] Anatomy, University of Kuopio, P.O. Box 1627, FIN-70211, Kuopio, Finland.

Introduction

The matrix of articular cartilage provides this tissue the ability to withstand large compressive stresses. The biomechanical properties of cartilage are largely determined by the abundance of proteoglycan (PG) aggregates within the collagen fibril network, synthesized and maintained by the articular chondrocytes. In osteoarthritis, the cartilage matrix is gradually eroded, compromising the function of the joint. The importance of joint motion and weight-bearing for the maintenance of normal, healthy articular cartilage has been shown in many studies. In vivo models have been useful in broadening our knowledge of cartilage tissue responses to the absence of joint movements, reduced or increased weight-bearing, and increased physical activity by running [1,2].

The composition of the extracellular matrix and the pattern of joint loading are important modulators of cartilage metabolism, including synthesis of new matrix, but the signals and transduction pathways mediating the modulation of chondrocyte metabolism are not well understood. The control of cartilage matrix synthesis is difficult to examine in vivo, while in vitro models offer a more direct way to study cellular responses to joint loading. The advantages of these models include experimentation under a defined environment, easy manipulation of the conditions, and determination of the effects of loading on chondrocyte metabolism. Our research has been focused on hydrostatic pressure because, together with mechanical loading and stretching, it is one of the environmental signals that control the metabolism of articular cartilage. We have investigated how hydrostatic loading affects the biosynthesis of PGs in terms of transcript levels, synthesis rate, and product structure. Changes in the Golgi apparatus and cytoskeleton caused by pressure have also been assessed as possible mediators of the metabolic response.

Articular Cartilage Matrix Components

Collagens and PGs are the major components of articular cartilage. As regards their expression during development, chondrocytes contain type I collagen mRNA only at the very early stages of chondrogenesis [3], while collagen type II transcripts are detectable in the chick limb bud slightly earlier than those of aggrecan and link protein, the latter two appearing at the stage when chondrogenesis begins morphologically [4]. During skeletal development, an identical pattern for aggrecan and link protein synthesis was noticed by in situ hybridization [5], and type IX collagen had an expression pattern very similar to that of aggrecan [6]. In the developing skeleton, high levels of biglycan mRNA were noticed in superficial chondrocytes, whereas decorin was strongly expressed in the deep zone of the cartilage [7]. In mature cartilage, expression of type II collagen is normally hardly detectable, while proteoglycans and their aggregates are more actively expressed by the chondrocytes, except that there are not yet data for the recently cloned hyaluronan synthases (for a review, see [8]).

In normal articular cartilage, the matrix components undergo a continuous and balanced turnover. Fibrillar collagen is very resistant to proteolytic cleavage and has a very slow turnover rate, while proteoglycans respond more quickly to the chemical and environmental alterations in the tissue. Serum, or growth factors such as insulin-like growth factor (IGF), stimulate proteoglycan synthesis and seem to be necessary for maintenance of the proteoglycan content in cartilage explants in vitro [9]. Hyaluronic acid (HA) and aggrecan have the same turnover time in explant cultures [10, 11] and they show coordinated regulation also in vivo [12]. Proteinase inhibitors decrease the loss of aggrecan and HA, and their catabolism also depends on metabolically active chondrocytes [11].

A net loss of large, aggregating PGs (aggrecans) and small PGs occurs in diseased cartilage [13]. In early osteoarthrosis [14] and chondromalacia [15], aggrecan molecules have a reduced molecular size, while in a more advanced stage they appear larger than those in a healthy tissue. This suggests increased degradation of PGs in early disease and a later repair process replacing the matrix PGs by a population of recently synthesized, larger molecules [13,14]. Increased PG [16] and collagen synthesis [17] occurs in early experimental osteoarthrosis.

Compression and Stretching Affect Cartilage and Chondrocytes

Cartilage explants and chondrocyte cultures have been exposed to direct mechanical compression [18–27] or stretching forces [28–30]. In general, the applied force and, importantly, the frequency of the loading cycle affect the metabolic response, the optimal frequency approaching that of a normal walking rhythm (for a review, see [31]).

In our previous studies, we used a mechanical loading apparatus with a nonporous loading head that cyclically compressed full-depth cartilage disks larger than the loading head [27]. In the directly loaded area, the highest stimulation in [^{35}S]sulfate incorporation during a short-term experiment was noticed with a 0.25-Hz cycle. The stimulation took place through the whole depth of the cartilage. Raising the pressure from 0.5 to 1 MPa, or increasing the frequency to 0.5 Hz, reduced the stimulation, particularly in the superficial parts of the articular cartilage.

As the strain of the cartilage in the directly loaded area was minimal (1%–2%) with the short peak- loading pulse (50 ms) used, the stimulation of [^{35}S]sulfate incorporation was probably caused by enhanced hydrostatic pressure. Because all these alterations were observed within 1.5 h from the beginning of loading, it appeared probable that the speed of posttranslational processing of the core protein was involved, including GAG assembly and sulfation in the endoplasmic reticulum and the Golgi apparatus, rather than enhanced transcription.

In the indirectly loaded area, the stimulation occurred with a faster (0.5-Hz) cycle, and only in the superficial zone [27]. The superficial zone aside of the loading head is mainly subject to stretching, suggesting that tensile forces are also an important stimulus for PG synthesis.

Influences of Hydrostatic Pressure on Matrix Synthesis

Hydrostatic pressure within articular cartilage is raised during each dynamic loading event of a joint. The loading creates hydrostatic pressure pulses that immediately spread into the underlying cartilage around the contact site. The hydrostatic pressure resulting from mechanical loading induces a flow of fluid through the matrix and creates streaming potentials and currents. Utilizing a pressure chamber, the effects of hydrostatic pressure can be investigated independently from other factors associated with mechanical loading.

Increased hydrostatic pressure influences various cell types such as bone-derived cells [32,33] and osteoblastoma cells [34]. It has clear influences on the cytoskeleton, integrins, and cell organelles [35–43]. Relatively few experiments have been carried out by applying hydrostatic pressure on cartilage explants or chondrocytes (for a review, see [31]), indicating that pressures at the physiological level tend to stimulate matrix synthesis, while higher values are inhibitory.

Effects of Hydrostatic Pressure on Proteoglycan Synthesis in Chondrocytes

To further investigate the role of hydrostatic pressure in the articular cartilage PG synthesis, we developed a special apparatus for this purpose. It is composed of a water-filled loading cylinder, a reference cylinder of the same size, and a computer-controlled hydraulic system to produce hydrostatic pressure, cyclic or continuous, in the loading cylinder [44]. The cartilage explants or monolayer cell cultures are exposed to pressure in culture dishes filled with medium and sealed by a membrane after excluding air from the dish. Labeled precursors and chemicals can be injected into the culture dishes to study the metabolic activities. The dishes are put into the chamber filled with prewarmed (37°C) distilled water [44].

First, cartilage explants and chondrocyte monolayers were subjected to short-term (1.5-h) or long-term (20-h) hydrostatic pressure. The response to hydrostatic pressure depended on the frequency of the pressure, the length of pressurization, and whether chondrocyte monolayer cultures or cartilage tissue explants were pressurized [44].

In short-term loading experiments (Fig. 1, open symbols), the [^{35}S]sulfate incorporation was stimulated in explants when a 0.5-Hz cycle was applied with 5-MPa pressure. In chondrocyte monolayers, however, [^{35}S]sulfate incorporation was inhibited with the same protocol and also with 0.25-Hz and 0.05-Hz loading cycles. In the longer pressurizations for 20h (Fig. 1, filled symbols), increased [^{35}S]sulfate incorporation in chondrocyte monolayers was found with the same cycles and pressures that were inhibitory in short-term experiments. When the pressurization frequency was further decreased under 0.0167Hz, there were no alterations in [^{35}S]sulfate incorporation [44].

A continuous, 30-MPa hydrostatic pressure remarkably inhibited sulfation, glycosylation, and protein synthesis as measured by incorporations of [^{35}S]sulfate, [^{3}H]glucosamine, and [^{14}C]leucine, respectively [45]. Aggrecan mRNA transcripts were also slightly decreased as related to glyceraldehyde 3-phosphate dehydrogenase (GAPDH) levels, while decorin and biglycan levels were elevated (Fig. 2A).

The structure of PGs secreted by chondrocyte cultures after exposure to continuous (5-MPa and 30-MPa) and cyclic hydrostatic pressures (5-MPa) was investigated. Two major bands were always noticed in autoradiography on agarose gels, the slow-mobility band representing aggrecan and the fast-mobility one the small interstitial PGs decorin and biglycan [45]. Both the control and pressurized cultures expressed abundantly mRNA transcripts of aggrecan, decorin, and biglycan (Fig. 2A), while no detectable expression of versican was detected (Fig. 2B), confirming the chondrocytic phenotype of the cultured cells. Smooth muscle cells served as a positive control for versican expression [45].

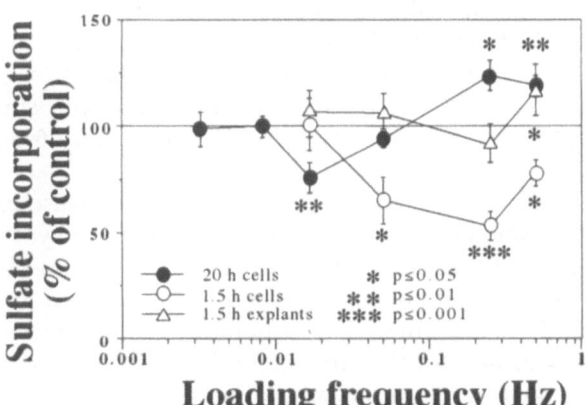

FIG. 1. [^{35}S]Sulfate incorporation vs. frequency of hydrostatic pressure on cartilage explants and chondrocyte cell cultures during cyclic hydrostatic pressurization in short-term (tissue and cell cultures) and long-term experiments (cell cultures)

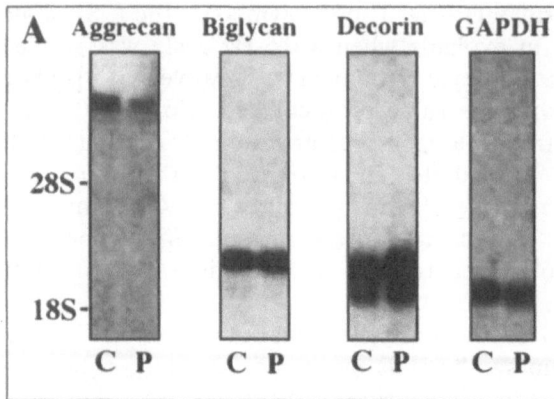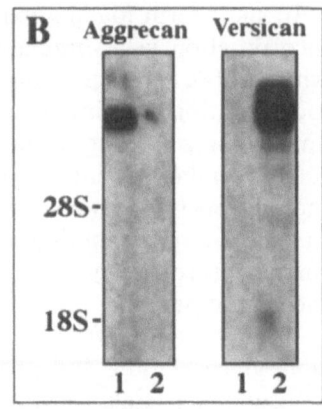

FIG. 2A,B. Northern blot analysis of proteoglycan (PG) mRNAs. **A** Total RNAs from control cultures (*C*) and from chondrocytes exposed to 30-MPa continuous hydrostatic pressure (*P*) were transferred onto a nylon membrane and hybridized with aggrecan, biglycan, decorin, and glyceraldehyde 3-phosphate dehydrogenase (GAPDH) cDNA probes. **B** Total RNAs from chondrocytes (*lane 1*) and human smooth muscle cells (*lane 2*) were separated by electrophoresis and hybridized with aggrecan and versican cDNA probes, respectively. The cDNA probes were generous gifts from Drs. V. Glumoff and E. Vuorio (aggrecan), Dr. L. Fisher (biglycan), and Dr. T. Krusius (decorin and versican)

Continuous 30-MPa hydrostatic pressure caused a retarded mobility of aggrecans in agarose gel electrophoresis [45]. This slowing was probably caused by the high magnitude of the pressure, and not by the static mode of the loading, because a 5-MPa continuous pressure did not have a similar effect. A change into a higher molecular weight aggrecan was in line with the finding that in Sephacryl S-1000 gel chromatography the peak of the monomeric large PGs shifted into a smaller K_{av} value. A slight increase in the average chain length of GAGs was observed in the chromatographic analysis on Sepharyl S-300. No similar observations were found after cyclic pressurizations [45].

The possibility that high hydrostatic pressure would cause excessive stress to the cells was examined by analyzing the PG pattern synthesized during 4-h labeling periods as much as 52h after the release of 30-MPa continuous pressure. The cultures continued active PG synthesis even after withdrawal of the pressure. However, there was a burst of [^{35}S]sulfate incorporation in samples labeled during 8–12h after loading and there was a simultaneous retardation in aggrecan migration on sodium dodecyl sulfate-(SDS-)agarose gels (Fig. 3). In addition, mRNA and protein levels of heat-shock protein 70 were determined. In line with previous results [46], increased heat-shock protein 70 mRNA levels were observed, peaking at 6h of continuous pressurization, and the protein level began to accumulate accordingly (Fig. 4).

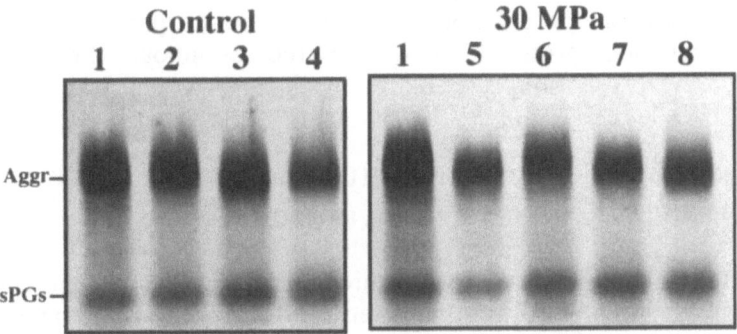

FIG. 3. Proteoglycans synthesized during 4-h labeling periods starting 0, 8, 24, or 48 h after release of continuous 30-MPa hydrostatic pressure (*lanes 5, 6, 7, 8*) and corresponding control cultures (*lanes 1, 2, 3, 4*). The migration positions of aggrecan (Aggr) and small PGs (sPGs) are marked in the figure

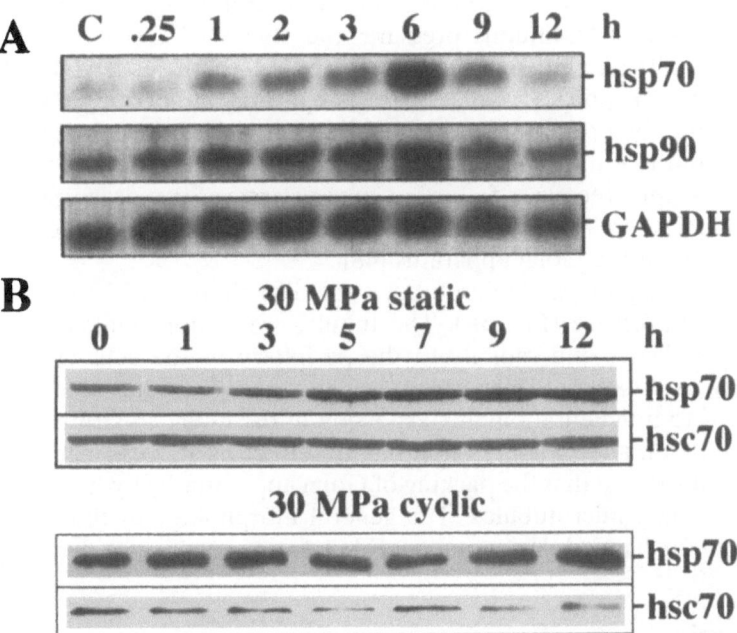

FIG. 4A,B. Expression of heat-shock proteins 70 (hsp-70) and 90 (hsp-90) during continuous and cyclic 30-MPa hydrostatic pressure. **A** The messenger RNA level of hsp-70 was increased during continuous 30-MPa pressure, while the hsp-90 level was relatively stable compared with the GAPDH level. **B** Accumulation of hsp-70 protein during 30-MPa static, but not cyclic, hydrostatic pressure was observed. Heat-shock cognate (hsc-70) was utilized in the normalization of the loadings

Cyclic 30-MPa loading did not stimulate heat-shock protein 70 synthesis, nor was heat-shock protein 90 induced by the continuous 30-MPa pressure (Fig. 4).

Changes in the Golgi Apparatus and Cytoskeleton of Chondrocytes Under High Hydrostatic Pressure

After 30-MPa continuous hydrostatic pressure for 2 h, the morphology of the chondrocytes was altered to a more retracted form. The stress fibers disappeared from the center of the cells, and only small punctually distributed material was stained (Fig. 5B). When 30-MPa pressure was applied cyclically, the number of the stress fibers was reduced and the remaining fibers were thinner than in control cells. Decreasing the continuous pressure level to 15 MPa resulted in a reduced number of thinner stress fibers. With lower levels of cyclic or continuous pressures, there were no changes in the organization of stress fibers; however, some individual cells had thinner fibers [47].

After 30-MPa continuous pressure, the stacks of Golgi apparatus were reversibly collapsed into a packed structure close to the nucleus (Fig. 5D). The normal stacked appearance of the Golgi apparatus was no longer visible in the electron microscopic preparation of the pressurized chondrocytes. Similar changes, but to a minor extent, were seen after 15-MPa continuous pressure. After a 60-min recovery following pressurization, the organization of the Golgi apparatus was fully reestablished. Lower pressures had no effects on the morphology of the Golgi apparatus [48].

The staining pattern of microtubules was also altered by 30-MPa continuous hydrostatic pressure (Fig. 5F). The tubules were more kinked and did not extend as clearly and radially to the periphery of the cells as in controls. Nocodazole treatment, which causes disassembly of chondrocyte microtubules, led to fragmentation and dispersion of the Golgi apparatus throughout the cytoplasm, and pressurization had no effect on its vesicular appearance. This result showed that the packing of Golgi apparatus by hydrostatic pressure required intact microtubules. The general morphology of the chondrocytes remained unchanged during nocodazole treatment.

Discussion

In cartilage, joint loading creates cell and matrix deformation, fluid flow, and electrical events induced by the flow of ions [49,50], in addition to the initial increase of hydrostatic pressure. Hydrostatic pressure has its most profound influences at the interphase between two phases, such as the lipid–water interface at membranes [51]. Thus, membrane structures such as ion channels could serve as a sensor of ambient hydrostatic pressure [52]. Another possible target is the conformation of proteins that can be influenced by hydrostatic pressure [36]. It is important to note that hydrostatic pressure spreads equally

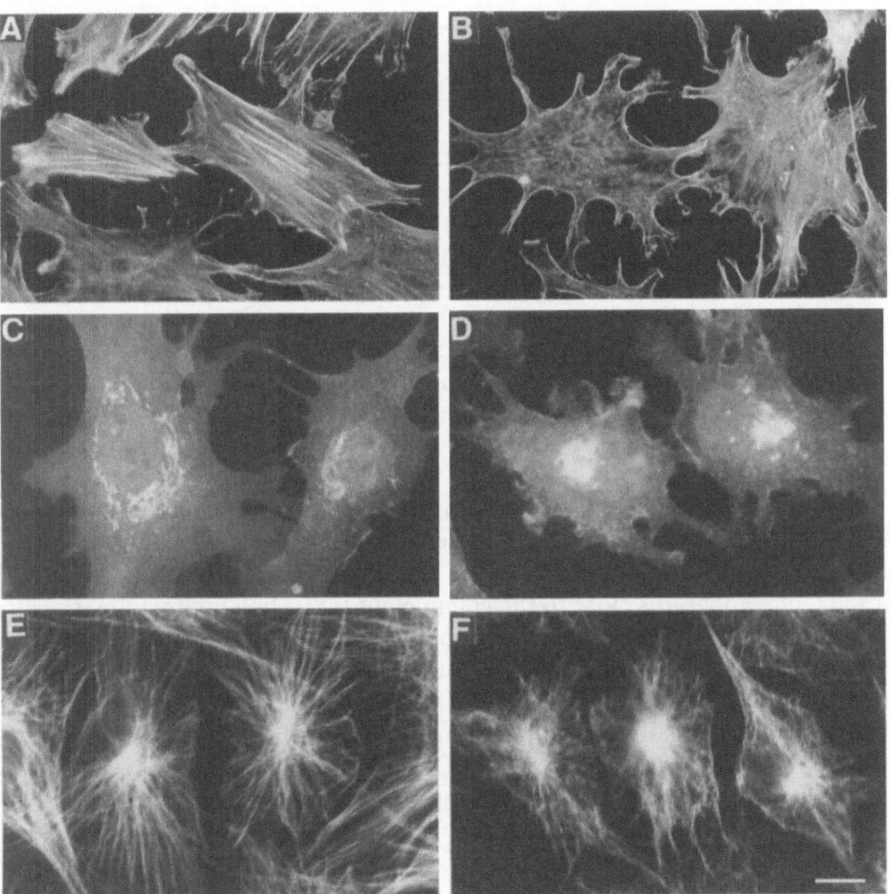

FIG. 5A–F. Effects of hydrostatic pressure on the chondrocyte cytoskeleton and Golgi apparatus. The cells were exposed to 30-MPA continuous pressure for 2h before fixation and staining for microfilaments with TRITC-phalloidin (**A,B**), for Golgi-associated carbohydrates with TRITC-WGA (wheat germ agglutinin) (**C,D**), and for microtubules with an antibody (**E,F**). Control cells (**A,C,E**); pressurized cells (**B,D,F**). *Bar*, 10μm

in intra- and extracellular fluids. Therefore, if a conceptual receptor for hydrostatic pressure is considered, it can exist not only in the pericellular or membrane position but also anywhere intracellularly. Thus, little is known about the primary mechanism of action of hydrostatic pressure, and likely sites include the membranes of the cell and perhaps specific proteins sensitive to hydrostatic pressure. Furthermore, it is probable that there are several "sensors" activated at different levels of hydrostatic pressure.

Influences of hydrostatic pressure on the metabolism of chondrocyte cultures were studied using an apparatus specially designed for this purpose. The experiments suggested that hydrostatic pressurization of articular cartilage and chondrocytes may influence the posttranslational processing of PGs, involving, for example, the GAG chain assembly and sulfation, as well as the intracellular transport of PGs and secretion into the extracellular space. Whether the simultaneous changes in the morphology of Golgi apparatus and cytoskeleton contribute to the altered PG synthesis remains to be elucidated. Regulation by hydrostatic pressure also involves mRNA levels of the PG core proteins [45,53].

Sulfation, glycosylation, and protein synthesis were all markedly inhibited by continuous high (30-MPa) hydrostatic pressure. In addition, retarded migration in SDS-agarose gel electrophoresis and earlier elution on Sephacryl S-1000 gel chromatography suggested a shift of aggrecans into a range of greater molecular weight. A slight increase observed in the relative length of GAG chains could explain this finding. Another explanation could be a higher substitution of the core protein serine residues with GAG chains, as in rat chondrosarcoma only 55% of the serine residues were substituted with carbohydrate [54].

High hydrostatic pressure had profound effects on the structural organization of microfilaments and microtubules in chondrocytes [48,55]. Along with the depolymerization of microtubules, high pressure caused a packed pattern of the Golgi apparatus close to the cell nucleus [48]. High hydrostatic pressure (causing depolymerization of microtubules) may slow down the intracellular traffic and thus the rate of the biosynthetic machinery. If the PG precursor molecule spends relatively more time in a compartment responsible for chain initiation and elongation, more and longer carbohydrate chains per core protein can be built, resulting in larger PG molecules. A microtubule disrupting agent, nocodazole, decreased [^{35}S]sulfate incorporation of chondrocyte cultures by 30%–40%, but the incorporation was further decreased if nocodazole-treated cultures were exposed to 30-MPa hydrostatic pressure (unpublished data). This result supports the idea that microtubules facilitate the synthesis or secretion of PGs, while high hydrostatic pressure influences other aspects of the synthesis, perhaps also transcription or translation.

The steady-state mRNA levels of aggrecan, decorin, and biglycan after continuous pressurization were also quantified. A decrease (25%) was noticed in aggrecan mRNA level, which is compatible with the reduced [^{35}S]sulfate incorporation rate. However, decorin and biglycan mRNA transcript amounts were increased (250%–500%), demonstrating the specific character of the regulation of the different PG mRNAs. In accordance with an earlier report on cartilage explants [56], mRNA levels did not consistently predict the rate of synthesis of the small PGs. At least certain mRNAs have been shown to associate with cytoskeletal elements [57], and disruption of cytoskeleton affects the stability of mRNAs [58]. Amino acid incorporation into PG core proteins was not specifically measured, so it remains to be determined whether there was a significant alteration in the rate of core protein biosynthesis.

Short-term pressurization (5 MPa, 0.5 Hz for 90 min) stimulated PG synthesis in explants but inhibited it in chondrocyte monolayer cultures [44]. This clearly demonstrates that normal extracellular matrix modulates the response of chondrocytes to hydrostatic pressure. Whether this involves specific bonds to, or molecular messengers from, the matrix is not known. While the 90-min pressurization of chondrocyte monolayers inhibited PG synthesis, a longer period of loading (20 h) in similar conditions brought about a synthesis stimulation [44], a finding underlining the importance of the time dependence of these phenomena.

After withdrawing the 30-MPa pressure treatment, the chondrocytes were quite viable, as suggested by a burst of PG synthesis 8–12 h after the end of loading. However, the enhanced expression of heat-shock protein 70 suggested that the treatment was to some extent stressful. No signs of cellular death were noticed at 30-MPa hydrostatic pressure, in line with recent observations in lymphoblasts [59].

Hydrostatic pressurization thus offers an interesting experimental model with which to study the regulation of chondrocyte matrix production by a naturally occurring environmental factor. At present, we do not know by which mechanism the change of hydrostatic pressure is sensed by the chondrocytes and how the pressure affects the transcription, translation, and glycosylation of the PGs. New, unknown genes might be involved, stressing the importance of the current methods used in molecular biology to aid us in our search for specific genes affected by the pressure.

Acknowledgments. The skillful and efficient technical assistance of Mrs. Elma Sorsa and Ms. Eija Antikainen is gratefully acknowledged. This work was financially supported by grants from the University of Kuopio, the North Savo Fund of the Finnish Cultural Foundation, the Finnish Cultural Foundation, the Academy of Finland, the Sigrid Juselius Foundation, and the Finnish Research Council for Physical Education and Sports, Ministry of Education.

References

1. Tammi M, Paukkonen K, Kiviranta I, et al (1987) Joint loading-induced alterations in articular cartilage. In: Helminen HJ, Kiviranta I, Tammi, M, et al (eds) Joint loading—Biology and health of articular structures. Wright & Sons, Bristol, pp 64–88
2. Helminen HJ, Kiviranta I, Säämänen A-M, et al (1992) Effect of motion and load on articular cartilage in animal models. In: Kuettner K, Schleyerbach R, Peyron JG, Hascall VC (eds) Articular cartilage and osteoarthritis. Raven Press, New York, pp 501–510
3. Sandberg M, Vuorio E (1987) Localization of types I, II and III collagen mRNAs in developing human skeletal tissues by in situ hybridization. J Cell Biol 104:1077–1084
4. Goetinck PF, Kiss I, Deák F, et al (1990) Macromolecular organization of the extracellular matrix of cartilage. Ann NY Acad Sci 599:29–38
5. Mundlos S, Meyer R, Yamada Y, et al (1991) Distribution of cartilage proteoglycan (aggrecan) core protein and link protein gene expression during human skeletal development. Matrix 11:339–346

6. Glumoff V, Savontaus M, Vehanen J, et al (1994) Analysis of aggrecan and tenascin gene expression in mouse skeletal tissues by Northern and in situ hybridization using specific cDNA probes. Biochim Biophys Acta 1219:613–622
7. Bianco P, Fisher LW, Young MF, et al (1990) Expression and localization of the two small proteoglycans biglycan and decorin in developing human skeletal and non-skeletal tissues. J Histochem Cytochem 38:1549–1563
8. Weigel PH, Hascall VC, Tammi M (1997) Hyaluronan synthases. J Biol Chem 272:13997–14000
9. Hascall VC, Handley CJ, McQuillan DJ, et al (1983) The effect of serum on biosynthesis of proteoglycans by bovine articular cartilage in culture. Arch Biochem Biophys 224:206–223
10. Morales TI, Hascall VC (1988) Correlated metabolism of proteoglycans and hyaluronic acid in bovine cartilage organ cultures. J Biol Chem 268:3632–3638
11. Ng CK, Handley CJ, Preston BN, et al (1992) The extracellular processing and catabolism of hyaluronan in cultured adult articular cartilage explants. Arch Biochem Biophys 298:70–79
12. Haapala J, Lammi MJ, Inkinen RI, et al (1996) Coordinated regulation of hyaluronan and aggrecan content in the articular cartilage of immobilized and exercised dogs. J Rheumatol 23:1586–1593
13. Mow VC, Ratcliffe A, Poole AR (1992) Cartilage and diarthrodial joints as paradigms for hierarchical materials and structures. Biomaterials 13:67–97
14. Rizkalla G, Reiner A, Bogoch E, et al (1992) Studies of the articular cartilage proteoglycan aggrecan in health and osteoarthritis. Evidence for molecular heterogeneity and extensive molecular changes in disease. J Clin Invest 90:2268–2277
15. Väätäinen U, Häkkinen T, Kiviranta I, et al (1995) Proteoglycan depletion and size reduction in lesions of early grade chondromalacia of the patella. Ann Rheum Dis 54:831–835
16. Sandy JD, Adams ME, Billingham MEJ, et al (1984) In vivo and in vitro stimulation of chondrocyte biosynthetic activity in early experimental osteoarthritis. Arthritis Rheum 27:388–397
17. Poole AR, Rizkalla G, Ionescu M, et al (1993) Osteoarthritis in the human knee: a dynamic process of cartilage matrix degradation, synthesis and reorganization. In: van den Berg WB, van der Kraan PM, van Lent PLEM (eds) Joint destruction in arthritis and osteoarthritis. Birkhäuser Verlag, Basel, pp 3–13
18. Palmoski MJ, Brandt KD (1984) Effects of static and cyclic compressive loading on articular cartilage plugs in vitro. Arthritis Rheum 27:675–681
19. Klämfeldt A (1985) Continuous mechanical pressure and joint tissue. Effect of synovial membrane products and indomethacin in vitro. Scand J Rheum 14:431–437
20. Schneiderman R, Keret D, Maroudas A (1986) Effects of mechanical and osmotic pressure on the rate of glycosaminoglycan synthesis in the human adult femoral head cartilage: an in vitro study. J Orthop Res 4:393–408
21. Gray ML, Pizzanelli AM, Grodzinsky AJ, et al (1988) Mechanical and physicochemical determinants of the chondrocyte biosynthetic response. J Orthop Res 6:777–792
22. Sah RL, Kim Y-J, Doong J-Y, et al (1989) Biosynthetic response of cartilage explants to dynamic compression. J Orthop Res 7:619–636
23. Guilak F, Meyer BC, Ratcliffe A, et al (1991) The effect of static loading on proteoglycan biosynthesis and turnover in articular cartilage explants. Trans Orthop Res Soc 16:50

24. Larsson T, Aspden RM, Heinegård D (1991) Effects of mechanical load on cartilage matrix biosynthesis in vitro. Matrix 11:388–394
25. Sah RL, Doong J-Y, Grodzinsky AJ, et al (1991) Effects of compression on the loss of newly synthesized proteoglycans and proteins from cartilage explants. Arch Biochem Biophys 286:20–29
26. Korver THV, van de Stadt RJ, Kiljan E, et al (1992) Effects of loading on the synthesis of proteoglycans in different layers of anatomically intact articular cartilage in vitro. J Rheum 19:905–912
27. Parkkinen JJ, Lammi MJ, Helminen HJ, et al (1992) Local stimulation of proteoglycan synthesis in articular cartilage explants by dynamic compression in vitro. J Orthop Res 10:610–620
28. Lee RC, Rich JB, Kelley KM, et al (1982) A comparison of in vitro cellular responses to mechanical and electrical stimulation. Am Surg 48:567–574
29. de Witt MT, Handley CJ, Oakes BW, et al (1984) In vitro response of chondrocytes to mechanical loading. The effect of short term mechanical tension. Connect Tissue Res 12:97–109
30. Uchida A, Yamashita K, Hashimoto K, et al (1988) The effect of mechanical stress on cultured growth cartilage cells. Connect Tissue Res 17:305–311
31. Parkkinen JJ, Lammi MJ, Tammi MI, et al (1994) Proteoglycan synthesis and cytoskeleton in hydrostatically loaded chondrocytes. In: Mow VC, Guilak F, Tran-Son-Tay R, Hochsmuth RM (eds) Cell mechanics and cellular engineering. Springer-Verlag, New York, pp 420–444
32. Imamura K, Ozawa H, Hiraide T, et al (1990) Continuously applied compressive pressure induces bone resorption by a mechanism involving prostaglandin E2 synthesis. J Cell Physiol 144:222–228
33. Ozawa H, Imamura K, Abe E, et al (1990) Effect of a continuously applied compressive pressure on mouse osteoblast-like cells (MC3T3-E1) in vitro. J Cell Physiol 142:177–185
34. Quinn RS, Rodan GA (1981) Enhancement of ornithine decarboxylase and Na^+, K^+ ATPase in osteoblastoma cells by intermittent compression. Biochem Biophys Res Commun 100:1696–1702
35. Goldinger JM, Kang BS, Choo YE, et al (1980) Effect of hydrostatic pressure on ion transport and metabolism in human erythrocytes. J Appl Physiol 49:224–231
36. Heremans K (1982) High pressure effects on proteins and other biomolecules. Annu Rev Biophys Bioeng 11:1–21
37. Varga S, Mullner N, Pikula S, et al (1986) Pressure effects on sarcoplasmic reticulum. J Biol Chem 261:13943–13956
38. Zimmerman AM, Tahir S, Zimmerman S (1987) Macromolecular synthesis under hydrostatic pressure. In: Jannasch HW, Marquis RE, Zimmerman AM (eds) Current perspectives in high pressure biology. Academic Press, London, pp 49–63
39. Heinemann SH, Conti F, Stuhmer W, et al (1989) Effects of hydrostatic pressure on membrane processes. J Gen Physiol 90:765–778
40. Kavecansky J, Dannenberg AJ, Zakim D (1992) Effects of high pressure on the catalytic and regulatory properties of UDP-glucuronosyltransferase in intact microsomes. Biochemistry 31:162–168
41. Acevedo AD, Bowser SS, Gerritsen ME, et al (1993) Morphological and proliferative responses of endothelial cells to hydrostatic pressure: role of fibroblast growth factor. J Cell Physiol 157:603–614

42. Haskin C, Cameron I (1993) Physiological levels of hydrostatic pressure alter morphology and organization of cytoskeletal and adhesion proteins in MG-63 osteosarcoma cells. Biochem Cell Biol 71:27–35
43. Crenshaw HC, Allen JA, Skeen V, et al (1996) Hydrostatic pressure has different effects on the assembly of tubulin, actin, myosin II, vinculin, talin, vimentin and cytokeratin in mammalian cells. Exp Cell Res 227:285–297
44. Parkkinen JJ, Ikonen J, Lammi MJ, et al (1993) Effects of cyclic hydrostatic pressure on proteoglycan synthesis in cultured chondrocytes and articular cartilage explants. Arch Biochem Biophys 300:458–465
45. Lammi MJ, Inkinen R, Parkkinen JJ, et al (1994) Expression of reduced amounts of structurally altered aggrecan in articular cartilage chondrocytes subjected to high hydrostatic pressure. Biochem J 304:723–730
46. Takahashi K, Kubo T, Kobayashi K, et al (1997) Hydrostatic pressure influences mRNA expression of transforming growth factor-1 and heat shock protein 70 in chondrocyte-like cell line. J Orthop Res 15:150–158
47. Parkkinen JJ, Lammi MJ, Inkinen R, et al (1995) Influence of short-term hydrostatic pressure on stress fiber organization in cultured chondrocytes. J Orthop Res 13:495–502
48. Parkkinen JJ, Lammi MJ, Pelttari A, et al (1993) Altered Golgi apparatus in hydrostatically loaded articular cartilage chondrocytes. Ann Rheum Dis 52:192–198
49. Frank EH, Grodzinsky AJ (1987) Cartilage electromechanics. I. Electrokinetic transduction and effects of electrolyte pH and ionic strength. J Biomech 20:615–627
50. O'Connor P, Orford R, Gardner DL (1988) Differential response to compressive loads of zones of canine hyaline articular cartilage: micromechanical, light and electron microscopic studies. Ann Rheum Dis 47:414–420
51. Jannasch HW, Marquis RE, Zimmerman AM (1987) Current perspectives in high pressure biology. Academic Press, London
52. Urban JPG, Hall AC, Gehl KA (1993) Regulation of matrix synthesis rates by the ionic environment of articular chondrocytes. J Cell Physiol 154:262–270
53. Smith RL, Rusk SF, Ellison BE, et al (1996) In vitro stimulation of articular chondrocyte mRNA and extracellular matrix synthesis by hydrostatic pressure. J Orthop Res 14:50–60
54. Lohmander LS, Shinomura T, Hascall VC, et al (1989) Xylosyl transfer to the core protein precursor of the rat chondrosarcoma proteoglycan. J Biol Chem 264:18775–18780
55. Parkkinen JJ, Lammi MJ, Pelttari A, et al (1993) Hydrostatic pressure modulates the organization of the cytoskeleton and Golgi apparatus in cultured chondrocytes. Trans Orthop Res Soc 18:617
56. Curtis AJ, Devenish RJ, Handley CJ (1992) Modulation of aggrecan and link-protein synthesis in articular cartilage. Biochem J 288:721–726
57. Bagchi T, Larson DE, Sells BH (1987) Cytoskeletal association of muscle-specific mRNAs in differentiating L6 rat myoblasts. Exp Cell Res 168:160–172
58. Symington AL, Zimmerman S, Stein J, et al (1991) Hydrostatic pressure influences histone mRNA. J Cell Sci 98:123–129
59. Takano KJ, Takano T, Yamanouchi Y, et al (1997) Pressure-induced apoptosis in human lymphoblasts. Exp Cell Res 235:155–160

Cyclic Tensile Stretch Inhibits Proteoglycan Synthesis by Downregulating Protein Kinase C Activity

Kanji Fukuda, Shigeki Asada, Kazuhiro Otani, Chiaki Hamanishi, and Seisuke Tanaka

Summary. We have reported the involvement of protein kinase C (PKC) in the development of osteoarthritis in vivo. In the current study, we examined the effect of mechanical stress on chondrocyte metabolism and the activity of PKC in vitro. Low frequency and magnitude of cyclic tensile stretch loaded on chondrocytes increased proteoglycan synthesis. However, high frequency and magnitude of stress decreased proteoglycan synthesis, and under this condition DNA synthesis was enhanced. PKC inhibitor and pretreatment with phorbol ester reversed the stress-inhibited proteoglycan synthesis. The PKC activity was reduced. We propose that PKC is involved in stress-mediated inhibition of proteoglycan synthesis.

Key Words. Chondrocytes, Osteoarthritis, Protein kinase C, Proteoglycan, Stress

Introduction

Articular cartilage consists of chondrocytes embedded in an extensive extracellular matrix containing structural macromolecules required for tissue functions. The matrix consists primarily of two components: collagen fibrils and glycosaminoglycans (GAGs). The sulfated GAGs in cartilage covalently bind to core protein, as an aggrecan (proteoglycan) aggregate [1].

Osteoarthrosis is a common pathway of joint deterioration, resulting from a physiological imbalance between mechanical stress on joint tissue and the ability to withstand the stress. Joint immobilization has been used to develop animal models of osteoarthrosis [2]. Conversely, moderate running increases aggrecan content in rabbit articular cartilage [3]. These studies show that loading on articular cartilage is required for physiological turnover of the

Department of Orthopaedic Surgery, Kinki University School of Medicine, 377-2 Ohno-Higashi, Osaka-Sayama, Osaka 589-8511, Japan.

extracellular matrix. However, excessive loading on the joint can also lead to deterioration of the articular cartilage [4–6]. Thus, mechanical stress is an essential factor in the regulation of aggrecan turnover in articular cartilage.

Protein kinase C (PKC) is an enzyme activated by inositol phospholipid hydrolysis and acts as a key enzyme for signal transduction in various physiological processes [7]. The role of PKC in cartilage tissue is unclear. We previously demonstrated the presence of PKC in cultured chondrocytes [8] and the expression in the cartilage of experimentally induced osteoarthritis [9]. Further, we recently reported the inhibitory effect in the progression of osteoarthritis of a PKC activator injected into rabbit knee joints [10]. These data suggested to us that PKC is involved in the development of osteoarthritis.

The purpose of this study was to examine the role of PKC in stress-mediated alteration of proteoglycan synthesis. A computerized, pressure-operated instrument (Flexercell Strain Unit; Flexercell, McKeesport, PA, USA) was used to induce deformation of cells [11].

Materials and Methods

Drugs and Chemicals

The materials used in this study were as follows: alpha-minimum essential medium (MEM) and fetal bovine serum (FBS) were obtained from Gibco (Grand Island, NY, USA) and HyClone (Logan, UT, USA), respectively; phorbol 12,13-dibutyrate (PDBu), 4α-phorbol 12,13-didecanoate (4α-PDD), and purified PKC from rat brain from Sigma (St. Louis, MO, USA); and [^{3}H]thymidine (37 MBq/ml) and [^{35}S]sulfate (Na$_2$^{35}SO$_4$, 17.1 GBq/ml) were from New England Nuclear (Boston, MA, USA).

Chondrocyte Culture

Articular cartilage slices were taken from the condylar ridge of the metacarpophalangeal joints of freshly slaughtered calves aged about 10 months. Care was taken to exclude the underlying marrow. Chondrocytes were obtained by enzymatic dissociation [8] and seeded in specially built, flexible-bottom culture plates coated with type I collagen (Flex I culture plates; Flexercell). Cells were seeded at a density of 2×10^5 cells/ml and cultured for 4 days before stretching.

For measurement of DNA synthesis, the cells were seeded at a density of 2×10^4 cells/ml and cultured for 2 days before stretching. As a control, cells were seeded in nondeformable surfaces made of the same substrate material (Flex II culture plate). The chondrocytes maintained a polygonal shape, not fibroblastic, that resembled a cobblestone shape. They were then placed in a vacuum-operated stress-inducing instrument [11]. The culture medium was

MEM, supplemented with penicillin-streptomycin-fungizone and 10% FBS at 37°C in a 5% CO_2 environment. To determine the effect of phorbol ester on proteoglycan synthesis, chondrocytes were seeded in 96-well plates (Becton Dickinson, Franklin Lakes, NJ, USA) at the same density.

In Vitro Application of Stretch

Cells were subjected to mechanical stretch using a pressure-operated instrument (Flexercell Strain Instrument; Flexercell) composed of a computer system controller and monitor, a control module containing pressure transducers, and solenoid valves with a vacuum baseplate and gasket on the plate. Frequency, stretch rate, and degree of elongation of the substrates were all controlled by computer. According to the supplier's manual, there is a linear relationship between the vacuum level (KPa) and maximum percent elongation of cells. Chondrocytes were stretched repeatedly for 3s and then relaxed (Fig. 1). For the lower stress level, the regimen was set at 10 cycles per hour; that is, every 6min chondrocytes were stretched for 3s to a maximum of 5% elongation followed by relaxation. For the higher stress level, the regimen was set at 10 cycles per minute, that is, 3 seconds of stretch to a maximum of 17% elongation followed by 3s of relaxation [12] (Table 1). To ensure that the cells adhering to the flexible membrane did not detach from the culture bottom, the

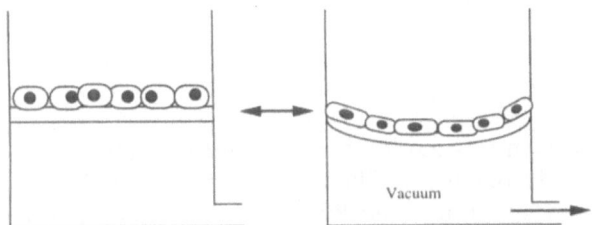

Vacuum

FIG. 1. Flexercell Strain Instrument. Isolated bovine chondrocytes were seeded on a flexible-bottom plate and allowed to attach. Cells were subjected to mechanical stretch using a pressure-operated instrument combined with a computer system

TABLE 1. Regimen of cyclic tensile stretch on chondrocytes

Level	Frequency (cycle)	Vacuum level (kPa)	Maximum elongation (%)
Low	10/h	2	5
High	10/min	10	17

Chondrocytes were seeded on flexible-bottom culture plates (Flex I culture plates; Flexercell). Frequency and vacuum level (kPa) were controlled by computer. Magnitude of maximum elongation of the cells was according to the supplier's instruction. Chondrocytes were repeatedly stretched for 3s followed by relaxation in both regimens.

medium was collected and centrifuged and the cell number counted. Even in the chondrocytes loaded for 24h under the higher stress level, the detachment rate of the chondrocytes was less than 1%.

Cell Morphology

After being cultured for 24h, with or without cyclic stretch loading, cells adherent to the surfaces were rinsed twice with phosphate-buffered saline (PBS), fixed with ethanol-acetone (50:50, v/v) for 5min, and stained with hematoxylin.

DNA Synthesis

Incorporation of [³H]thymidine was used to measure DNA synthesis. Chondrocytes were seeded at a density of 5×10^4 cells/ml in flexible-bottomed culture plates and allowed to attach to the membrane for 2 days. After incubation under cyclic tensile stretch for 18h, $40\,\mu l$ for [³H]thymidine (1.875MBq/ml in MEM) was added, and the cells were incubated for another 6h. The cell layers were then washed three times with cold PBS and treated successively with 5% trichloroacetic acid (TCA) and ethanol/ethyl ether (3:1, v/v). The residual materials in the wells were solubilized with 0.3M NaOH, the solution was neutralized with 6M HCl, and radioactivity was measured in a liquid scintillation counter [13].

Proteoglycan Synthesis

Cyclic tensile stretch was loaded for 24h, and [³⁵S]sulfate (0.74KBq/ml) was added in the last 4h of culture. The media were collected and cell layers were washed three times with ice-cold PBS. The cells were then placed in 1ml of PBS using a rubber policeman, sonicated for 30s at 0°C, and the proteoglycan present within the media and cells was then measured by assessing the incorporation of [³⁵S]sulfate into the cetylpyridinium chloride (CPC) precipitable material [14].

PKC Activity

Enzyme activity was measured using a Biotrak kit (Amersham, Little Chalfont, England). This assay system is based on the PKC-catalyzed transfer of the γ-phosphate group of adenosine-5'-triphosphate to a peptide that is specific for PKC. All assay components were thawed to 25°C before initiating the assay. Cyclic tensile stretch was loaded at the indicated time, and cell layers were washed with MEM and sonicated for 30s at 0°C in 50mM Tris/HCl pH 7.5 containing 5mM ethylenediaminc tetraacetic acid (EDTA), 10mM ethyleneglycol tetraacetic acid (EGTA), 0.3% w/v β-mercaptoethanol, 10mM benzamidine, and $50\mu g/ml$ phenylmethylsulfonyl fluoride, according to the supplier's recommendation. After $25\mu l$ of cell lysate was collected, an equal volume of component mixture was added that contained $12mM$ calcium acetate in a buffer containing $8mole\%$ Lα-phosphatidyl-L-serine, $24\mu g/ml$ phorbol 12-myristate 13-acetate, $900\mu M$ peptide, and $30mM$ dithlothreitol in $50mM$ Tris/HCl pH 7.5 and 0.05% w/v sodium azide. Then $25\mu l$ of magnesium ATP buffer was added containing $150\mu M$ ATP, $45mM$ magnesium acetate, and $10\mu Ci/ml$ of $[^{32}P]ATP$ in $50mM$ Tris/HCl, pH 7.5, and 0.05% w/v sodium azide. This preparation was mixed and incubated at $25°C$ for $15min$, followed by binding paper separation. Purified PKC from rat brain was used as the standard, and phosphate transferred per $15min$ was calculated according to the supplier's manual.

Statistical Analysis

Student's t-test was used to determine statistical significance.

Results

Proteoglycan Synthesis

Isolated bovine chondrocytes were seeded at a density of 2×10^5 cells/ml placed under cyclic tensile stretch. We first measured the proteoglycan synthesis in the cell layer using a radiolabeled precursor with two different regimens of stretch (see Table 1). There was no significant difference in cell number after 24h of stretch. Under conditions of low frequency and percent of stretch, proteoglycan synthesis was clearly enhanced. However, higher stress reduced proteoglycan synthesis in the cell layer (Fig. 2). We then focused on the higher stress condition to determine the underlying mechanisms in the inhibition of proteoglycan synthesis. Although higher stress enhanced the incorporation of a radiolabeled precursor present in the medium, the total amount of newly synthesized proteoglycan was inhibited (Table 2).

Morphological Change

After 24h of incubation, control chondrocytes (no stretch) remained round or polygonal and showed no particular orientation. Chondrocytes exposed to cyclic tensile stretch also had no apparent morphological changes.

DNA Synthesis

Chondrocytes were seeded at a density of 5×10^4 cells/ml followed by incorporation of $[^3H]$thymidine. Higher stress conditions of cyclic tensile stretch significantly enhanced DNA synthesis (Fig. 3).

40   K. Fukuda et al.

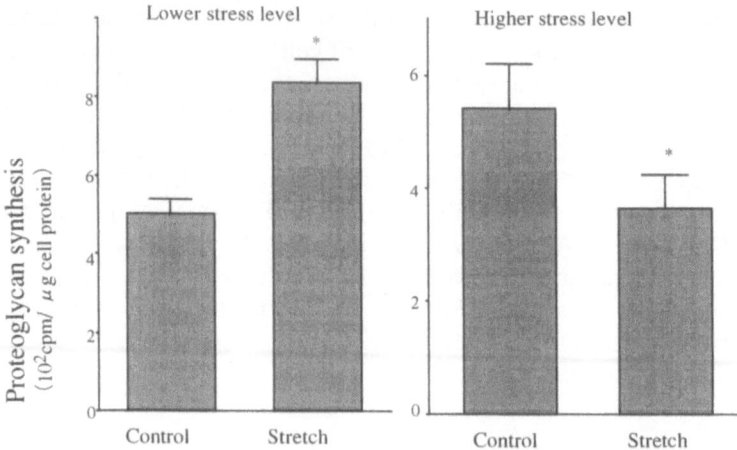

FIG. 2. Effect of cyclic tensile stretch on proteoglycan synthesis in bovine articular chondrocytes. Cells were seeded at a density of 2 × 10⁵ cells/ml in specially built, flexible-bottom culture plates. The stretch regimens are given in Table 1. Proteoglycan synthesis was measured based on [^{35}S]sulfate incorporation. Data are expressed as the mean ± SD of 6 wells. *, $P < .01$. Results were similar in three additional experiments

TABLE 2. Effect of higher stress conditions of cyclic tensile stretch on proteoglycan synthesis ($^{35}SO_4$ cpm/well)

Condition	Cell-associated	Medium	Total
No stress	6487 ± 497	1525 ± 331	9013 ± 458
Stress	4769 ± 479*	2486 ± 305*	7253 ± 358*

Cells were cultured in the absence or presence of a higher cyclic tensile stretch (see Table 1). Data are expressed mean ± SD of 6 wells.
*, $P < .01$. Results were similar in two additional experiments.

Involvement of PKC

When chondrocytes were cultured for 24h in the presence of phorbol ester, which directly activates cellular PKC, proteoglycan synthesis was enhanced (Fig. 4). When an inactive phorbol ester, 4α-PDD, was used, proteoglycan synthesis was unchanged. Coadministration of the PKC inhibitor H-7 [15] clearly reversed the stretch-induced inhibition of aggrecan synthesis (Fig. 5). Staurosporine, another PKC inhibitor [16], also reversed stretch-induced actions. These inhibitors had no significant effect on base-line aggrecan synthesis (data not shown). To deplete PKC, chondrocytes were cultured for 2h with or without a phorbol ester (100nM PDBu). The cell layer was then washed three times with PBS, and a further 48h of incubation with cyclic tensile stretch was carried out. Although proteoglycan synthesis was inhibited by stretch, this

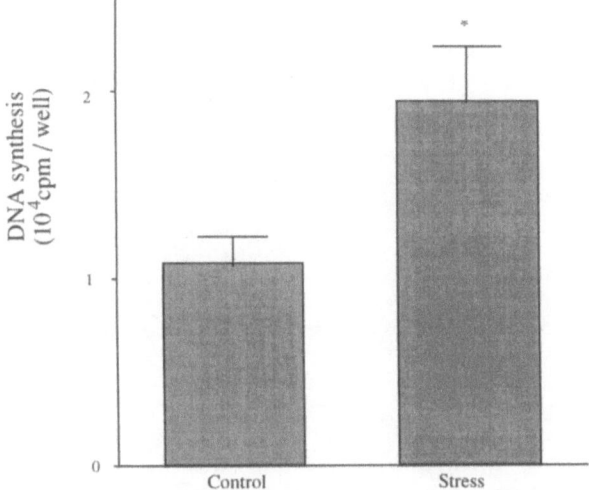

FIG. 3. Effect of cyclic tensile stretch on DNA synthesis in bovine articular chondrocytes. Cells were seeded at a density of 5×10^4 cells/ml in specially built, flexible-bottom culture plates. DNA synthesis was measured based on [^{3}H]thymidine incorporation. Data are expressed as the mean ± SD of 6 wells. *, $P < .01$

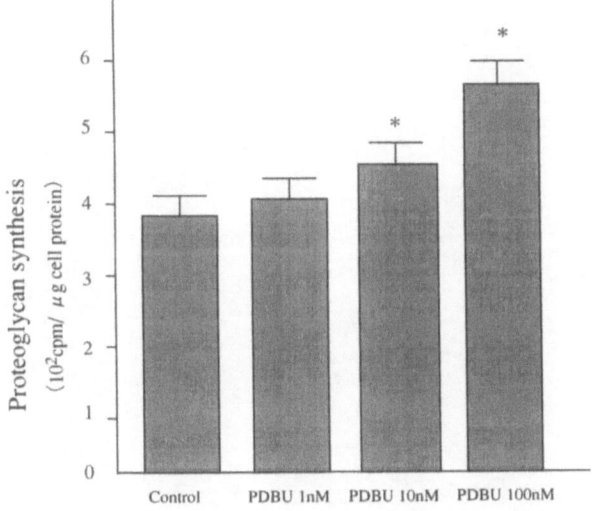

FIG. 4. Effect of phorbol ester on proteoglycan synthesis. Cells were seeded at a density of 2×10^5 cells/ml in 96-well plates. Different concentrations of phorbol ester (PDBu) were added for 24 h. Data are expressed as the mean ± SD of 6 wells. *, $P < .01$. Results were similar in two additional experiments

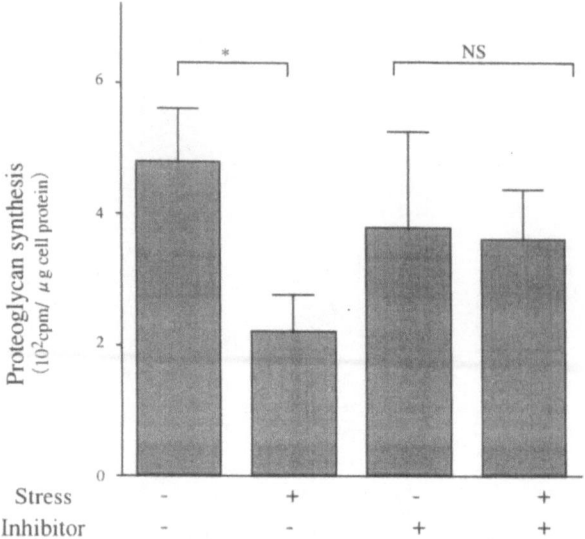

FIG. 5. Effect of a protein kinase C inhibitor on stress-mediated inhibition of proteoglycan synthesis. Cyclic tensile stretch (stress) was loaded on the chondrocytes in the absence (−) or presence (+) of a protein kinase C inhibitor (H7, 1μM) for 24h. Data are expressed as the mean ± SD of 6 wells. *, $P < .01$. NS, not significant

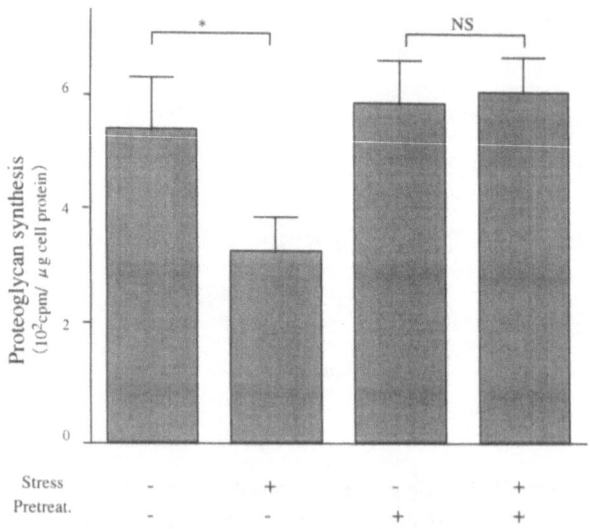

FIG. 6. Effect of pretreatment with phorbol ester on stress-mediated inhibition of proteoglycan synthesis. Chondrocytes were pretreated with phorbol ester (PDBu, 100nM) for 2h and cyclic tensile stretch (stress) was loaded for 24h. Data are expressed as the mean ± SD of 6 wells. *, $P < .01$. NS, not significant

TABLE 3. Effect of cyclic tensile stretch on protein kinase C (PKC) activity

Time	Exp. 1	Exp. 2	Exp. 3
3 min	80 ± 12	68 ± 12	n.d.
1 h	64 ± 11	56 ± 10	56 ± 12
24 h	43 ± 12	48 ± 11	42 ± 11

n.d., not determined.
Cells were cultured in the basence or presence of a higher cyclic tensile stretch (see Table 1). Enzyme activity was measured using a Biotrak kit, and phosphate transferred per 15 min was compared with nonstretched controls at the indicated time. Data are expressed as percent of control (mean ± SD of 6 wells). Three experiments are shown, using different preparations of bovine chondrocytes.

inhibition was completely blocked by PDBu pretreatment (Fig. 6). PKC activity was measured in the presence or absence of cyclic tensile stretch at the indicated time. This assay system is based on PKC-catalyzed transfer of the γ-phosphate group of adenosine-5'-triphosphate to a peptide that is specific for PKC. Usually, 20–40 pmole phosphate/15 min per well was transferred in the absence of cyclic tensile stretch. Cyclic tensile stretch significantly decreased PKC activity. Even 3 min of stretch loaded on the chondrocytes, the shortest time for detection after cyclic stretch, reduced PKC activity (Table 3).

Discussion

The effect of loading on articular cartilage generally has been studied in experimental animals. Although alterations of articular cartilage can be quantified reliably in these in vivo models, the cellular mechanisms controlling the changes are difficult to examine and thus have remained largely obscure. In this study, we used an apparatus for loading mechanical stress on isolated chondrocytes in vitro. Because the chondrocytes are rounded and surrounded with a matrix of normal cartilage, the physiological significance of this apparatus is questionable; that is, flat cells attach to only one surface where the cells are elongated. In this context, cartilage slices have been used for in vitro studies [17]. Furthermore, chondrocytes cultured in agarose gel, which synthesizes a mechanically functional extracellular matrix [18], may provide a more useful model system [19]. The Flexercell Strain Instrument used in this study makes it feasible to observe alterations in chondrocyte metabolism, at the cellular level, especially in the signal transduction pathway.

We detected an increase and decrease in proteoglycan synthesis by chondrocytes under lower and higher stress, respectively. In vitro studies have shown that static and dynamic loading of cartilage slices leads to an increase or decrease in matrix synthesis, depending on the magnitude and duration of the applied load [20–24]. Recently, Kin et al. tested several conditions using cartilage disk explants to determine the effect of physical stimuli [25]. There is still a need to carefully determine the effective threshold for increased synthesis using this apparatus.

In this report, we focused on the inhibition of proteoglycan synthesis elicited by higher stress, because it is a characteristic feature observed under conditions in which there is an advanced degeneration of articular cartilage, such as osteoarthrosis [26]. Our results show that inhibition of proteoglycan synthesis with cyclic stress is not the result of cell toxicity, as DNA synthesis was enhanced with this stress. We also observed enhanced DNA synthesis of an osteoblast-like cell, using the same regimen of cyclic tensile stretch [12]. Increased DNA synthesis has been demonstrated in aortic smooth muscle cells as well [27].

Previously we demonstrated the presence of PKC on chondrocytes, using [^{3}H]PDBu binding [8]. Recently, we noted the appearance and changes in distribution of PKC-positive chondrocytes in rat knee joints with mechanically induced osteoarthritis [9]. These data clearly suggest the involvement of PKC in the development of osteoarthritis. Accordingly, we examined the involvement of PKC with cyclic tensile stretch in vitro. In this study, two separate experiments were done, that is, using PKC inhibitors and downregulation of the response. We found that a PKC inhibitor, H-7, reversed stress-suppressed aggrecan synthesis. Because depletion or downregulation of PKC by phorbol esters has been shown to result in a reduction in response to subsequent phorbol ester treatment [18], we also pretreated cells with a phorbol ester before cyclic stretch. Proteoglycan synthesis was not inhibited under these conditions. These results demonstrate the involvement of PKC in stress-mediated inhibition of proteoglycan synthesis.

Recent observations indicate the presence of strain-sensitive ion channels in the membrane [28,29] and stretch-induced increases in intracellular calcium [30]. Calcium signaling is coupled to phosphoinositide turnover, which results in the increased production of diacylglycerol, a second messenger of PKC [31]. Accordingly, activation of PKC could be present in the stress-loaded chondrocytes.

However, phorbol ester treatment, which activates cellular PKC directly, enhances proteoglycan synthesis in the absence of cyclic tensile stretch, as we have reported elsewhere [8]. To explain this discrepancy, we measured PKC activity directly in the absence or presence of mechanical stress and noted downregulation of the enzyme activity in cyclically stretched chondrocytes. These data are consistent with our recent observation, in which experimental osteoarthritis was induced in the knee joints of rabbits by resection of the anterior cruciate ligament. At 4 weeks after the operation, osteoarthritic changes were observed. When PKC activator was administered intraarticularly, cartilage structures were preserved almost completely [10].

One possible explanation is the depletion of PKC with mechanical stress. Mechanical stress on chondrocytes may distort the membrane or cytoskeleton and lead to the inhibition of PKC activity. Parkkinen demonstrated a total disappearance of stress fibers with a hydrostatic pressure load on chondrocytes [32]. Recent observations indicate the involvement of PKC in the synthesis of stress fibers for focal adhesion [33,34]. The stress fibers may be involved in the regulation of proteoglycan synthesis in chondrocytes [35].

Various factors are probably involved in this action, and future research will focus on the precise signal transduction mechanisms leading to the inhibition of PKC. In this context, we will examine the free radical family, especially superoxide anion [36] and nitric oxide [37]. In addition, alteration in the size of proteoglycan synthesized must be investigated, as Smith et al. demonstrated recently [38].

Osteoarthrosis can be caused by mechanical stress loaded on articular cartilage. We have shown here a downregulation of PKC with cyclic tensile stretch in vitro.

Acknowledgments. We thank M. Ohara for helpful comments. This work was supported by a research grant from a Scientific Research Fund from the Ministry of Education, Science, Sports and Culture of Japan and by a grant from the Japan Rheumatism Foundation.

References

1. Heinegard D, Sommarin Y (1987) Proteoglycans: an overview. Methods Enzymol 144:305–319
2. Videman T, Eronen I, Friman C (1981) Experimental osteoarthritis in the rabbit. Acta Orthop Scand 52:11–22
3. Saamanen A-M, Tammi M, Kiviranta I, et al (1988) Running exercise as a modulator of proteoglycan matrix in the articular cartilage of young rabbits. Int J Sports Med 9:127–132
4. Juvelin J, Kiviranta I, Saamanen A-M, et al (1990) Indentation stiffness of canine knee articular cartilage— influence of strenuous joint loading. J Biomech 23:1239–1246
5. Palmoski MJ, Brandt KD (1981) Running inhibits the reversal of atrophic changes in canine knee cartilage after removal of a leg cast. Arthritis Rheum 24:1329–1337
6. Setton LA, Mow VC, Muller FJ, et al (1994) Mechanical properties of canine articular cartilage are significantly altered following transection of the anterior cruciate ligament. J Orthop Res 12:451–463
7. Nishizuka Y (1986) Studies and perspectives of protein kinase C. Science 233:305–312

8. Fukuda K, Yamasaki H, Nagata Y, et al (1991) Histamine H1-receptor-mediated keratan sulfate production in rabbit chondrocytes: involvement of protein kinase C. Am J Physiol 261:C413–C416

9. Satsuma H, Saito N, Tanaka S, et al (1996) Alpha and epsilon isozymes of protein kinase C in the chondrocytes in normal and early osteoarthritic cartilage. Calcif Tissue Int 58:192–194

10. Hamanishi C, Hashima M, Tanaka S, et al (1996) Protein kinase C-activator inhibits progression of osteoarthritis-induced rabbit knee joints. J Lab Clin Med 127:540–544

11. Sumpio BE, Banes AJ, Levin LG, et al (1987) Mechanical stress stimulates aortic endothelial cells to proliferate. J Vasc Surg 6:252–256

12. Nishioka S, Fukuda K, Tanaka S (1993) Cyclic stretch increases alkaline phosphatase activity of osteoblast-like cells: a role for prostaglandin E_2. Bone Miner 21:141–150

13. Fukuda K, Ohtani K, Tanaka S, et al (1993) Keratan sulfate inhibits its release in rabbit chondrocyte. Connect Tissue Res 30:75–83

14. Fukuda K, Matsumura F, Tanaka S (1993) Histamine H2 receptor mediates keratan sulfate secretion in rabbit chondrocytes: role of cAMP. Am J Physiol 265:C1653–C1657

15. Hidaka H, Inagaki M, Kawamoto S, et al (1984) Isoquineline-sulphonamides, novel and potent inhibitors of cyclic nucleotide dependent kinase and protein kinase C. Biochemistry 23:5036–5041

16. Conquer JA, Kandel RA, Cruz TF (1992) Interleukin 1 and phorbol 12-myristate 13-acetate induce collagenase and PGE_2 production through a PKC-independent mechanism in chondrocytes. Biochim Biophys Acta 1134:1–6

17. Sah R, Grodzinsky A, Plaas A, et al (1992) Effect of static and dynamic compression on matrix metabolism in cartilage explants. In: Kuettner K, Schleyerbach R, Peyron, Hascall V (eds) Articular cartilage and osteoarthritis. Raven Press, New York, pp 373–392

18. Buschman MD, Gluzband YA, Grodzinsky AJ, et al (1992) Chondrocytes in agarose culture synthesize a mechanically functional extracellular matrix. J Orthop Res 10:745–758

19. Freeman PM, Natarajan RN, Kimura JH, et al (1994) Chondrocyte cells respond mechanically to compressive load. J Orthop Res 12:311–320

20. Urban JPG (1994) The chondrocyte: a cell under pressure. Br J Rheumatol 33:901–908

21. Gray ML, Pizzanelli AM, Grodzinsky AJ, et al (1988) Mechanical and physicochemical determinations of the chondrocyte biosynthetic response. J Orthop Res 6:777–792

22. Palmoski MJ, Brandt KD (1984) Effects of static and cyclic compressive loading on articular cartilage plugs in vitro. Arthritis Rheum 27:675–681

23. Sah RL-Y, Kim YJ, Doong J-YH, et al (1989) Biosynthetic response of cartilage explants to dynamic compression. J Orthop Res 7:619–636

24. Hall AC, Urban JPG, Gehl KA (1991) The effect of hydrostatic pressure on matrix synthesis in articular cartilage. J Orthop Res 9:1–10

25. Kim YJ, Sah R, Grodzinsky A, et al (1994) Mechanical regulation of cartilage biosynthetic behavior: physical stimuli. Arch Biochem Biophys 311:1–12

26. Mankin HJ, Lippiello L (1970) Biochemical and metabolic abnormalities in articular cartilage from osteoarthritic human hips. J Bone Joint Surg 52A:424–434

27. Sumpio BE, Banes AJ (1988) Response of porcine aortic smooth muscle cells to cyclic tensional deformation in culture. J Surg Res 44:696–701
28. Lansman JB, Hallam TJ, Rink TJ (1987) Single stretch-activated ion channels in vascular endothelial cells as mechanotransducers. Nature (Lond) 325:811–813
29. Duncan R, Misler S (1989) Voltage-activated and stretch-activated Ba^{2+} conducting channels in an osteoblast-like cell line (UMR 106). FEBS Lett 251:17–21
30. Reich KM, Frangos JA (1991) Effect of flow on prostaglandin E_2 and inositol triphosphate levels in osteoblasts. Am J Physiol 261:C428–C432
31. Davis MJ, Meininger GA, Zawieja DC (1992) Stretch-induced increases in intracellular calcium of isolated vascular smooth muscle cells. Am J Physiol 32:H1292–H1299
32. Parkkinen J, Lammi M, Inkinen R, et al (1995) Influence of short-term hydrostatic pressure on organization of stress fibers in cultured chondrocytes. J Orthop Res 13:495–502
33. Tang D, Tarrien M, Dobrzynski P, et al (1995) Melanoma cell spreading on fibronectin induced by 12(S)-HETE involves both protein kinase C- and protein tyrosine kinase-dependent focal adhesion formation and tyrosine phosphorylation of focal adhesion kinase (pp125FAK). J Cell Physiol 165:291–306
34. Barry S, Critchley D (1994) The RhoA-dependent assembly of focal adhesions in Swiss 3T3 cells is associated with increased tyrosine phosphorylation and the recruitment of both pp125FAK and protein kinase C-δ to focal adhesion. J Cell Sci 107:2033–2045
35. Newman P, Watt FM (1988) Influence of cytochalasin D-induced changes in cell shape on proteoglycan synthesis by cultured articular chondrocytes. Exp Cell Res 178:199–210
36. Fukuda K, Dan H, Tanaka S, et al (1994) Superoxide dismutase inhibits interleukin-1-induced degradation of human cartilage. Agents Actions 42:71–73
37. Fukuda K, Kumano M, Tanaka S, et al (1995) Zonal difference of nitric oxide synthesis with interleukin-1 in bovine chondrocytes. Inflamm Res 44:434–437
38. Smith R, Donlon B, Gupta M, et al (1995) Effects of fluid-induced shear on articular chondrocyte morphology and metabolism in vitro. J Orthop Res 13:824–831

Muscarinic Receptor-Mediated Ca^{2+} Control, Protein Kinase C Activity, and Proteoglycan Release and Synthesis in Articular Chondrocytes

Makoto Hashima, Chiaki Hamanishi, and Seisuke Tanaka

Summary. To determine the presence and role of muscarinic receptors on articular chondrocytes, Scatchard analysis of muscarinic antagonist binding to membrane fragments of rabbit articular chondrocytes, and analysis of the changes in the intracellular calcium ion concentration, protein kinase C (PKC) activity, and the synthesis and release of glucoseaminoglycan (GAG) induced by the muscarinic agonists and antagonists were carried out. Scatchard analysis of the muscarinic antagonist [^{3}H]quinuclidinyl benzilate (QNB) revealed a single class of binding sites with a K_D of 3.2 ± 0.12nM and a B_{max} of 83.19 ± 2.73fmol/mg of protein. The addition of the muscarinic agonist oxotremorine elevated the intracellular calcium ion concentration and protein kinase C activity, increased the release, and decreased the synthesis of GAG. The specific M1 receptor antagonist inhibited all these stimulative or inhibitory effects of oxotremorine almost completely, although specific M2 and M3 receptor antagonists did not. This is the first study, to our knowledge, documenting the presence and role of muscarinic receptors on articular chondrocytes.

Key Words. Muscarinic receptor, Articular chondrocyte, Proteoglycan, Protein kinase C, Calcium

Introduction

Cholinergic muscarinic receptors have been mainly found on cells in neural tissue [1–4], on smooth muscle or secreting cells in the gastrointestinal system [5–7], and on adrenal gland cells [8]. The muscarinic M1 receptor subtype was reported to be linked to phosphoinositide turnover [3] in cultured brain cells. Muscarinic receptors have not been found in articular cartilage. We examined muscarinic receptors on chondrocytes in connection with intracellular calcium

Department of Orthopaedic Surgery, Kinki University School of Medicine, 377-2 Ohno-Higashi, Osaka-Sayama, Osaka 589-8511, Japan ions, protein kinase C (PKC) activity, and glucoseaminoglycan (GAG) release and synthesis.

Materials and Methods

Drugs and Chemicals

Dulbecco's modified Eagle's medium (DMEM), HAM's F-12, and neomycine were obtained from Gibco (Grand Island, NY, USA), fetal bovine serum (FBS) from HyClone (Logan, UT, USA), atropine, oxotremorine, pirenzepine, and 1-(5-isoquinolinylsulfonyl)-2-methyl-pirenzepine (H7) from Sigma (St. Louis, MO, USA), and [^{3}H]quinuclidinyl benzilate ([^{3}H]QNB, 33.1 Ci/mmole) from DuPont (Boston, MA, USA). AF-DX116 (AFDX) was obtained from Boehringer Ingelheim (Ingelheim, Germany), 1,1-dimethyl-4-diphenylacetoxypiperidinium (4-DAMP) from Cosmo Bio (Tokyo, Japan), shark-derived chondroitin sulfate from Seikagaku (Tokyo, Japan), and Fura 2-AM from Wako Pure Chemical (Tokyo, Japan). The PKC assay kit was obtained from Amersham (Buckinghamshire, England), 1,9-dimethylmethylene blue (DMB) from Serva (Heidelberg, Germany), [^{35}S]sulfate from New England Nuclear (Boston, MA, USA), and pronase E from Kaken Kagaku (Tokyo, Japan).

Chondrocyte Culture

Cartilage was removed aseptically from the shoulder and knee joints of male Japanese white rabbits, chopped into fine pieces, and digested with 0.2% collagenase [9] for 3 h. DMEM and HAM's F-12 were mixed at a ratio of 1:1 [10]. The chondrocytes were cultured in 75-cm^2 tissue culture plates in DMEM supplemented with penicillin-streptomycin-amphotericin B and 10% FBS at 37°C in a 5% CO_2 atmosphere. When the cells had reached confluency, they were seeded at a density of 1×10^5 cells/ml in 24- or 96-well plates. The cells were allowed 48 h to attach.

Binding of Ligands to Chondrocyte Membranes

When the cells had again reached confluency, they were harvested in the manner described next. After rapid shaking of the flasks, the cells were separated from the growth medium by centrifugation at $1000 \times g$ for 5 min, and the resulting pellet was then washed three times with Dulbecco's phosphate-buffered saline by centrifugation at $1000 \times g$ for 2 min. The cell number was determined with a hemocytometer. Subsequently, the cells were rewashed with 10 mM NaKPO$_4$ buffer (Na$_2$HPO$_4$, 8.1 mM; KH$_2$PO$_4$, 1.9 mM, pH 7.5). The pelleted intact cells were rapidly frozen in liquid nitrogen and stored at −80°C until assayed.

To provide cell membranes for the muscarinic receptor binding assays, the frozen cells were thawed and suspended in 10 mM NaKPO$_4$ buffer. The cell homogenate was prepared by homogenizing with a Handy Sonic UR-20P (Tomy Seiko, Tokyo, Japan) and centrifuged at 48000 × g for 15 min. The resulting pellet was resuspended in the same buffer and rehomogenized. Microscopic examination of the homogenate revealed that all the cells had ruptured into fine membrane particles.

Specific [^{3}H]QNB Binding Assay

Specific [^{3}H]QNB binding was determined using the filtration assay. The cell homogenate (~10^6 cells) was incubated briefly with [^{3}H]QNB (1.6–21.0 nM) in a final volume of 1.0 ml of 10 mM NaKPO$_4$ buffer at 25°C for 90 min. The final concentration of protein per assay tube (1 ml) was 0.3–0.4 mg. Nonspecific [^{3}H]QNB binding was determined in the presence of 20 μM atropine sulfate, and all assays were performed in triplicate. The reaction was terminated by rapid filtration through Whatman glass fiber filters. The filters were rinsed three times with 5 ml of ice-cold 10 mM NaKPO$_4$ buffer to remove excess free [^{3}H]QNB and dried.

The ligand was extracted from the filters into 5 ml of scintillation fluid and measured in a scintillation counter. Saturation and inhibition data were analyzed by nonlinear least squares regression analysis. The averaged data from independent experiments was weighted or unweighted to obtain the best fitted curves. Protein was determined using bovine serum albumin as a standard.

Calcium Ion Assay

Cells (1 × 10^4) were monolayer cultured, and Fura 2-AM (5 μM) was added to the cells. Oxotremorine (10^{-5} M) was added to the cells and the intracellular calcium ion concentration was measured periodically (ARGUS-50/CA; Hamamatsu Photonics, Hamamatsu, Japan). The calcium ion concentration was measured after challenge with QNB (10^{-5} M) or with the nonselective muscarinic agonist oxotremorine (10^{-5} M) after 15 min of pretreatment with QNB (10^{-5} M), the M1 antagonist pirenzepine (10^{-5} M), the M2 antagonist AFDX (10^{-5} M), the M3 antagonist 4DAMP (10^{-5} M), and the phospholipase C-blocker neomycine (300 μM).

PKC Activity

Chondrocytes were cultured for 24 h in a serum-free medium, washed three times, and homogenized with a Handy Sonic UR-20P. The protein volume was corrected, and the PKC activity was measured using the PKC assay kit. Oxotremorine (10^{-5}–10^{-8} M) challenge was followed by addition of 10^{-5} M of QNB.

GAG Assay

Reacting fluid was prepared with 16 mg of DMB, which was dissolved with 5 ml of ethanol, 2 ml of acid buffer, and 993 ml of distilled water. The standard solution was made using shark-derived chondroitin sulfate. The chondrocytes were challenged with 10^{-5} M of oxotremorine alone, oxotremorine and several concentrations of QNB, 10^{-5} M of the M1 antagonist pirenzepine, 10^{-5} M of the M2 antagonist AFDX, 10^{-5} M of the M3 antagonist 4DAMP, and the PKC antagonist H7 for 48 h. Using photoabsorptiometry at a wavelength of 525 nm, the concentration of chondroitin sulfate in $100 \mu l$ of the supernatant of each cell culture was mixed with $100 \mu l$ of reacting fluid, and measured.

GAG Synthesis

Chondrocytes were cultured for 24 h in serum-free medium, washed three times, challenged for 24 h by several of the ligands described in the foregoing GAG assay, and then exposed for 8 h to 1500 kBq/ml of $Na_2{}^{35}SO_4{}^{2-}$. The cell layers were washed three times; then, 1.4 ml of ice-cold 0.15 N NaOH was added and the cells were immediately scraped off with a rubber policeman (Falcon cell scraper, Becton Dickinson, Lincoln Park, NJ, USA). Equal volumes of the medium and cell fraction were combined and neutralized with 6 N HCL. To 1 ml of the mixture was added 2 ml of Tris-HCl buffer (pH 7.8), containing 5 mM $CaCl_2$ and 4 mg of pronase E (1000 tyrosine units), and the mixture was incubated for 12 h at 55°C. Then, $50 \mu l$ of water containing $5 \mu g$ of chondroitin sulfate and 1.0 ml of 2 mM $MgSO_4$ were added. Polysaccharides were precipitated by the addition of 1.0 ml of 1% cetylpyridinium chloride (CPC) at 37°C for 1 h, and the precipitate was collected on a Milipore filter (Whatman GF/F) and washed five times with 1% CPC-0.02 M NaCl, 1 ml. The filter was air dried and solubilized in 10 ml of Econo Fluor-2, and the radioactivity was measured in an Aloka scintillation spectrometer.

Results

$[^3H]QNB$ Binding Assay

Saturation experiments were performed to determine the equilibrium dissociation constant (K_D) for $[^3H]QNB$ and the number of receptor sites in the cultures (B_{max}). Total $[^3H]QNB$ binding increased rapidly and reached its maximum after 1 h of incubation. When $20 \mu M$ of atropine was added, total radioligand binding decreased acutely to the level of nonspecific binding, which was defined as radioligand binding in the presence of $20 \mu M$ atropine (Fig. 1). The binding of $[^3H]QNB$ in the cultures was well characterized by a single site with a K_D of 3.2 ± 0.12 nM and a linear Scatchard plot (Fig. 2). The protein content of the cultures was determined, and the B_{max} was expressed as 83.19 ± 2.73 fmol/mg of protein.

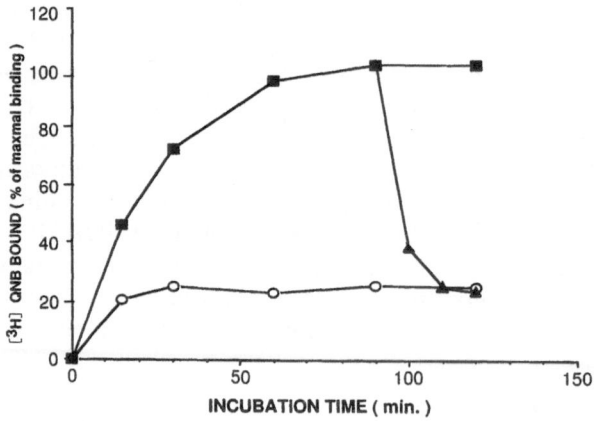

FIG. 1. Total [³H]QNB ([³H]quinuclidnyl benzilate) binding increased rapidly and reached its maximum after 1 h of incubation. When 20 μM of atropine was added (*triangles*), total radioligand binding (*squares*) decreased acutely to the level of non-specific binding (*circles*)

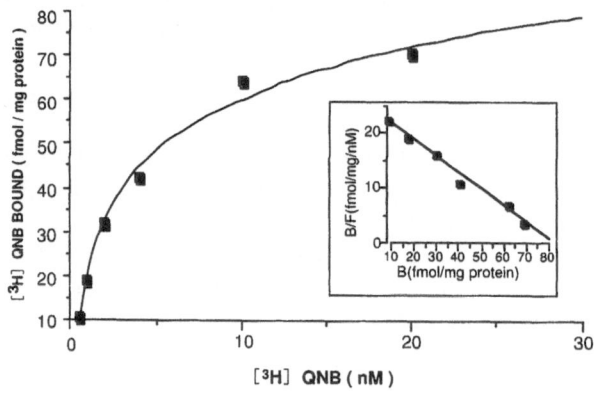

FIG. 2. Specific binding of [³H]QNB to cultured articular chondrocytes. *Inset,* Scatchard plot of the specific binding of [³H]QNB; *B/F*, bound/free; *B*, bound

Intracellular Calcium Ion Concentration

The intracellular calcium ion concentration increased to fourfold 15 s after being challenged with oxotremorine (Fig. 3). The calcium ion concentration did not increase on challenge with QNB alone or with oxotremorine after 15 min of pretreatment with QNB, the M1 antagonist pirenzepine, or with the phospholipase C-blocker neomycine. The M2 antagonist AFDX and the M3 antagonist 4DAMP did not inhibit the increase in the calcium ion concentration induced by oxotremorine (Table 1).

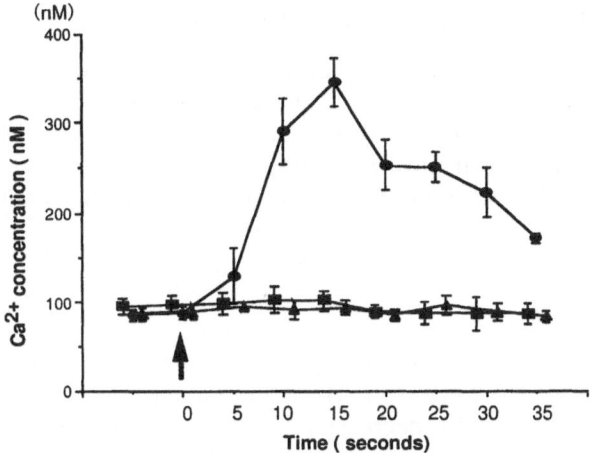

FIG. 3. Calcium ion concentration in the cultured articular chondrocytes after challenge with oxotremorine alone (*circles*), QNB alone (*triangles*), or both (*squares*)

TABLE 1. Calcium ion concentrations, protein kinase C (PKC) activity, and release and synthesis of glucoseaminoglycan (GAG) after challenge with oxotremorine with 15 min of pretreatment with [^{3}H]quinuclidinyl benzilate (QNB), pirenzepine, AF-DX116 (AF-DX), 1,1-dimethyl-4-diphenyl acetoxy piperidinium (4DAMP), 1-(5-isoquinolinyl sulfonyl)-2-methyl-pirenzepine (H7), or neomycine

	[Ca^{2+}], (nM)	PKC (ng/ml)	GAG release (% control)	GAG synthesis (% control)
Control	90.3 ± 4.2	123.1 ± 9.4	100.0 ± 1.7	100.0 ± 6.7
OXO	346.0 ± 28.2*	178.6 ± 11.2*	129.0 ± 1.4*	45.7 ± 8.2*
OXO + QNB	102.0 ± 15.2	126.3 ± 6.8	100.8 ± 5.3	70.3 ± 4.1
OXO + PZ	112.0 ± 22.7	129.0 ± 7.3	108.7 ± 1.5	68.7 ± 1.9
OXO + AF-DX	327.0 ± 22.7	175.0 ± 10.1	128.2 ± 1.4	46.2 ± 4.9
OXO + 4-DAMP	331.0 ± 24.3	172.9 ± 8.9	127.8 ± 1.6	45.5 ± 4.3
OXO + H7		122.7 ± 10.8	107.9 ± 2.3	89.6 ± 9.3
OXO + neomycine	103.1 ± 9.8			

OXO, oxotremorine; PZ, M1 antagonist, pirenzepine; AF-DX, M2 antagonist; 4-DAMP, M3 antagnoist; H7, PKC antagonist; neomycine, phospholipase C-blocker.
$n = 4$; *, $P < .05$.

PKC Activity

The PKC activity increased on challenge with oxotremorine dose dependently and significantly at concentrations of 10^{-5}M and 10^{-6}M. The addition of 10^{-5}M of QNB, or the M1 antagonist pirenzepine, inhibited the increase in PKC almost completely, although addition of the M2 antagonist AFDX, the M3 antagonist 4DAMP, and the PKC antagonist H7 did not (Table 1).

Release of GAG and Chondroitin Sulfate

The concentration of chondroitin sulfate in the culture medium was increased significantly 48h after the addition of oxotremorine at a concentration of 10^{-5}M. The addition of 10^{-5}M of QNB, 10^{-5}M of the M1 antagonist pirenzepine, or 10^{-5}M of the PKC antagonist H7 significantly inhibited this increase but the M2 antagonist AFDX and the M3 antagonist 4DAMP did not (Table 1).

GAG Synthesis

GAG synthesis decreased on challenge with oxotremorine dose dependently, and the addition of 10^{-5}M of QNB, the M1 antagonist pirenzepine, or the PKC antagonist H7 inhibited this decrease in synthesis although addition of the M2 antagonist AFDX and the M3 antagonist 4DAMP did not (see Table 1).

Discussion

This is the first study to demonstrate that muscarinic receptors are a single class of membrane-bound receptors found on chondrocytes. Stimulation of muscarinic receptor by the nonselective muscarinic agonist oxotremorine elevated the intracellular calcium ion concentration, stimulated PKC activities, increased the release of GAG, and inhibited GAG synthesis in a dose-dependent manner. The dominant subtype of muscarinic receptor (MR) on chondrocytes seemed to be MR-1, because the specific MR-1 receptor antagonist pirenzepine inhibited the stimulative effects of oxotremorine almost completely whereas the specific MR-2 receptor antagonist AF-DX and the MR-3 receptor antagonist 4DAMP did not.

Because muscarinic receptors are cholinergic, the mechanism of stimulation might involve acetylcholine or acetylcholine-like substances entering the matrix from the synovial fluid, from vascular buds that traverse the tidemark in arthritic conditions [11], or from the chondrocytes themselves. Skin keratocytes reportedly produce and secrete acetylcholine by themselves and express several types of muscarinic receptors [12]. Whether chondrocytes produce acetylcholine, or what types of external stimulation increase the concentration of acetylcholine or acetylcholine-like substances in the cartilage matrix in either normal or pathological joints, needs to be determined. Once the muscarinic receptors were activated, stimulated phosphoinositide turnover [3] increased calcium ion concentrations and activated not only calcium-independent subtypes but also calcium-dependent subtypes of PKC.

In our in vivo experiments using rat early osteoarthritic joints, we have found that one form of calcium-dependent PKC, α-PKC, newly appeared in chondrocytes, calcium-independent ε-PKC was activated [13], chondroitin sulfate levels were increased both intra- and extracellularly, keratane sulfate was increased in the cartilage matrix, and dermatan sulfate was also depicted in the osteoarthritic cartilage matrix (in preparation).

We have also recently reported that an intra-articularly injected PKC activator markedly inhibited the progression of osteoarthritis induced in rabbit knee joints [11]. In this in vitro study, muscarinic stimulation eventually increased GAG release from the chondrocytes and inhibited GAG synthesis. It should thus be elucidated whether these in vitro events also take place in the articular cartilage in vivo, and whether activation or inhibition of muscarinic receptors affects the onset and progression of osteoarthritis.

References

1. Lin S-C, Olson KC, Okazaki H, Richelson E (1986) Studies on muscarinic binding sites in human brain identified with [3H]pirenzepine. J Neurochem 46:274–279
2. Ashkenazi A, Ramachandran J, Capon DJ (1989) Acetylcholine analogue stimulates DNA synthesis in brain-derived cells via specific muscarinic receptor subtypes. Nature (Lond) 340:146–150
3. Atkins PT, Surmeier D, Kitai ST (1990) M1 muscarinic acetylcholine receptors in cultured rat neostriatum regulates phosphoinositide hydrolysis. J Neurochem 54:266–273
4. Ellis J, Huyler JH, Kemp DE, Weiss S (1990) Muscarinic receptors and second-messenger responses of neurons in primary culture. Brain Res 511:234–240
5. Wada K, Sakamoto C, Motozaki T (1992) M3 muscarinic receptors mediate pepsinogen secretion via polyphosphoinositide hydrolysis in guinea pig gastric chief cells. Gastroenterol Jpn 27:473–481
6. Zhang L, Buxton ILO (1993) Protein kinase regulation of muscarinic receptor signalling in colonic smooth muscle. Br J Pharmacol 108:613–621
7. Honda K, Takano Y, Kamiya H (1993) Pharmacological profiles of muscarinic receptors in the longitudinal smooth muscle of guinea pig ileum. Jpn J Pharmacol 62:43–47
8. Akaike A, Sasa M, Tamura Y, Ujihara H, Takaori S (1993) Effects of protein kinase C on the muscarinic excitation of rat adrenal chromaffin cells. Jpn J Pharmacol 61:145–148
9. Benya P, Padilla S, Nimni M (1977) The progeny of rabbit articular chondrocytes synthesize collagen type I, III and type I trimer, but not type II. Biochemistry 16:865–872
10. Glaser JL, Conrad HE (1984) Properties of chick embryo chondrocytes grown in serum-free medium. J Biol Chem 259:6766–6772
11. Hamanishi C, Hashima M, Satsuma H, Tanaka S (1996) Protein kinase C-activator inhibits progression of osteoarthritis induced in rabbit knee joints. J Clin Lab Med 127:540–544
12. Grando SA, Zelickson BD, Kist DA, Weinshenker D, Bigliardi PL, Wendelschafer-Crabb G, Kennedy WR, Dahl MV (1995) Keratinocyte muscarinic acetylcholine receptors: immunolocalization and partial characterization. J Invest Dermatol 104:95–100
13. Satsuma H, Saitou N, Hamanishi C, Hashima M, Tanaka S (1996) Alpha and epsilon isozymes of protein kinase C in the chondrocytes in normal and early osteoarthritic articular cartilage. Calcif Tissue Int 58:192–194

B. Functional Diagnosis of Osteoarthritis

Physical Diagnostics of Cartilage Degeneration

STEVEN TREPPO[1,2], SCOTT I. BERKENBLIT[1,2], DAVID L. BOMBARD[1], ELIOT H. FRANK[1], and ALAN J. GRODZINSKY[1,2]

Summary. We have focused on a new technology for nondestructive measurement of electrical and mechanical properties of articular cartilage via electrodes placed on the tissue surface. The long-term goal of this research is to enable detection of early stages of cartilage degradation based on the sensitivity of cartilage electromechanical properties to damage of the aggrecan-collagen network and loss of the highly charged aggrecan molecules. Ultimately, this technique may find application in early in vivo detection of cartilage degradation via arthroscopy. Experimental and theoretical results [1,2] have shown that an electric current applied to the articular surface of cartilage will produce a current-generated mechanical stress within the bulk of the tissue, via electrokinetic mechanisms, measurable at the surface. Based on this principle, a surface probe has been developed containing electrodes for applying current to the cartilage surface and an overlying piezoelectric sensor for measuring the resulting stress. Small sinusoidal currents applied to cartilage produce sinusoidal surface stresses at the same frequency. Such responses have been observed using disks of bovine articular cartilage, cartilage on intact bovine knee joint surfaces, and, recently, in preliminary in vivo studies in a canine knee joint model. The frequency response of the current-generated stress was found to agree well with trends predicted by poroelastic theory [1]. Because the depth to which current penetrates into the tissue is proportional to the imposed spatial wavelength (twice the electrode spacing), we have developed a multiple wavelength probe to test the possibility that measurement using multiple wavelengths and frequencies could be used to image depth-dependent partial thickness degradation, as occurs in early osteoarthritis.

---

[1] Continuum Electromechanics Group, Center for Biomedical Engineering, Department of Electrical Engineering and Computer Science, Masschusetts Institute of Technology, Cambridge, MA 02139, U.S.A.
[2] Harvard–M.I.T. Division of Health Sciences and Technology, Massachusetts Institute of Technology, 77 Massachusetts Avenue, Cambridge, MA 02139, U.S.A.

Key Words.   Cartilage, Diagnostic, Electrokinetic, Degeneration, Surface probe

Introduction

Current clinical diagnosis of osteoarthritis (OA) and methods for monitoring disease progression are based on external physical examination and roentgenographic criteria. However, these methods reveal cartilage and bone involvement only in the later stages of disease [3]. A major need is for early quantitative assessment of degenerative changes in the physical as well as biochemical properties of cartilage. This need has motivated the ongoing development of magnetic resonance imaging (MRI) techniques [4] and improved methods for arthroscopic evaluation of cartilage [5]. While specialized NMR/MRI techniques have been applied to assessment of cartilage composition [6], current clinical MRI methods have limited resolution and do not focus on tissue physical properties [7]. Arthroscopic evaluation has been routinely based on visual inspection [8] and qualitative mechanical probing. Thus, we have focused on quantitative diagnostics of tissue physical properties that may complement observations using other imaging modalities.

The failure of cartilage in OA is ultimately defined as a failure of the tissue's biomechanical properties and the inability of the tissue to withstand high levels of mechanical stress in the joint. Therefore, quantitative assessment of tissue physical properties in vivo is needed, along with correlative MR imaging [9], to best understand and evaluate disease progression. A more sensitive and specific measure of cartilage degradation than is currently available might help to determine whether treatment or altered activity could change the course of the early pathological changes of OA [10]. This knowledge could significantly reduce health care costs of OA and improve the quality of life for those patients [11]. In addition, there is a great need for methods to rapidly assess the efficacy of therapeutic interventions being developed to prevent cartilage destruction [12] or induce cartilage repair [13].

One of the early events in OA is a molecular-level alteration of the cartilage extracellular matrix and the loss of certain highly charged macromolecules (aggrecan) from the matrix. These molecular-level changes often occur in localized regions of cartilage along the joint surface and occur nonuniformly with depth into the tissue. (With visual inspection, the cartilage surface might still appear normal.) Investigators have hypothesized that such molecular changes should cause changes in the tissue's functional biomechanical properties. However, there have been few direct quantitative studies of the material properties of human cartilage in vivo.

We have observed that cartilage exhibits electromechanical transduction properties that change in a manner very sensitive to matrix alterations [14–18]. These studies showed that alterations or loss of tissue proteoglycans (PGs) caused early changes in tissue electromechanical properties. While PG loss also affected cartilage biomechanical properties, the changes in electromechanical behavior were often far more dramatic. These results provided the basis for an in vivo surface electromechanical spectroscopic approach to detect cartilage degeneration. We summarize here our recent progress with this new diagnostic modality and our initial in vivo canine studies using the spectrometer.

In Vivo Probes of Cartilage Mechanical Behavior

Early degradative changes in human OA cartilage include increased fibrillation of collagen with an accompanying increase in tissue water content (swelling) [19], as well as loss of aggrecan. These matrix changes occur initially in the superficial zone and nonuniformly with depth from the articular surface [20]. The resulting changes in cartilage material properties in animal models of OA have been well documented in studies in vitro (see [21] for review). However, there are fewer studies of physical changes in human OA cartilage. Knowledge of such changes at the molecular and tissue level could help to provide a differential diagnostic measurement. The tracking of in vivo cartilage physical properties would also aid in longitudinal studies of OA progression, allowing pharmaceutical companies to evaluate the efficacy of a pharmacological intervention. In addition, in situ physical diagnostics could provide an objective measurement of the quality of repair cartilage as tissue-engineered cartilage develops toward a clinical reality.

To date, the few studies of human cartilage physical properties have focused on tissue mechanical behavior assessed using handheld probes. In one study of the structural properties of cartilage from the lateral femoral condyle surface, Tkaczuk measured load-deformation curves in 25 autopsy specimens and during 35 open procedures [22]. The cartilage was classified as healthy or diseased based on X-ray examination. The measurements were taken with a blunt probe connected firmly to the joint with a custom fixing device; cartilage thickness was assessed as the distance between the articular surface and the point where the probe pierced the subchondral bone in a test to failure. Tkaczuk found that cartilage stiffness depended on age, but that there was no significant difference in stiffness between healthy and diseased cartilage. Any differences that existed may have been masked by the cartilage thickness evaluation.

After many years of experience with a blunt arthroscopic probe to subjectively assess the integrity of cartilage from the medial facet of the patella, Dashefsky [23] designed a more objective arthroscopic measurement apparatus. He used an instrumented indentor attached to a force transducer to study the mechanical properties of patellar cartilage in patients with chondromalacia. In a group of 107 knees with patellofemoral symptoms and signs, 90% were evaluated as "soft," but more than half of these soft cartilages showed no detectable visual changes of the articular surface of the patella. Interestingly, of 58 patients with no signs or symptoms, 50% showed softening of the cartilage. These results suggested that physical property changes may not correlate with the patient symptoms until an irreversible threshhold of damage occurs with the chronic wear and tear of cartilage.

More recently, Lyyra et al. [24], developed an arthroscopic indentor instrumented with strain gauges for measurement of tissue stiffness in vivo (Artscan 1000; Artscan Medical Innovations, Helsinki, Finland). A constant deformation is imposed on the cartilage by the indentor, and the "instantaneous" load response during a 1-s measurement interval is used to evaluate the tissue stiffness before appreciable stress relaxation has occurred. To compute an effective dynamic modulus, an independent measurement of tissue thickness is necessary, as with any indentation technique. The device was able to detect differences in the stiffness of cartilage in different regions of normal knees. Interestingly, however, the indentor detected only 30%–40% decreases in cartilage stiffness in the most severely affected regions of the patellar cartilage of patients with known chondromalacia [25].

From these studies, it is important to note that early OA cartilage may appear normal by visual inspection. Given that arthroscopy is one of the most common orthopaedic procedures [26], visual inspection alone during arthroscopy may not be sufficient for diagnostic purposes, suggesting the need for quantitative approaches. In addition, these studies suggest that purely mechanical tests alone (e.g., indentation tests) may not provide a sufficiently sensitive index of early degenerative changes in cartilage. This, in part, has motivated the incorporation of cartilage's electromechanical transduction properties into a surface diagnostic probe [2], as described next.

Electromechanical Surface Spectroscopy

Cartilage exhibits electromechanical transduction properties that change in a sensitive manner following the loss of negatively charged proteoglycans [27]. We hypothesized that the application of a small electric current at the cartilage surface via a surface electrode array would produce a mechanical stress within the tissue bulk that could be detected at the surface by a sensor array. The electrical (input) and mechanical (output) signals are periodic in both space and time, and the imposed temporal frequency and spatial wavelength can be independently varied by circuitry or probe construction, respectively [1,28].

Electrode Fabrication for Surface Sensor/Transducer

To form the surface sensor, a silver sheet is bonded to a Mylar film using a urethane epoxy (Tycel 7000/7200; Lord, Erie, PA, USA). The opposite side of the Mylar film (metallized with a thin film of aluminum) is bonded with a phenolic rubber adhesive (Plymaster 212; Norwood, Frazier, PA, USA) to a 52-μm polyvinylidene flouride (PVDF) piezoelectric film with a NiCu alloy metallization (KYNAR; AMP, Philadelphia, PA, USA). The sensor and excitation electrode patterns are etched from their respective metallizations using standard photofabrication techniques. The silver (excitation) electrodes are chlorided electrolytically to form Ag/AgCl electrodes to obtain a well-defined

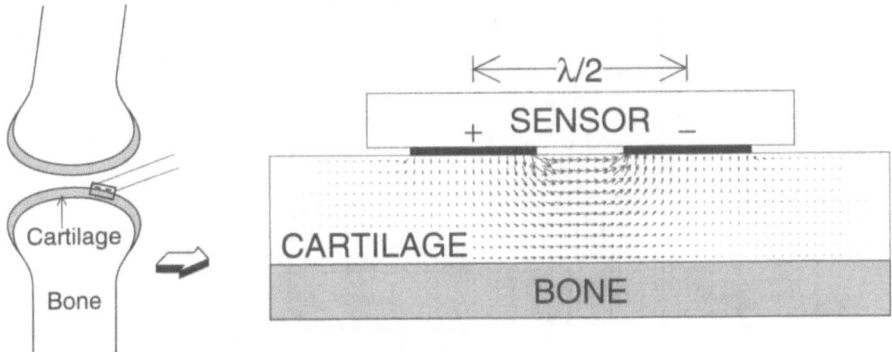

FIG. 1. Surface probe consists of excitation electrode array and mechanical surface stress sensor mounted on cartilage. Theoretical analysis has shown that current-generated stress can be measured by applying a standing wave of current to the cartilage surface of an intact joint, allowing for a nondestructive measurement. The current-generated stress in the bulk tissue is complex but related to the intratissue current density profile shown by the *arrows* [1]. This field can have an independently imposed temporal frequency and spatial wavelength (λ). The penetration depth of the measurement is proportional to the spatial wavelength (λ) and also increases with decreasing frequency [1]

interfacial electrode impedance on contact with the cartilage. A two-electrode probe in contact with cartilage is shown schematically in Fig. 1; the current-driving electrodes and mechanical stress sensor are depicted in a configuration for arthroscopic or in vitro testing.

Probe Sensitivity to Cartilage Fixed-Charge Density

The high negative fixed-charge density of cartilage is associated with the aggrecan molecules of the extracellular matrix (ECM). The glycosaminogly-can (GAG) chains attached to aggrecan core protein contain many sulfate and carboxyl groups that are ionized at physiological pH [29]. These charge groups give rise to the associated electromechanical and physiochemical properties of the tissue under physiological loading conditions [20,29]. The loss of aggrecan is one of the hallmarks of early cartilage degeneration. Thus, the ability to sensitively measure changes in matrix aggrecan and corresponding changes in physical properties is an important feature for a useful diagnostic probe. We first tested the sensitivity of our electromechanical surface probe to changes in cartilage fixed-charge density by pH-induced alteration of the ionization state of GAG charge groups.

Our tests were motivated by previous studies of streaming potential and current-generated stress measured on individual disks of cartilage in uniaxial confined compression in vitro. In those studies, a decrease in bath pH, which neutralized the GAG negative charge groups in situ, caused a concomitant

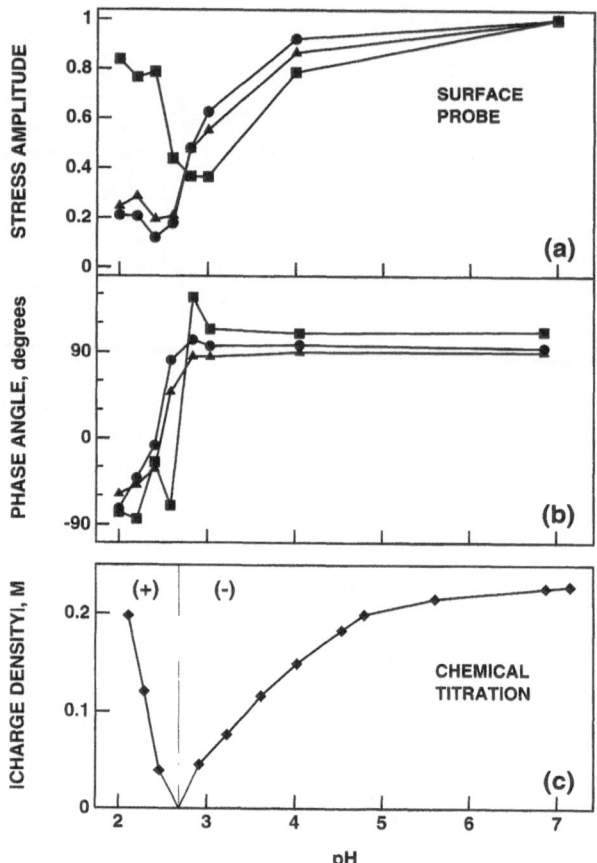

FIG. 2. **a** Current-generated stress amplitude vs. bath pH for adult bovine cartilage normalized to response at pH 7; **b** phase of the stress with respect to the applied current density of $1\,mA/cm^2$ at 0.025 (*circles*), 0.1 (*triangles*), and 1.0 Hz (*squares*). **c** Magnitude of the fixed-charge density of adult bovine cartilage measured by chemical titration [31]. The net charge changes sign as it passes through the isoelectric point (IEP) in the pH range 2.4–2.8. Minimum stress amplitude (**a**) and a 180° phase shift (**b**) occur close to the IEP

decrease in the electrokinetic responses [15,30]. The effect of bath pH on adult bovine cartilage fixed-charge density is shown in Fig. 2c [31]. As with human cartilage [20], lowering bath pH below pH 7 leads to a decrease in fixed-charge density as GAG (and protein) carboxyl groups become increasingly neutralized. At the isoelectic pH of cartilage, typically in the range pH 2.4–2.8 [29], there is zero net charge; below the isoelectric pH, there is increasing net positive charge associated predominantly with the ionized amino groups of collagens, as sulfate and carboxyl groups are further neutralized.

The effect of bath pH on the current-generated stress induced by the surface probe configuration of Fig. 1 is shown in Fig. 2a,b [2]. As bath pH is lowered below pH 7, the stress amplitude decreased substantially to a minimum value in range pH 2.4–2.8 (Fig. 2a). This minimum decreased monotonically with decreasing frequency (increasing penetration depth of the poroelastic deformation profile [1]). The amplitude of the stress closely tracked the measured changes in charge density. When the pH was lowered below the isoelectric pH, the stress amplitude began to increase again, and the phase angle changed abruptly by 180° (Fig. 2b), indicating that the direction of the current-generated stress has been reversed. At and below the isoelectric pH, the 180° phase shift and the increase in stress amplitude indicate that the positively charged amino groups on the collagen molecules were beginning to dominate the electrokinetic transduction. Taken together, these data show the sensitivity of probe measurements to molecular-level changes associated with aggrecan charge.

Variable Wavelength Imaging of Current-Generated Stress Following Loss of Aggrecan

Both the frequency and wavelength of the applied current density affect the depth of penetration of the current-induced poroelastic deformation within the tissue. The characteristic depth of penetration of the current density itself is approximately one-third the spatial wavelength of the current [2]. This wavelength, λ, is determined by the electrode excitation pattern at the cartilage surface. Therefore, a probe with six independently addressable electrodes was constructed (Fig. 3) such that connection to each electrode could be varied externally, thereby enabling multiple wavelengths to be applied using a single device. Applied current densities having a short wavelength compared to cartilage thickness are confined to the superficial region of the tissue; the associated current-generated stress therefore reflects the properties of the superficial zone. In contrast, long-wavelength excitations penetrate the full depth of the tissue and thereby reflect the average properties of full-thickness cartilage. Thus, combinations of short- and long-wavelength excitations enable the probe to "image" depth-dependent focal lesions.

To test the ability of the probe to spatially localize matrix damage, calf cartilage-bone plugs were subjected to trypsin digestion in a specialized diffusion chamber that allowed the enzyme to contact the tissue only at the articular surface. Hence, enzymatic digestion resulted in increased loss of tissue aggrecan starting at the surface and penetrating deeper into the tissue with increasing duration of treatment. The multiple wavelength probe was used to measure the long- and short-wavelength stress response of cartilage disks before and after trypsin digestion, as a model of aggrecan degradation. In normal tissue, the short-wavelength response was approximately one-half the long-wavelength response (Fig. 4 [32]), consistent with the spectroscopic nature of the poroelastic response. After a 2-h trypsin treatment, the short-wavelength response decreased significantly compared to the long-wavelength response, shown in Fig. 4 as the ratio of short- to long-wavelength signals (Berkenblit et al., in manuscript).

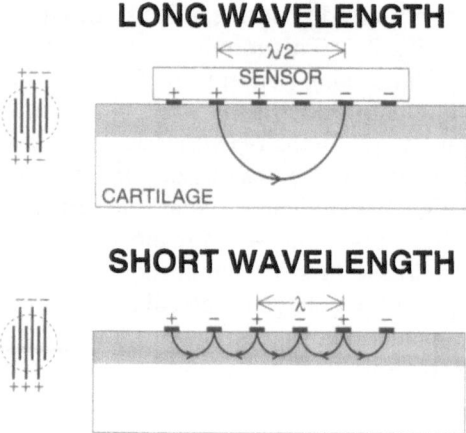

FIG. 3. Schematic of a probe with six independently addressable electrodes. By varying the external connections to each electrode, multiple wavelengths λ can be applied using a single device. Depicted is a "long" and "short" wavelength pattern (related to the electrode spacing, λ), where the relative depth of penetration of the current is represented by the arrows. If the *shaded region* represents degraded cartilage, examination of short- and long-wavelength responses enable spatial imaging of the pattern degradation

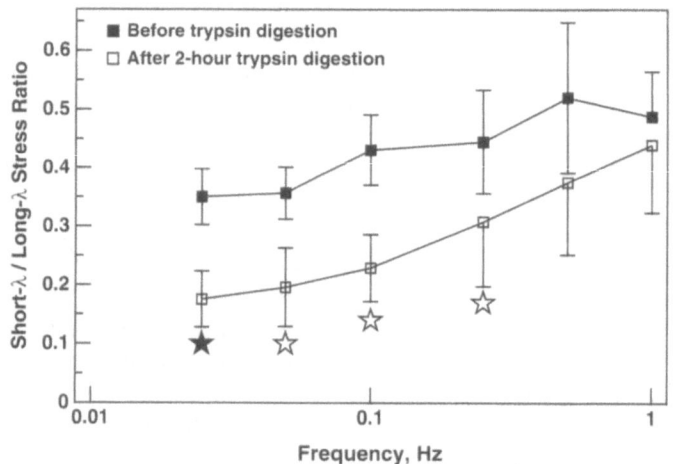

FIG. 4. Ratio of short-wavelength to long-wavelength stress response measured in full-thickness calf cartilage-bone plugs, both before (*filled squares*) and after (*open squares*) 2 h of surface trypsin digestion to remove proteoglycans (PGs) from the extracellular matrix ($n = 4$, mean ± SEM). Current-generated stress was measured using the multiple wavelength probe of Fig. 3. Stress ratios after trypsin treatment were significantly different from controls (*filled star*, $P \leq .01$; *open star*, $P \leq .05$ by ANOVA) up to frequencies of 0.25 Hz

This in vitro model system provided controlled PG loss from the tissue and resulted in a significant decrease in the stress compared to controls. Biochemical and histological analyses showed a progressive loss of aggrecan constituents from the ECM and correlated well with the time dependence of changes in the short to long wave response. These results further confirmed the sensitivity of the current-generated stress to molecular-level degradation of cartilage, and showed the ability for spatial imaging using this diagnostic approach.

Effect of Degradation of Matrix Collagens on Current-Generated Stress and Tissue Impedance

Because cartilage degradation in early OA involves alterations in the collagen network as well as the PGs, it is also important to understand the extent to which surface probe measurements may reflect the status of the collagen network. The electrokinetic surface probe was used to investigate the response to collagen network damage induced by recombinant human collagenase 1 and 3 (rhMMP-1 and rhMMP-13). Adult bovine cartilage-bone plugs were subjected to 24-h treatment with MMP-1 or MMP-3 in the same diffusion chamber as that for trypsin. Immunohistochemical staining for collagen cleavage sites using monoclonal antibody 9A4 was absent in control tissue and was most intense in the superficial layer of MMP-1- and MMP-13-treated tissue.

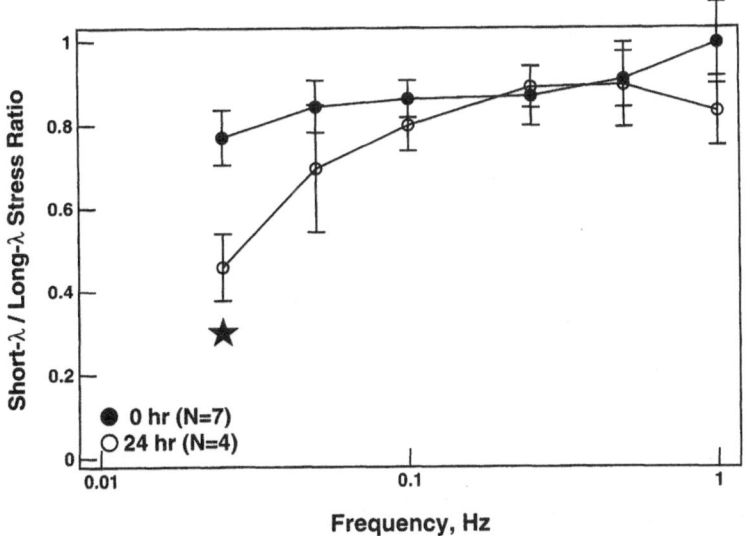

FIG. 5. Ratio of short-wavelength to long-wavelength stress response measured in adult bovine cartilage disks, both before (*filled circles*) and after (*open circles*) 24h of treatment with recombinant human MMP-1 to disrupt the collagen network (*filled star*, $P \leq .05$)

MMP-1 cleaved to an increasing depth with time; staining was apparent to a depth of 0.8 mm by 24 h, while staining for MMP-13 appeared confined to the surface. The release of proteoglycan and collagen constituents (as a percent of total) increased with time of treatment by MMP-1 and was greater than that released by MMP-13 treatment by 24 h [32]. Figure 5 shows the short- to long-wavelength stress response ratio (SR) for control disks (0-h) and disks after 24 h of MMP-1 treatment. The resulting MMP-1-induced degradation caused a decrease in this ratio by 24 h, significantly different at 0.025 Hz ($P \le .01$) [32]. In contrast, there were no significant differences between controls and disks treated with MMP-13 by 24 h. As in OA, cleavage and fibrillation of superficial collagen can result in loss of tissue PG; additional PG loss may have resulted from nonspecific collagenase activity. Nevertheless, we clearly observed changes in probe response after damage to the collagen–PG matrix.

We also measured changes in cartilage impedance via the surface probe interdigitated electrode array, as an additional physical property that may be related to matrix integrity and fixed-charge density. The cartilage electrical impedance, measured while current was applied to the probe excitation electrodes, was assessed using the system of Fig. 6. Figure 7 shows the impedance of disks measured in the long-wavelength configuration before and after 24-h treatment with MMP-13 [32]. The impedance increased significantly after treatment, particularly at the higher frequencies ($P \le .05$). Similar trends in impedance were observed after MMP-1 treatment (not shown). Cartilage electrical impedance increases after loss of GAG fixed-charge density or increased swelling at constant GAG density. Thus, damage to collagen or PG could increase the impedance as seen in Fig. 7 [32].

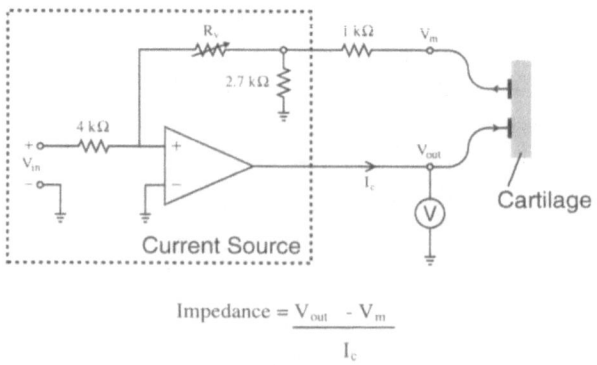

$$\text{Impedance} = \frac{V_{out} - V_m}{I_c}$$

FIG. 6. Schematic of the current source used for impedance measurements. A sinusoidal input voltage (V_{in}) to the current source resulted in a current I_c to the cartilage. The voltage difference $V_{out} - V_m$, between electrodes on the cartilage, divided by the current I_c, is the measured impedance, Z_{meas}. This purely electrical measurement can be made simultaneously with the current-generated stress response at the prescribed input frequencies (as in Fig. 7) or sequentially at any other frequency

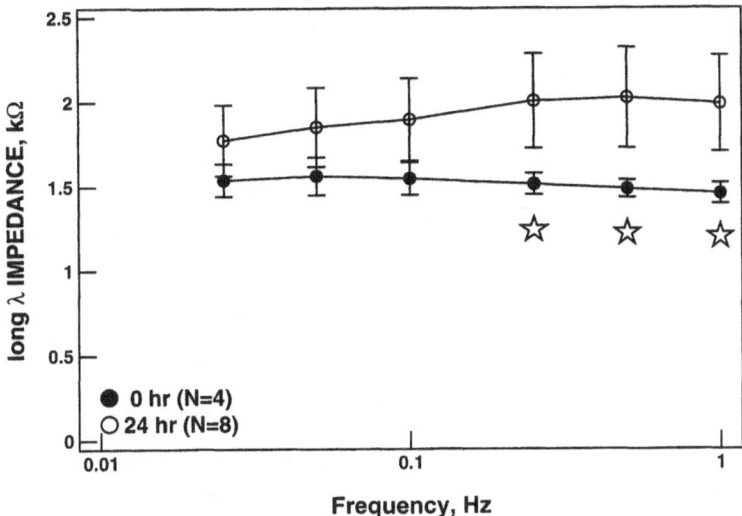

FIG. 7. Long-wavelength impedance measured in adult bovine cartilage disks [32], both before (*filled circles*) and after (*open circles*) 24 h of treatment with recombinant human (rh) MMP-13. The impedance increased post treatment, especially at high frequencies (*open star*, $P \leq .05$). Similar results were seen with rhMMP-1

Fabrication of Handheld In Vivo Probe

To be usable arthroscopically, the previously characterized surface sensor/transducer must be incorporated into a handheld probe that can be used in conjunction with a cannula into the knee joint. The probe must fulfill certain design criteria: (1) the outer body dimension and shape should fit down an arthroscopic cannula; (2) the functional circuitry of the probe must be appropriately sealed to perform in aqueous media; and (3) the PVDF piezo-film output electrodes must be shielded from the excitation electrodes and other sources of electromagnetic fields to maximize signal to noise on the stress signal. A recently developed prototype of such a probe embodiment is shown in Fig. 8, with a schematic of the internal connections and circuitry in the inset of Fig. 9a. Typical frequency-response measurements using the handheld probe are compared with that using the in vitro chamber-mounted probe in Fig. 9a. Normalization of probe output response to that observed at 0.025 Hz shows identical trends, providing validation that the handheld probe is detecting the same poroelastic phenomena seen with the chamber-mounted in vitro probes.

The ease of use of the handheld probe has allowed us to begin testing cartilage during open joint surgery in a mature canine model. After the femeropatellar groove was uncovered by displacing the patella, the handheld probe was applied to the facets of the condyles (shaded area in the inset of Fig. 9b), and the current-generated stress was measured. The results from three

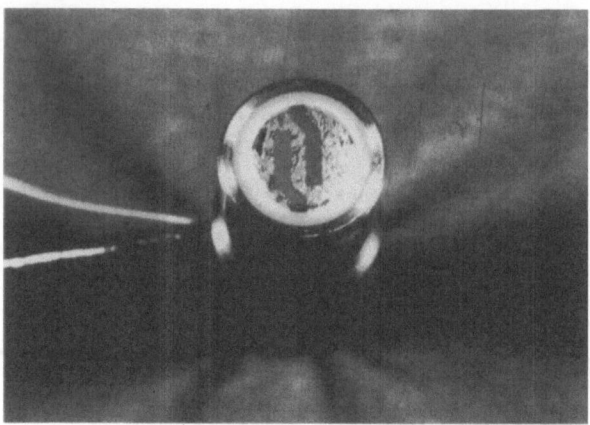

FIG. 8. Fully assembled handheld arthroscopic-like probe for measurements with intact joint surfaces. Rectangular Ag/AgCl electrodes can be used, or half-circles for enhanced signal output. Current-carrying wires and output voltage wires from the piezoelectric film can be seen emanating from the probe body. The outer body casing for this prototype is 1 cm in diameter; the most recent version is 6 mm in diameter and has a multiple wavelength configuration

normal joint surfaces are compared in Fig. 9b with data from normal adult bovine cartilage in vitro; the frequency response trends are in close agreement.

The feasibility of in vivo diagnostics with the handheld probe has been shown, but limitations still remain: (1) movement of the handheld probe during in vivo testing by a surgeon (found to be about 0.05 Hz) can contaminate the stress output below 0.1 Hz, restricting measurements to be done from 0.1 to 1.0 Hz; and (2) a compromise must be achieved whereby maximal signal is obtained using acceptable low-amplitude applied currents; that is, currents in the range reported here.

Future

A new prototype handheld probe is being completed to improve on the design short-comings of previous version. The present instrument has an outer body diameter of 6 mm, and has four electrodes to enable multiwavelength imaging of depth-dependent degradation associated with cartilage lesions.

Acknowledgments. This research has been supported in part by an NIH SBIR grant, NSF grant BCS-9111401, and a grant from Pfizer. The authors greatly acknowledge the contributions of Dr. Ivan Otterness, Dr. A.J Malici, Emerson Quan, Nikhil Batra, and Jeffery Tsay.

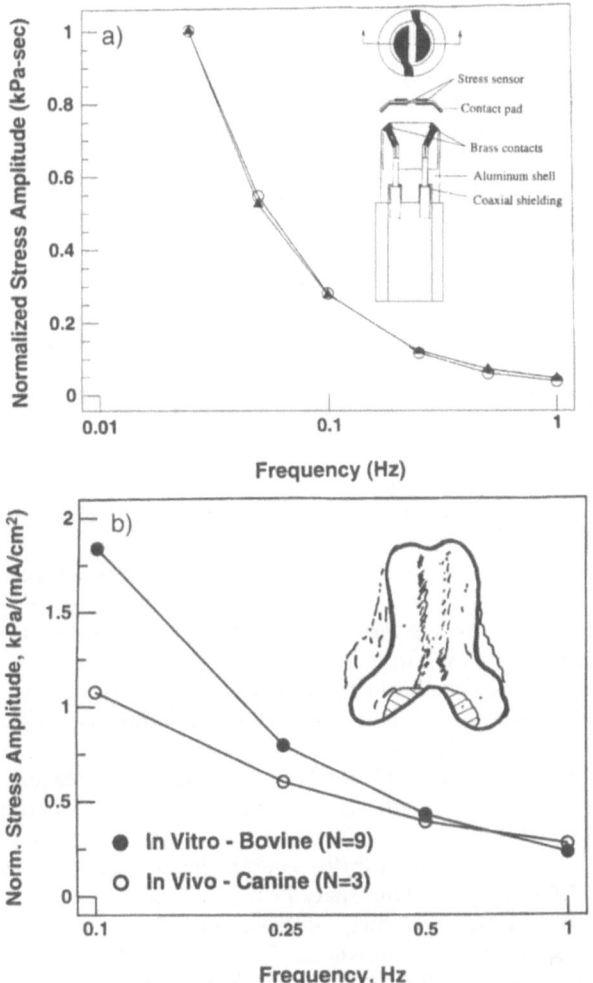

FIG. 9. **a** To compare the output of the two-electrode handheld (*filled triangles*) and chamber-mounted (*open circles*) probes, the output of the probes was normalized to that of 0.025 Hz. There is good agreement between the devices, validating the handheld probe with respect to the chamber-mounted variable wavelength probe. The *inset* shows a schematic of a cut section of the handheld probe. A connection is made between the contact pads on the PVDF stress sensor through brass contacts to cables for recording. Not shown are contacts that bring the external current to the Ag/AgCl electrodes shown. **b** The handheld probe has been used to make in vivo measurements with a canine model during an open joint procedure (*open circles*). The data are in close agreement with output acquired from adult bovine cartilage (*closed circles*) with the same device. The *inset* shows a diagram of the canine femeropatellar groove; the measurements were taken from the intact joint (shown as *shaded regions*)

72   S. Treppo et al.

References

1. Sachs JR, Grodzinsky AJ (1989) An electromechanically coupled poroelastic medium driven by an applied electric current: surface detection of bulk material properties. Phys-Chem Hydrodyn 11:585–614
2. Berkenblit SI, Frank EH, Salant EP, Grodzinsky AJ (1994) Nondestructive detection of cartilage degeneration using electromechanical surface spectroscopy. J Biomech Eng 116:384–392
3. Moskowitz RW, Howell DS, Goldberg VM, Mankin HJ (eds) (1992) Osteoarthritis: diagnosis and medical/surgical management, 2nd edn. Saunders, Philadelphia
4. Hall LD, Watson PJ, Tyler JA (1997) Magnetic resonance imaging and the progression of osteoarthritis, osteoporosis and aging. In: Osteoarthritis: public health implications for an aging population. Johns Hopkins University Press, Baltimore
5. Dieppe P (1995) The classification and diagnosis of osteoarthritis. In: Osteoarthritic disorders. American Academy of Orthopaedic Surgeons, Rosemont, IL
6. Bashir A, Paley D, Davidson SA, Gray ML, Burstein D (1997) Mri measurements of fixed charge density as a measure of cartilage proteoglycan content. In: Transactions of the 43rd annual meeting, vol 22. Orthopaedic Research Society, San Francisco, CA, p 217
7. Mink JH, Reicher MA, Crues JV III (1992) Magnetic resonance imaging of the knee. Raven, New York
8. Ewing JW (1990) Articular cartilage and knee joint function: basic science and arthroscopy. Raven, New York
9. Lohmander S (1993) Osteoarthritis: a major cause of disability of the elderly. In: Musculoskeletal soft-tissue aging: impact on mobility. American Academy of Orthopaedic Surgeons, Rosemont, IL
10. Sabiston CP, Adams ME, Li DKB (1987) Magnetic resonance imaging of osteoarthritis: correlation with gross pathology using an experimental model. J Orthop Res 5:164–172
11. Hamerman D (1997) Osteoarthritis: public health implications for an aging population. Johns Hopkins University Press, Baltimore
12. Cawston T (1993) Blocking cartilage destruction with metalloproteinase inhibitors: a valid therapeutic target? Ann Rheum Dis 52:769–770
13. Kuettner KE, Goldberg VM (1995) Osteoarthritic disorders. American Academy of Orthopaedic Surgeons, Rosemont, IL
14. Hoch DH, Grodzinsky AJ, Koob TJ, Albert ML, Eyre DR (1983) Early changes in material properties of rabbit articular cartilage after meniscectomy. J Orthop Res 1:4–12
15. Frank EH, Grodzinsky AJ, Eyre DR, Koob TJ (1987) Streaming potential: a sensitive index of enzymatic degradation in articular cartilage. J Orthop Res 5:497–508
16. Frank EH, Grodzinsky AJ (1987) Cartilage electromechanics I: electrokinetic transduction and the effects of electrolyte pH and ionic strength. J Biomech 20:615–627
17. Frank EH, Grodzinsky AJ (1987) Cartilage electromechanics II: a continuum model of cartilage electrokinetics. J Biomech 20:629–639
18. Bonasser LJ, Sandy JD, Lark MW, Plaas AHK, Frank EH, Grodzinsky AJ (1997) Inhibition of cartilage degradation and changes in physical properties induced by IL-1β and retinoic acid using matrix metalloproteinases. Arch Biochem Biophys 334:404–412

19. Maroudas AI (1976) Balance between swelling pressure and collagen tension in normal and degenerate cartilage. Nature (Lond) 260:808–809
20. Maroudas A (1979) Physicochemical properties of articular cartilage. In: Adult articular cartilage. Pitman Medical, Kent, England, pp 215–290
21. Mow VC, Setton LA, Guilak F, Ratcliffe A (1995) Mechanical factors in articular cartilage and their role in osteoarthritis. In: Osteoarthritic disorders. American Academy of Orthopaedic Surgeons, Rosemont, IL
22. Tkaczuk H (1986) Human cartilage stiffness. In vivo studies. Clin Orthop 206:301–312
23. Dashefsky JH (1987) Arthroscopic measurement of chondromalacia of patella cartilage using a microminiature pressure transducer. Arthroscopy 3:80–85
24. Lyyra T, Jurvelin J, Pitkanen P, Väätäinen U, Kiviranta I (1995) Indentation instrument for the measurement of cartilage stiffness under arthroscopic control. Med Eng Phys 17:395–399
25. Kiviranta I, Lyyra T, Väätäinen U, Seuri R, Jeroma H, Tammi M, Jurvelin J (1995) Knee joint articular cartilage shows general softening in patients with chondromalacia of patella. In: Transactions of the 41st annual meeting, vol 20. Orthopaedi Research Society, Orlando, FL, p 197
26. Chang RW, Falconer J, Stulberg SD, Arnold WJ, Manheim LM, Dyer AR (1993) A randomized, controlled trial of arthroscopic surgery versus closed-needle joint lavage for patients with osteoarthritis of the knee. Arthritis Rheum 36:289–296
27. Bonassar LJ, Frank EH, Murray JC, Paguio CG, Moore VL, Lark MW, Sandy JD, Wu JJ, Eyre DR, Grodzinsky AJ (1995) Changes in cartilage composition and physical properties due to stromelysin degradation. Arthritis Rheum 38:173–183
28. Sachs JR, Grodzinsky AJ (1994) Theory of electromechanical spectroscopy in poroelastic media: surface detection of bulk properties. In: Transactions of the 16th International Conference, IEEE Engineering in Medicine and Biology Society, Baltimore, MD, pp 752–753
29. Grodzinsky AJ (1983) Electromechanical and physicochemical properties of connective tissues. CRC Crit Rev Biomed Eng 9:133–199
30. Grimshaw PE, Eisenberg SR, Grodzinsky AJ, Koob TJ, Eyre DR (1983) The kinetics of in vitro neutralization and enzymatic extraction of cartilage charge groups: characterization by isometric compressive stress. In: Transactions of the 29th Annual Meeting, vol 8. Orthopaedic Research Society, Anaheim, CA, p 122
31. Frank EH, Grodzinsky AJ, Philips SL, Grimshaw PE (1990) Physiochemical and bioelectric determinants of cartilage material properties. In: Biomechanics of diarthrodial joints. Springer, Heidelberg Berlin New York, p 147
32. Treppo S, Otterness IG, Malici AJ, Berkenblit SI, Grodzinsky AJ (1998) Effects of Mmp-1 and Mmp-13 induced matrix degradation on electrokinetic and dielectric properties of adult articular cartilage by surface spectroscopy. In: Transactions of the 45th Annual Meeting, vol 23. Orthopaedic Research Society, New Orleans, LA, p 153

Applications of MRI for Evaluating Osteoarthritis

CHARLES G. PETERFY

Summary. Magnetic resonance imaging (MRI) provides a unique opportunity to explore osteoarthritis in ways that were unimaginable in the past. While MRI has not replaced radiography in clinical practice, it has many advantages for exploring the cause of pain and dysfunction in diarthroidal joints, and for following the course of therapy. MRI offers three principal advantages over conventional radiography for evaluating the health of joints: a multiplanar tomographic viewing perspective, unparalleled soft tissue contrast, and digital image format. MRI techniques that have been developed harness different tissue characteristics in cartilage and surrounding structures to allow examination of all components of the joint simultaneously. This capability for whole-organ imaging of the joint is unprecedented in medical imaging and cogent to the current view of osteoarthritis as a disease of organ failure. MRI is thus a valuable tool with unprecedented and unparalleled capabilities for evaluating osteoarthritis and its progress and provides a unique opportunity for exploration of this highly prevalent and debilitating disease.

Key Words. MRI, Osteoarthritis, Arthritis, Cartilage, Imaging

Introduction

The past two decades have seen remarkable advances in medical imaging. The development of magnetic resonance imaging (MRI), in particular, has brought unprecedented power to the study of joint disease and its causes, and has offered a unique opportunity to explore osteoarthritis in ways not imaginable in the past. This chapter reviews the advantages of MRI over radiography for this application. I also point out ways that MRI can be used as a tool for

Department of Radiology, University of California San Francisco, Osteoporosis and Arthritis Research Group, 505 Parnassus Ave, Suite M392, San Francisco, CA 94143-0628, U.S.A.

exploring the causes of pain and dysfunction in diarthroidial joints and for testing the efficacy and safety of new therapies.

How MRI Works

Magnetic resonance imaging creates images by causing hydrogen nuclei (protons) to align themselves with the strong magnetic field within the bore of a MRI magnet, much as a compass needle aligns with the magnetic field of the earth [1–3]. When these protons are exposed to an additional alternating or rotating magnetic field perpendicular to the static main magnetic field and tuned to the resonant frequency of the protons (i.e., application of a "radiofrequency pulse"), the protons realign with this new field. Rotation of these proton fields against the main magnetic field induces an alternating electrical current in receiver wires in an imaging coil placed near the patient. The magnitude of this current and, therefore, the signal intensity on an MR image depend not only on regional variations in the amount of hydrogen protons in a sample but also on micromagnetic influences exerted on these protons by other substances in the sample, as well as the type and timing of the radiofrequency pulses used during imaging. It is this multiplicity of factors affecting the MR signal that gives MRI its unparalleled range in tissue contrast.

Fundamental Advantages of MRI

MRI offers three principal advantages over conventional radiography for evaluating diarthroidial joints: (1) multiplanar tomographic viewing perspective, (2) unparalleled soft tissue contrast, and (3) digital image format.

Tomographic Viewing Perspective

Radiography is a projectional imaging technique that casts two-dimensional shadows of three-dimensional (3-D) anatomy on a flat receptor, the radiographic film [4] (Fig. 1). This method allows relatively large amounts of anatomy to be depicted as a single image but causes morphological distortion and magnification. These factors generally do not impact heavily on clinical interpretations, but can interfere with efforts to make accurate dimensional measurements, such as joint-space width. A far greater problem of the projectional viewing perspective is that overlapping structures are superimposed upon one another, because this can obscure even large structural abnormalities on otherwise high-quality radiographs (Fig. 2). Projectional superimposition is generally handled by comparing several different views of the same anatomy. However, this is only a partial solution to the fundamental problem.

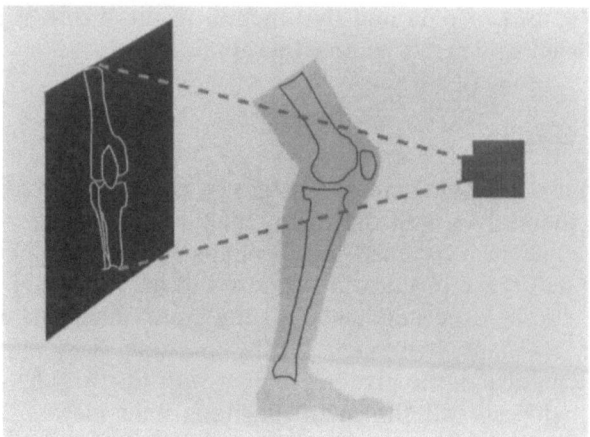

FIG. 1. Projectional viewing perspective. Projectional radiographs generate two-dimensional (2-D) images with morphological distortion, magnification, and superimposition. Although these images are adequate for most routine clinical applications, accurate morphological measurements are not readily achieved. (From [26], with permission)

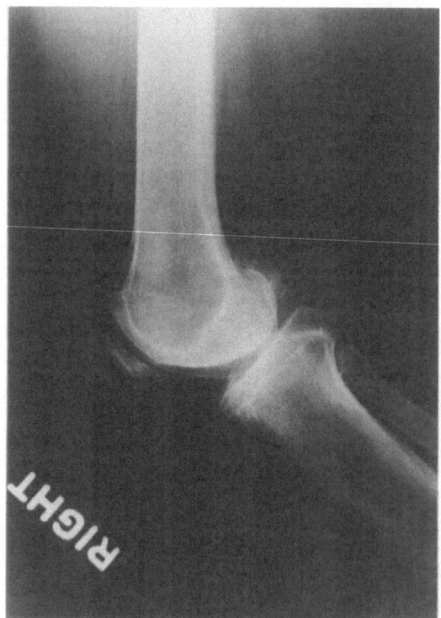

FIG. 2. Projectional superimposition. Lateral projection of the knee shows superimposition of articular contours and confuses efforts to identify the appropriate surfaces across which to measure the width of the patellofemoral joint. The medial and lateral femoral condyles are similarly superimposed, obscuring osteophytes along their margins. (From [26], with permission)

Tomographic imaging techniques, such as MRI, produce cross-sectional images of the anatomy without morphological distortion or magnification (Fig. 3). Therefore, although the images acquired with most clinical MRI systems generally show lower spatial resolution than do radiographs, dimensional measurement is more straightforward with MRI. Tomography also obviates the problem of superimposition. Thus, despite lower two-point discrimination, MRI can disclose morphological abnormalities that are completely occult on radiographs. In patients with rheumatoid arthritis, for example, MRI has been found to be twice as sensitive as conventional radiography for detecting bone erosions [5,6], which contrasts with the misconception held by many clinicians that MRI is insensitive to bone abnormalities. In fact, MRI is currently the most sensitive method available for detecting bone trauma, osteomyelitis, osteonecrosis, and bone neoplasms. This special sensitivity of MRI for bone pathology relates not only to its tomographic viewing perspective but also to its unique capacity for visualizing the marrow tissue. In particular, MRI is extremely responsive to changes in marrow water content.

Not only is MRI tomographic, it is capable of acquiring sections in any plane. In contrast, X-ray computed tomography (CT) is restricted to the transaxial (axial) plane (transverse to the bore of the gantry). Accordingly,

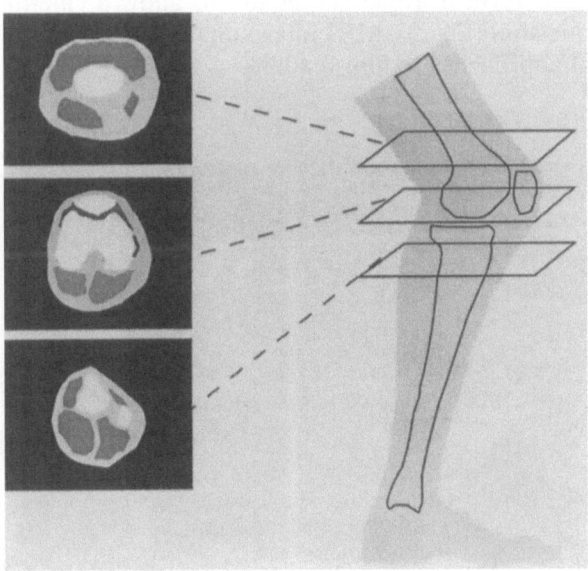

FIG. 3. Tomographic viewing perspective. Tomographic sections provide cross-sectional images of the anatomy free of morphological distortion, magnification, and superimposition, which facilitates morphometric analysis despite somewhat lower two-point resolution. (From [26], with permission)

only transverse sections of the knee, hip, and spine can be acquired directly with CT. Small structures, such as the hand and wrist, can be positioned sideways in the gantry and thus imaged in other planes, but sagittal CT images of the knee can only be generated by reformatting a stack of slices originally acquired in the transverse plane (Fig. 4). Because the minimum slice thickness used in clinical CT does not approach the typical in-plane resolution, reformation is generally associated with some degree of image degradation. Also, even minor movement between individual CT slices results in steplike distortions that can mimic fracture (Fig. 4). Direct multiplanar tomography of MRI is, therefore, a significant advantage.

One consequence of cross-sectional imaging is that a significantly larger number of individual images is required to cover the same anatomy than would be necessary with projectional radiography. This number is multiplied when several pulse sequences are acquired to harness different tissue characteristics for image contrast (see following). For example, comparison of single 3-D MRI examinations of the knee acquired at three different timepoints may require review of 180–360 individual images (Fig. 5). This number of images printed on hard copy film (20–40 films with 9-on-1 configuration) can cover an entire wall of view boxes and pose a significant challenge to visual coordination (similar to viewing individual frames from a movie). However, because the image data are originally stored in digital format, individual images from each examination can be stacked in separate windows on a workstation and scrolled back and forth in rapid succession to allow a cine-like view of the structures in question (Fig. 5). MRI image analysis does not, therefore, emulate traditional approaches to film reading.

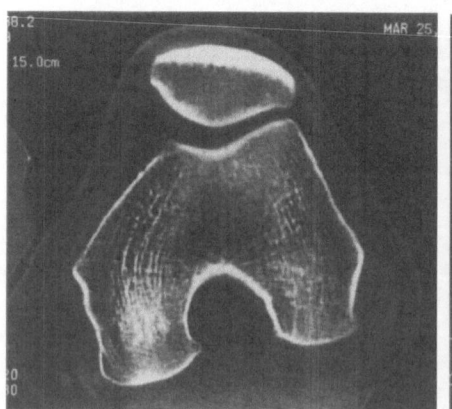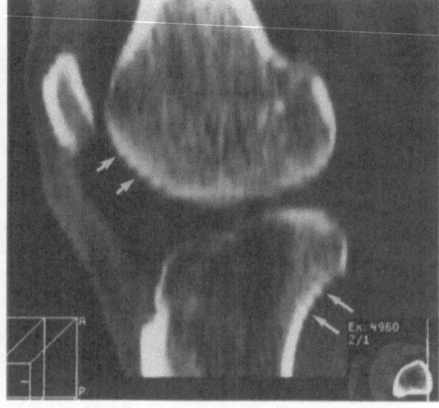

a   b

FIG. 4a,b. Multiplanar reformation of axially acquired computed tomography (CT) images. **a** Axial image shows high spatial resolution of bony structure. **b** Sagittal reformations from original data show the step artifacts (*arrows*). (From [26], with permission)

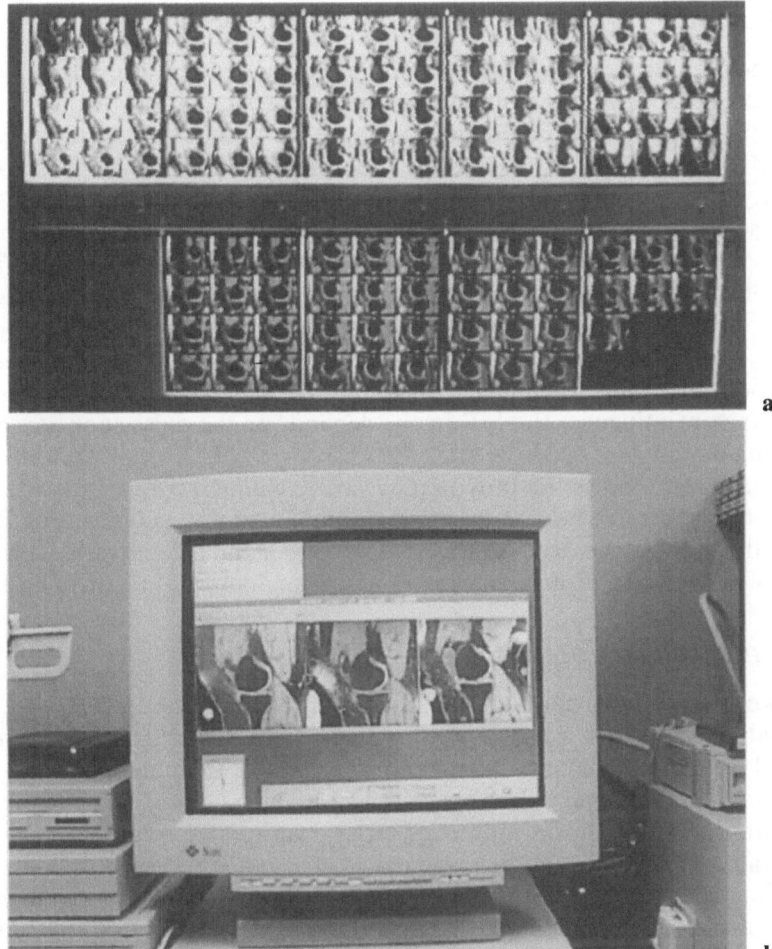

a

b

FIG. 5a,b. Handling large numbers of cross-sectional images. **a** Two serially acquired three-dimensional (3-D) magnetic resonance imaging (MRI) data sets of a knee, composed of 60 cross-sectional images each, occupy a large amount of wall space and are difficult to coordinate visually when viewed on conventional film. **b** Three similar 3-D MRI data sets can be viewed more easily on a workstation monitor as stacks of sections. This approach allows side-by-side comparison of anatomically matched serial images to maximize visual sensitivity to change, while at the same time allowing the reader to rapidly survey the anatomy, adjust image contrast, pan and zoom the images, and perform a variety of computer analyses, including simple dimensional measurements as well as more sophisticated analyses, such as volumetric quantification, geometric modeling, and parametric mapping

Soft Tissue Contrast

The most fundamental quality of an image is contrast. It is contrast with the background or adjacent structures that makes a lesion visible on any image. Of all the modalities available today, none have the breadth of soft tissue contrast that MRI has. This is because, unlike other imaging techniques such as radiography, CT, ultrasonography, and scintigraphy for which the image gray scale is generally linked to only one or two tissue characteristics (e.g., physical density and atomic number for radiography; physical density for CT; acoustic impedance mismatch for ultrasonography; differential uptake of radiotracer for scintigraphy), as many as six tissue characteristics (proton density, T_1 relaxation, T_2 relaxation, proton diffusion, magnetization transfer, and magnetic susceptibility) affect the image contrast on MRI. The degree to which each of these factors influences the MR image depends on the pulse sequence and the imaging parameters used.

Regardless, MRI is the only noninvasive technique with which all components of a diarthroidial joint can be examined simultaneously. For the first time, the joint can be evaluated as a whole organ and osteoarthritis, therefore, can be viewed as a disease of organ failure, analogous to heart failure.

Digital Image Format

Unlike conventional film-based radiography, which has an analogue image format, MRI images are digital [4]. As mentioned, storage of image data in digital form offers a number of advantages. First, large numbers of images can be stored in a relatively small space (e.g., on optical disk, magnetic tape, etc.) and transmitted electronically over large distances, and hard copies can be generated as needed. Digital image data can also be processed by computer to alter the characteristics of the image (e.g., noise reduction, contrast modification, edge enhancement, and image subtraction), as well as to obtain quantitative information, such as the distance between morphological structures (e.g., joint-space width) or the mean pixel value within a specified region of interest (ROI). More sophisticated morphometric analyses, such as determination of the volume or 3-D geometry of an anatomical structure, are also possible.

Imaging Changes in Joint Tissues in Osteoarthritis Using MRI

Imaging Bone

Because of its relative lack of hydrogen nuclei, bone tissue does not generate any signal on conventional MRI. Cortical and trabecular bones are, therefore, depicted as curvilinear signal voids silhouetted on either side by signal-producing tissues, such as marrow and adipose (Fig. 6). MRI thus has an inherent contrast for bone. Despite this, the contours of individual cortices and

FIG. 6. MRI of bone. Coronal T_1-weighted image of the knee shows cortical bone as a curvilinear signal void silhouetted by high signal intensity marrow fat and adipose tissue

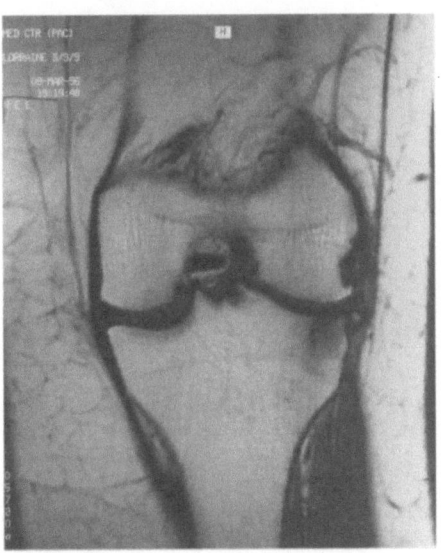

trabeculi are generally less sharp on conventional MR images than on routine clinical radiographs because clinical MRI typically has lower spatial resolution than does clinical radiography (at least, along the two dimensions of the radiographic film). This potential advantage of radiography, however, must be balanced against its problem with projectional superimposition, which can transform a complex 3-D network of trabeculi in the cancellous bone into an incomprehensible haystack of overlapping linear shadows. The relative weakness of MRI in two-point discrimination is, thus, offset by the advantages of its tomographic viewing perspective.

As was just stated, despite a lower spatial resolution, MRI can disclose abnormalities that are often obscured on conventional radiographs because of their location. The exception to this is any irregularity along the small fraction of the osseous cortex that happens to be tangential to the X-ray beam. Here, radiography outperforms MRI. However, that portion usually represents less than 10% of the total surface of the bone. MRI is, therefore, well suited for examining the marginal osteophytes (Fig. 6) in osteoarthritis, and is especially helpful in delineating central osteophytes (Fig. 7), which can be extremely difficult to see with conventional radiographs and that may have different reasons for developing than do marginal osteophytes and thus different implications to the disease.

The most intriguing capability of MRI in regard to the bones is its capacity for detecting abnormalities involving the marrow space. Conditions arising in this compartment generally remain occult on radiographs until the cortical and trabecular bones themselves are affected. MRI, on the other hand, can directly visualize any excess water in the marrow space, and thus identify hemorrhage

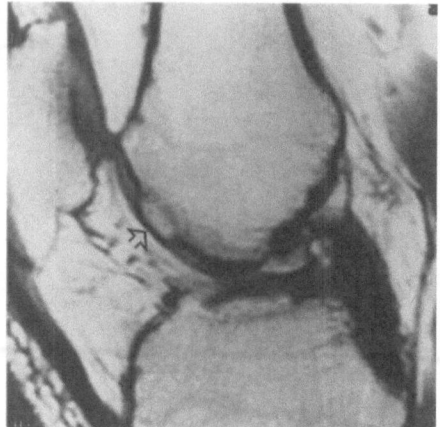
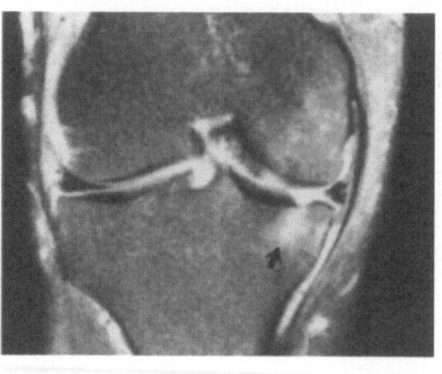

7

8

Fig. 7. Central osteophytes. Sagittal MRI of the knee shows a central osteophyte (*arrow*) of the femoral trochlea. (From [26], with permission)

Fig. 8. Bone marrow edema in osteoarthritis. Fat-suppressed T_2-weighted fast spin-echo image of a knee with osteoarthritis shows water signal (*arrow*) in the marrow subjacent to an articular cartilage defect

and edema from even mild bone trauma, as well as exudate from early osteomyelitis and cellular material from infiltrating neoplasms. Areas of "marrow edema" are often seen in joints with osteoarthritis (Fig. 8). Usually, these areas develop beneath defects in the articular surface, presumably from pulsion of synovial fluid through the defect or from microtrauma associated with biomechanical incompetence of the load-bearing surface. Occasionally, however, epiphyseal marrow edema is seen some distance from the articular surface or at entheses. There is speculation that the development of marrow edema in osteoarthritis is associated with local pain, but this hypothesis has never been carefully tested. Whether areas of marrow edema correlate directly with increased uptake of technetium-labeled radiotracer in bone scintigraphy or accelerated disease progression, or inversely with the response to treatment, has yet to be determined. Nevertheless, this is a feature of osteoarthritis that only MRI can elucidate.

Imaging Articular Cartilage

Clinical MRI derives its signal almost exclusively from hydrogen nuclei (protons) in fat and water. The high water content, or proton density, of hyaline articular cartilage forms the basis for MRI signal in this tissue. To date, there has been no systematic study of the relative water contents of different articular cartilages in the body, but in general, the weight fraction of water in normal cartilage is approximately 0.7 [7]. This value is determined by a subtle balance between the Donnan osmotic pressure produced by negatively charged proteoglycans in cartilage and the resistance to swelling exerted by a fine meshwork of collagen fibrils radiating from the deep calcified zone of cartilage to the articular surface [7]. Disruption of this collagen matrix can result in elevation of the water content, but typically only by a few percent. The potential for altering cartilage signal by this mechanism is, therefore, theoretically limited.

Another important determinant of MRI signal intensity is the microenvironment in which the tissue water molecules reside. The actual signal intensity of cartilage is, therefore, modulated through a variety of mechanisms by the proteoglycan-collagen matrix. These mechanisms include T_1 relaxation, T_2 relaxation, water diffusion, magnetization transfer, and magnetic susceptibility [8]. The degree to which each of these affect the final signal intensity on an MR image depends on the type of pulse sequence and the specific imaging parameters used.

T_2 relaxation represents a loss of MRI signal over time caused by protons falling out of phase with each other because of the heterogeneous environment produced by their own micromagnetic fields. Freely mobile water molecules (e.g., in synovial fluid) show relatively little of this type of interaction and thus retain MRI signal over long periods of time. Accordingly, the signal intensity of synovial fluid remains high on MR images acquired with a long echo time (TE) (Fig. 9). Collagen, by virtue of its highly regular structure, tends to immobilize water molecules and promote internuclear interactions

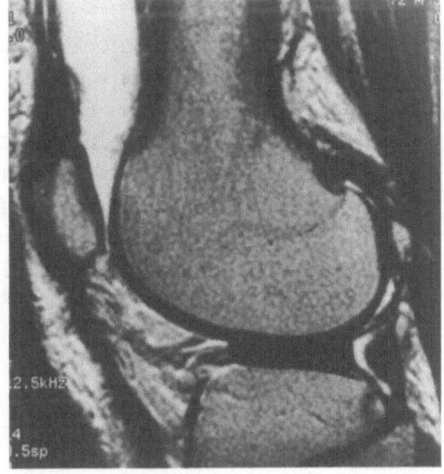

FIG. 9. Differences in water signal in synovial fluid and cartilage on T_2-weighted MR images. Synovial fluid contains freely mobile water protons that show slow T_2 relaxation and, therefore, retain signal on long-TE (echo time) images. In contrast, water protons in cartilage are immobilized by collagen and loose signal rapidly. Cartilage therefore appears dark on long-TE images

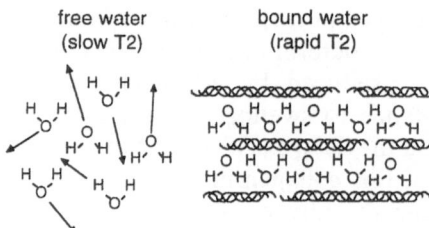

free water
(slow T2)

bound water
(rapid T2)

FIG. 10. Immobilization of cartilage water protons by collagen promotes T_2 relaxation

among their protons, thus accelerating T_2 relaxation [9] (Fig. 10). Collagen-containing tissues, such as cartilage (also tendons, ligaments, menisci, labrum, scar, and fibrous neoplasms) lose signal rapidly on MRI. Therefore, in contrast to synovial fluid, cartilage shows a low signal intensity on long-TE (T_2-weighted) MR images despite having a relatively high proton density (~70% that of synovial fluid) (Fig. 9).

Water diffusion in cartilage also contributes to signal loss on T_2-weighted MR images [10,11] because water molecules that have changed positions during a portion of the MRI acquisition can no longer be brought back into phase properly and so do not contribute maximally to the net signal. This loss of phase coherence is proportional to the distance traveled by the diffusing water protons and is, therefore, worse on long-TE images. The presence of proteoglycans, particularly chondroitin sulfate, in normal cartilage inhibits water diffusion and keeps this effect relatively small; however, with very strong gradients and specialized phase-sensitive pulse sequences, water diffusion can be demonstrated and even quantified in normal articular cartilage [10,11]. With cartilage degeneration and proteoglycan loss, however, water diffusion has been shown to increase considerably. Accordingly, diffusion may play a more significant role in cartilage signal modulation in osteoarthritic joints.

Another collagen-dependent mechanism of signal loss in cartilage is magnetization transfer [12–14]. This change is caused by a transfer of magnetization from protons in tissue water to protons in collagen that have been selectively suppressed, either deliberately with a specialized pulse sequence or inadvertently during conventional multislice imaging. Signal loss from cartilage water by this mechanism is, therefore, indirectly mediated by collagen and proportional to the concentration of this protein in the cartilage. This effect increases with the number of slices used and is most pronounced on fast spin-echo images because of the multiple 180° rephasing pulses employed in this technique.

Disruption or loss of the collagen matrix in cartilage results not only in a modest elevation in proton density but also removal of the signal-modulating effects of collagen-dependent T_2 relaxation and magnetization transfer. Collectively, these effects increase the signal intensity in areas of matrix damage, or early chondromalacia (Fig. 11). Various patterns of signal abnormality

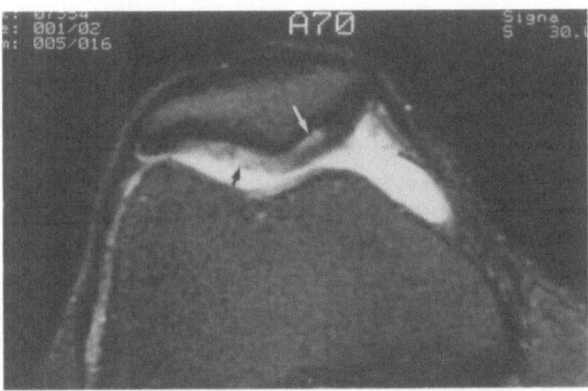

FIG. 11. Elevated T_2 signal (*arrows*) in chondromalacic cartilage

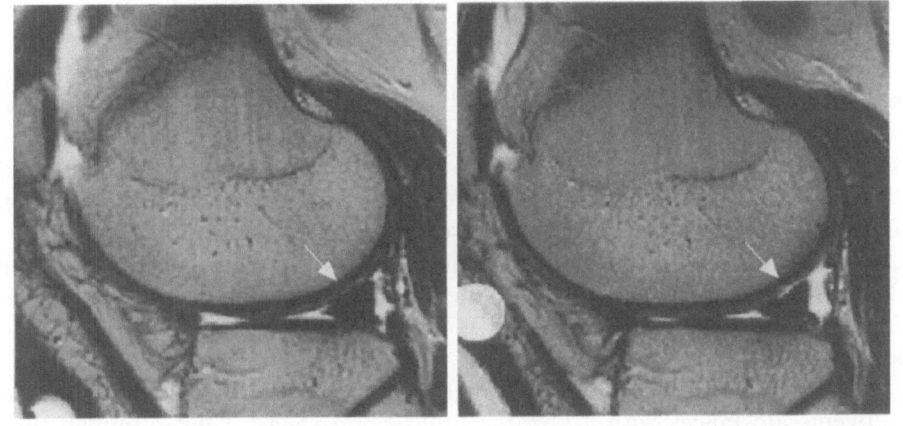

a   b

FIG. 12a,b. Cartilage attrition is preceded by elevated T_2 signal. **a** Sagittal T_2-weighted fast spin-echo image of the knee of a patient 2 months after partial lateral meniscectomy shows a focus of elevated signal intensity (*arrow*) in the articular cartilage immediately adjacent to the operated meniscus. **b** Nine months later, there is a focal cartilage defect (*arrow*) in this location

have been described in chondromalacic cartilage [8,15]. Although there is anecdotal evidence to show that these abnormalities can develop rapidly, longitudinal investigations of their natural history in cartilage are lacking (Fig. 12).

In addition to subjectively monitoring these abnormalities in articular cartilage, it is possible to quantify T_2 changes using widely available techniques. By combining the data from images of the same cartilage acquired with several different TEs, it is possible to estimate the T_2 of the cartilage by fitting an exponential curve to the observed signal intensity values for each pixel. The T_2

can be estimated in this way for a specific region of interest in the cartilage, or depicted in image mode as a map of the entire cartilage in which the signal intensity of each pixel corresponds to the T_2 at that site [16]. This approach, although widely available and relatively easy to use, tends to underestimate T_2, partly because of increased diffusion-related effects with increasing TE [9]. Underestimation of T_2 is greatest in chondromalacic cartilage, where water diffusion is increased. Unless special techniques are employed, the potential increase in T_2 measurable with this technique in chondromalacic cartilage is slightly suppressed by diffusion-related effects. Nevertheless, large changes of T_2 might still be demonstrable.

T_2-weighted spin-echo and fast spin-echo images are useful, therefore, for evaluating articular cartilage because they offer high contrast between the cartilage and adjacent synovial fluid, are sensitive to early matrix damage, and may yield quantitative information about the status of the intercellular matrix. One limitation of these techniques, however, is spatial resolution. The minimum slice thickness achievable with such two-dimensional (2-D) pulse sequences using most clinical systems available today is only 3 mm. Although thinner slices are already possible on many MRI scanners, the majority of systems cannot support this. It is possible to combine high in-plane resolution with thin slices using 3-D MRI. With 3-D MRI, instead of exciting multiple single slices one at a time (2-D MRI), a very thick slice (slab) is excited and then partitioned in the slice-select direction with additional phase encoding. Because imaging time is directly proportional to the number of phase-encoding steps, 3-D MRI requires longer acquisition times than conventional 2-D MRI. Because of this, rapid gradient-echo methods are typically used for 3-D MRI, although fast spin-echo techniques are also being developed to support 3-D MRI.

One problem with gradient-echo methods is that they offer poor T_2 contrast between substances with T_2s in the millisecond range. Thus, although they adequately differentiate the meniscus ($T_2 < 1$ ms) from synovial fluid ($T_2 \simeq 200$ ms), gradient echo only poorly differentiates cartilage ($T_2 \simeq 15$ ms) from synovial fluid (Fig. 13). Accordingly, tissue characteristics other than T_2 must be harnessed to generate contrast on 3-D gradient-echo images.

One option for contrast generation is magnetization transfer, which under appropriate conditions selectively reduces the signal intensity of tissues that contain both water and collagen. Addition of a magnetization-transfer pulse to a 3-D gradient-echo sequence selectively suppresses signal in the articular cartilage, but not in the synovial fluid or in fat in bone marrow or adipose tissue (Fig. 13). Subtraction of images acquired with and without the magnetization-transfer pulse produces a map of the tissue distribution of magnetization transfer in the joint and depicts the articular cartilage as an isolated band of high signal intensity sharply delimited from adjacent structures, which show low signal intensity (Fig. 13).

Similar contrast can also be achieved with T_1-weighted 3-D gradient-echo images in which T_1 contrast has been augmented by the use of fat suppression

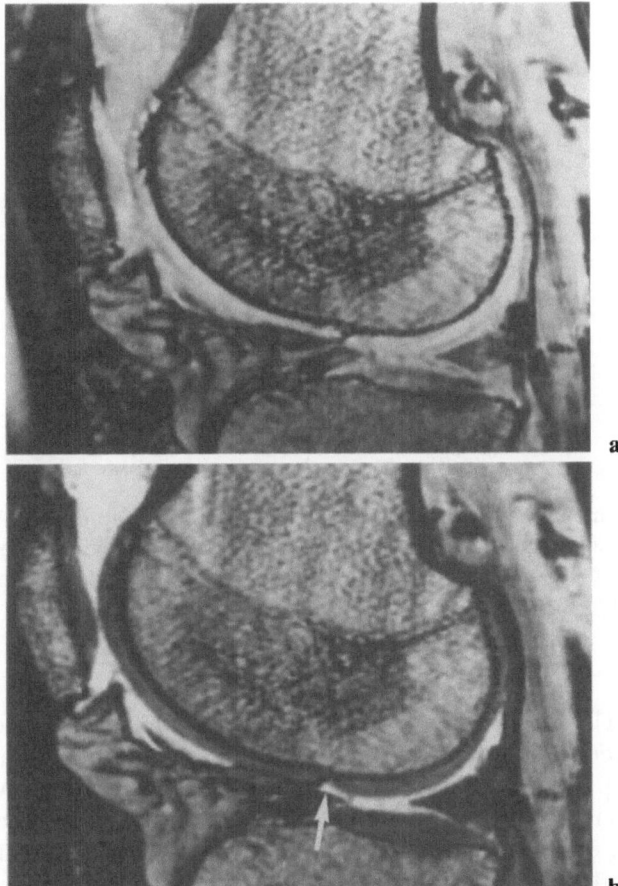

Fig. 13a,b. Harnessing magnetization-transfer contrast in articular cartilage. **a** Sagittal T_2*-weighted gradient-echo image of the knee shows poor contrast between the articular cartilage and synovial fluid. **b** The same scan following a magnetization-transfer pulse shows selective loss of signal intensity from the articular cartilage, thus revealing a focal defect (*arrow*) not visible on the previous scan shown in **a**. (From [13], with permission)

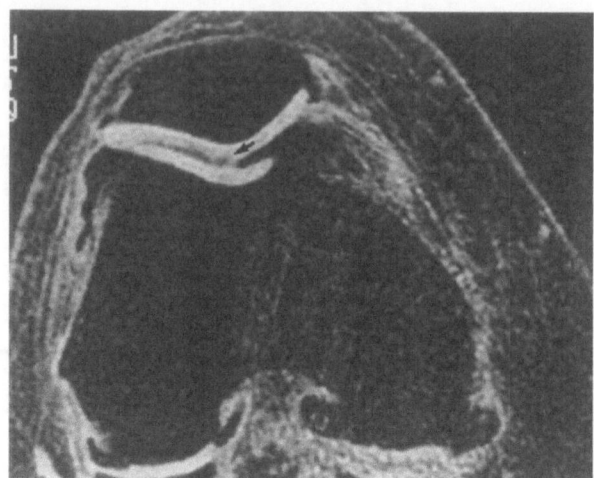

FIG. 14. Augmenting T_1 contrast in cartilage using fat suppression. Axial fat-suppressed, T_1-weighted 3-D gradient-echo image shows cartilage as an isolated band of high signal intensity adjacent to low signal intensity subchondral bone and synovial fluid. Note the surface fibrillation of the patellar ridge (*arrow*)

[13,14,17–21] (Fig. 14). This technique is widely available, easy to use, and can be performed in only half the time required for magnetization-transfer subtraction [14]. Several studies have demonstrated the high sensitivity and specificity of this technique for detecting cartilage defects in the knee [18–20]. In a comparison of T_1-weighted gradient echo with and without fat suppression, T_2*-weighted gradient-echo, and conventional T_1-weighted, proton-density-weighted, and T_2-weighted spin-echo sequences in ten elderly cadaver knees, Recht et al. [20] found fat-suppressed, T_1-weighted gradient echo (flip angle = 60°; TE = 10 ms; voxel size = $469 \times 938 \times 1500 \mu m$) to have the greatest sensitivity (96%) and specificity (95%) for demonstrating patellofemoral cartilage lesions visible on pathological sections. Others [18,19] have reported similar results using the same technique in vivo and arthroscopic correlation. Accordingly, fat-suppressed 3-D gradient echo has become the method of choice for detailed evaluation of cartilage morphology using clinical MRI technology.

In addition to subjective evaluation of focal defects and generalized thinning of articular cartilage, a number of techniques have been developed for quantifying various morphological parameters, such as the thickness, volume, geometry, and surface topography of cartilage. By summing the voxels contained within segmented 3-D images of individual cartilage plates, it is possible to determine the exact volume of these complexly shaped structures. In a study of whole amputated knees and patellar specimens obtained from total knee arthroplasty, the volume of articular cartilage over the femur, tibia, and patella

FIG. 15. Quantifying cartilage volume with MRI. The graph depicts cartilage volumes determined from fat-suppressed, T_1-weighted 3-D gradient-echo images (*open circles*) and magnetization-transfer subtraction images (*closed circles*) plotted against volumes measured directly by water displacement. A total of 12 cartilage plates (6 patellar, 3 tibial, 3 femoral) from 6 knees were included. The *line* represents theoretical 100% accuracy. (From [14], with permission)

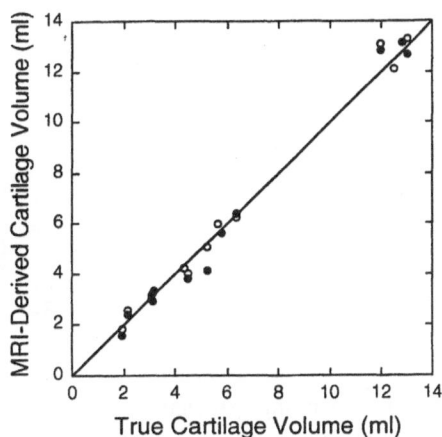

determined by MRI correlated well with the corresponding volumes determined by scraping the cartilage off the bones and measuring their displacement of water in graduated cylinders (Fig. 15) [14]. The reproducibility of this technique was also high: the coefficient of variation for volumes determined from repeated acquisitions of the same knee was approximately 4%. Others have reported similar findings using slightly different image-processing methods [22].

One problem with measuring cartilage volume in this way is that it currently demands considerable human input. Accurate segmentation of the articular cartilage, especially in patients with osteoarthritis, requires special expertise and perceptual skills on the part of the reader. Although many techniques available today are at least semi-automated, an experienced eye is still necessary to confirm and, not uncommonly, to edit manually the primary segmentation so as to assure its accuracy. Improvements in the degree of automation of this process would be extremely useful but are not easy to achieve.

Total volume measurements offer little information about the distribution of cartilage changes in the joint. Total cartilage volume is accordingly insensitive to focal change. Theoretically, a loss of cartilage in one region could be balanced by an equivalent increase in volume elsewhere in the joint and thereby elude detection by this method. By subdividing 3-D reconstructions of the articular cartilage into several smaller regions [23], it is possible to evaluate the volume at specific sites, such as the weight-bearing surfaces of the femorotibial joints. However, the reproducibility of such measurements decreases as the subdivisions are made smaller. Ultimately, extremely high spatial resolution is necessary to maintain precision. If sufficient resolution can be achieved within a reasonable imaging time, the prospect of mapping the cartilage thickness in vivo becomes feasible [24,25] (Fig. 16). Cartilage thickness maps may render insight into the importance of the location of cartilage lesions to the progression of osteoarthritis.

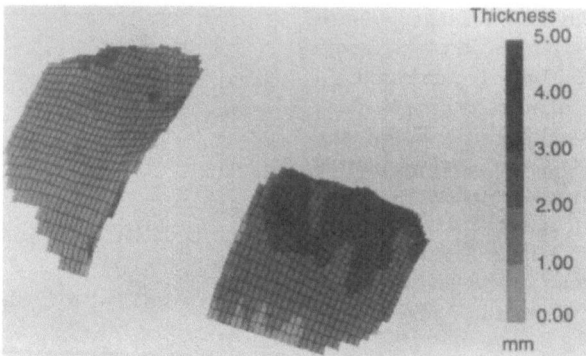

Fɪɢ. 16. Mapping articular cartilage thickness with MRI. Geometric models of the tibial cartilage were generated from a fat-suppressed T_1-weighted 3-D gradient-echo image data set. Regional cartilage thickness (perpendicular to the cartilage–bone interface) is depicted in intervals of 1 mm as different shades of gray. (From [26], with permission)

Imaging Other Articular Structures

The utility of MRI for evaluating other important intraarticular structures, such as the menisci and cruciate ligaments, has long been known to clinicians, but only recently have the implications of injury to these structures been viewed in light of more than just their immediate impact on joint function and comfort. Using methods similar to those described for the articular cartilage, the volume of synovial effusion can be accurately and precisely determined and monitored with serial MRI. Intravenous gadolinium-containing contrast material can disclose the amount and distribution of inflamed synovial tissue in both osteoarthritic and rheumatoid joints. And, finally, the integrity of periarticular muscles and tendons can be assessed with relative ease using conventional MRI pulse sequences. Even conventional MRI thus provides a richer and more comprehensive picture of what is going on in the arthritic joint, and can assist in the development of better models of joint pathophysiology with which to guide the search for new therapies for arthritis.

Considerations for Multicenter Clinical Studies

Many of the techniques described here can be performed with most clinical MRI systems currently in use around the world. At present there are more than 4000 systems in the United States and 9000 systems worldwide. Conducting multicenter clinical studies with MRI is, therefore highly feasible, so long as proper steps are taken to ensure quality.

It is important, first of all, that only imaging centers with competent and motivated personnel and that utilize the appropriate hardware and software be used. On-site training may be necessary at some of these centers, particularly those not experienced in conducting this type of research. Once the technical parameters for an imaging protocol are fully specified and programmed into the computers of the various MRI systems used in a study, images generated by the different centers are usually indistinguishable. Special expertise and experience are required to design an appropriate MRI protocol for a specific clinical trail, as well as to interpret the images. Centralized expert analysis in addition to study coordination are, therefore, essential to the success of any clinical study utilizing MRI. Provided adequate quality assurance is firmly in place, MRI is likely to reduce the number of patients and centers required to demonstrate drug efficacy, as well as the cost and time necessary to complete the study.

In conclusion, MRI provides a tool of unprecedented power for evaluating arthritis and its causes, and may offer more reliable measures of disease progression and treatment response than are currently attainable by other methods. Thus, both the assessment of new therapies for osteoarthritis and investigations of the pathophysiology in this disorder can be facilitated. Investigators concerned with osteoarthritis and other articular disorders should become more knowledgeable about MRI so that they can take full advantage of its unique capabilities and play a more active role in directing its development.

References

1. Budinger T, Lauterbur P (1984) Nuclear magnetic resonance technology for medical studies. Science 226:288–298
2. Young S (1988) Magnetic resonance imaging: basic principles. Raven, New York
3. König S, Brown R (1984) Determinants of proton relaxation in tissue. Magn Reson Imaging 1:437–449
4. Peterfy C (1997) Imaging techniques. In: Klippel J, Dieppe P (eds) Rheumatology, 2nd edn. Mosby, Philadelphia, pp 14.1–14.18
5. Palmer WE, Rosenthal DI, Shoenberg OI, et al (1995) Quantification of inflammation in the wrist with gadolinium-enhanced MR imaging and PET with 2-[F-18]-fluoro-2-deoxy-D-glucose. Radiology 196:645–655
6. Gindele A, Peterfy CG, Häckl F, et al (1996) MR imaging evaluation of arthritis in the wrist using a low-field, dedicated extremity system (Artoscan™). Presented at the 96th annual meeting of the American Roentgen Ray Society, May, 1996, San Diego, CA
7. Mow VC, Ratcliffe A, Poole AR (1992) Cartilage and diarthroidial joints as paradigms for hierarchical materials and structures. Biomaterials 13:67–97
8. Peterfy CG, Genant HK (1996) Emerging applications of magnetic resonance imaging for evaluating the articular cartilage. Radiol Clin North Am 34:195–213
9. Xia Y, Farquhar T, Burton-Wurster N, Lust G (1997) Origin of cartilage laminae in MRI. J Magn Reson Imaging 7:887–894

10. Xia Y, Farquhar T, Burton-Wurster N, Ray E, Jelinski LW (1994) Diffusion and relaxation mapping of cartilage-bone plugs and excised disks using microscopic magnetic resonance imaging. Magn Reson Med 31:273–282
11. Burstein D, Gray ML, Hartman AL, Gipe R, Foy BD (1993) Diffusion of small solutes in cartilage as measured by nuclear magnetic resonance (NMR) spectroscopy and imaging. J Orthop Res 11:465–478
12. Woolf SD, Chesnick S, Frank JA, Lim KO, Balaban RS (1991) Magnetization transfer contrast: MR imaging of the knee. Radiology 179:623–628
13. Peterfy CG, Majumdar S, Lang P, van Dijke CF, Sack K, Genant H (1994) MR imaging of the arthritic knee: improved discrimination of cartilage, synovium and effusion with pulsed saturation transfer and fat-suppressed T_1-weighted sequences. Radiology 191:413–419
14. Peterfy CG, van Dijke CF, Janzen DL, et al (1994) Quantification of articular cartilage in the knee by pulsed saturation transfer and fat-suppressed MRI: optimization and validation. Radiology 192:485–491
15. Rose PM, Demlow TA, Szumowski J, Quinn SF (1994) Chondromalacia patellae: fat-suppressed MR imaging. Radiology 193:437–440
16. Dardizinski B, Mosher T, Li S, Van Slyke M, Smith M (1997) Spatial variation of T_2 in human articular cartilage. Radiology 205:546–550
17. Disler D (1997) Fat-suppressed three-dimensional spoiled gradient-recalled MR imaging: assessment of articular and physeal hyaline cartilage. A J R 169:1117–1123
18. Disler DG, McCauley TR, Kelman CG, et al (1996) Fat-suppressed three-dimensional spoiled gradient-echo MR imaging of hyaline cartilage defects in the knee: comparison with standard MR imaging and arthroscopy. A J R 167:127–132
19. Disler DG, McCauley TR, Wirth CR, Fuchs MC (1995) Detection of knee hyaline articular cartilage defects using fat-suppressed three-dimensional spoiled gradient-echo MR imaging: comparison with standard MR imaging and correlation with arthroscopy. A J R 165:377–382
20. Recht MP, Pirraino DW, Paletta GA, Schils JP, Belhobek GH (1996) Accuracy of fat-suppressed three-dimensional spoiled gradient-echo FLASH MR imaging in the detection of patellofemoral articular cartilage abnormalities. Radiology 198:209–212
21. Chandnani VP, Ho C, Chu P, Trudell P, Resnick D (1991) Knee hyaline cartilage evaluated with MR imaging: a cadaveric study involving multiple imaging sequences and intraarticular injection of gadolinium and saline solution. Radiology 178:557–561
22. Dupuy DE, Spillane R, Rosol M, et al (1996) Quantification of articular cartilage in the knee with three-dimensional MR imaging. Acad Radiol 3:919–924
23. Pilch L, Stewart C, Gordon D, et al (1994) Assessment of cartilage volume in the femorotibial joint with magnetic resonance imaging and 3D computer reconstruction J Rheumatol 21:2307–2321
24. Eckstein F, Sitteck H, Gavazzenia A, Milz S, Putz R, Reiser M (1995) Assessment of articular cartilage volume and thickness with magnetic resonance imaging (MRI). Trans Orthop Res Soc 20:194
25. Ateshian GA, Kwak SD, Soslowsky LJ, Mow VC (1994) A stereophotogrammetric method for determining in situ contact areas in diarthroidial joints, and a comparison with other methods. J Biomech 27:111–124
26. Peterfy C, Howard D (1997) Imaging the patellofemoral joint: current status and future directions. Am J Knee Surg 10:110–120

Development of Quantitative Magnetic Resonance Imaging for Assessment of Cartilage Damage and Repair In Vivo

Jenny A. Tyler[1], Laurance D. Hall[2], and Paul J. Watson[2]

Summary. This chapter describes the computerized analysis of quantitative magnetic resonance (MR) parameters of water protons within articular cartilage. Those parameters were found to be consistently within a defined range for normal healthy cartilage and altered in a reproducible manner when the cartilage was fibrillated or the matrix degraded. T_1 and T_2 relaxation rates and magnetization transfer characteristics (T_1sat and Msat/M_0) of water in distal interphalangeal (DIP) joints were analyzed from a set of MR images acquired in vivo with a total scan time of 35 min, slice thickness of 1.5 mm, and resolution of $150 \mu m^2$. A significant two- to threefold increase in the T_2 and Msat/M_0 ratio was found in DIP cartilage from asymptomatic volunteers compared to patients with nodal osteoarthritis. A similar increase was identified in 3-mm-diameter, full-depth biopsy samples from osteoarthritic (OA) femoral cartilage representative of different stages in cartilage degeneration compared to values obtained from processing images of the knee of normal volunteers with a slice thickness of 2 mm and resolution of $600 \mu m^2$. This technology therefore provides an objective and quantitative means of identifying and monitoring cartilage degradation and repair within joints in vivo.

Key Words. Magnetic resonance imaging, Articular cartilage, Osteoarthritis, T_2 relaxation rate, magnetization transfer

Introduction

Posttraumatic knee problems pose a considerable challenge for the clinician whether they arise from traumatic injuries or pathology such as osteoarthritis (OA) or osteochondritis dissecans (OCD). Cartilage lesions are frequently

---

[1] Strangeways Research Laboratory, Worts' Causeway, Cambridge CB1 4RN, U.K.
[2] Herchel Smith Laboratory for Medicinal Chemistry, Cambridge University School of Clinical Medicine, University Forvie Site, Robinson Way, Cambridge CB2 2PZ, U.K.

seen at arthroscopy; they do not heal naturally and often undergo progressive degeneration [1,2]. These are a source of great morbidity in young people. The treatment most commonly available for the resulting pain and disability in a hip or knee is removal of both damaged and healthy cartilage from the affected joint and replacement with a prosthesis. The procedure restores a fairly normal range of pain-free motion and is considered to be very successful for elderly patients [3]. However, total joint arthroplasties have a limited life span and will not support unlimited heavy loading or the vigorous use required to provide the quality of life demanded by younger patients [4]. Alternative treatments are therefore eagerly sought.

Several novel procedures have been described that aim to promote the regeneration of repair cartilage that is hyaline in nature so as to provide a more durable matrix and eventually true regeneration of this specialized tissue (for detailed review, see [5]). One approach is to increase the number of cells with chondrogenic potential at the site of repair by isolating suitable cells, replicating them in culture, and implanting them at high density directly into the cartilage defect in vivo; many experimental and a few clinical studies have been reported using either committed, fully differentiated chondrocytes [6–11] or mesenchymal, prechondrogenic cells derived from periosteum or bone marrow [12–14]. An alternative method has been to avoid cell transplantation by implanting a biodegradable matrix containing growth factors into the defect, which promotes migration and supports chondrogenesis of endogenous stem cells from within the joint [5,15,16].

All these novel methods show great promise and could be appropriate for different applications. However, it is essential that they be rigorously tested in clinical trials to establish whether there is indeed a significant advantage over the techniques of arthroscopic debridement currently used [17,18], Pridie drillholes [19], or osteochondral grafts [20,21]. At present, the success of cartilage repair is evaluated clinically by various types of scoring based on visual assessment of the joint following examination by arthroscopy, radiography, or magnetic resonance imaging (MRI), and occasionally by histology of very small biopsy samples that usually represent less than 1% of the total repair tissue. Those methods are subjective, time consuming, and qualitative, and there is a clear need to find a noninvasive, objective, and quantitative means of monitoring the regenerative process that takes into account the heterogeneous nature of the newly formed cartilage.

Magnetic Resonance Imaging

All protons within living tissues have an inherent magnetic moment and spin randomly, giving rise to no net magnetization or direction. When a finger or knee is placed within the magnetic field of the MR scanner, the protons continue to spin but align themselves parallel or antiparallel to the direction of the field (B_0), corresponding to low and high energy states, respectively. In the course of an MR examination, a radiofrequency (RF) pulse (B_1) is applied to the sample from a transmitter coil orientated perpendicular to B_0, and the protons are momentarily tilted out of alignment; the precession of the induced net transverse magnetization around the axis of the static B_0 field produces a voltage across the ends of the receiver coil that is detected as the MR signal. The degree of contrast between, for example, bone and cartilage in the MR image can be varied by varying the timing of the pulse. As a result of random thermal motion, the spins lose coherence with one another and the signal decays. The time for the MR signal to return to zero depends on many factors. One is the rate at which the energized spins lose their excess energy to their immediate environment, called spin-lattice or T_1 relaxation, which affects mainly magnetization parallel to B_0 and leads to a net loss of energy from the spin system; another is the slight difference in frequency in the spins of neighboring protons that tend to drift out of alignment with one another, losing their phase coherence, which is called the spin-spin or T_2 relaxation. This change therefore affects the transverse component of the magnetisation but does not cause a net loss of energy (for a comprehensive review, see [22]).

Spatial Resolution

The digital resolution in a two-dimensional MR image is determined by the slice thickness, typically 1–4 mm, and the pixel size, typically 100–1000 μm. The pixel size is predetermined at the start of the experiment by choosing the field of view (FOV) for the object of interest and the size of the matrix, for example, 128, 256, or 512. There are now many examples in the literature of attempts that have been made to measure cartilage dimensions of thickness or volume from an MR image [23–32]. In such cases, or where images are to be scored visually, the highest possible resolution that provides enough signal in the allocated scan time is recommended. However, if quantitative values are to be acquired, it may be appropriate to gain increased signal to noise per pixel at the expense of a lower resolution image.

MR Scanner

In the following experiments, all MRI measurements were made using an Oxford Instruments (Oxford, U.K.) 31-cm horizontal bore 2.4-tesla magnet operated by a modified Bruker Biospec II console with a purpose-designed 8-strut quadrature RF probe (internal diameter, 26 mm) and gradient coils that provided a maximum magnetic field gradient of 0.15 T m^{-1}. Magnetic field gradients were produced using Golay and Maxwell coils on a 10-cm-internal-diameter former. All data were transferred via a fast data transfer unit to a network of computer workstations operating CaMReS software developed in the Herchel Smith Lab using the UNIX and X-window systems for image processing, display, and archiving.

Quantitative Magnetic Resonance Imaging

Any variation in the environment of the water protons within cartilage caused by compression or changes in matrix concentration, hydration, or amounts of interfibrillar water within the collagen fibrils leads to altered rates of relaxation of the induced MR signal. For example, it is known that the signal intensity in a T_1-weighted MR image appears decreased in degenerative cartilage compared to healthy cartilage [33–38]. As described earlier, the MR parameters that give rise to this altered contrast can be expressed as a quantitative value (quantitative MRI, qMRI). Importantly, using this system, T_1, T_2, and MT values can be fitted on a pixel-by-pixel basis to single or multiple exponential models with appropriate error and statistical analyses. The objective of the present work was therefore to investigate whether it was possible to acquire MR parameters from an MR image of a joint in vivo that accurately reflects discrete changes in cartilage composition.

Measurement of T_1 and T_2 Relaxation

There are many methods of measuring T_1 and T_2 relaxation times [25,39–41]. To assess the T_2 component of signal decay, the repetition time (TR, time interval between one RF pulse and the next) is kept constant and the echo time (TE, time interval between the RF pulse and sampling the MR signal) is varied. One example of an experiment to measure T_2 relaxation rates in cartilage in vivo is shown in Fig. 1. Each image from left to right was of the same distal interphalangeal (DIP) joint of an asymptomatic volunteer (45-year-old woman) scanned at a repetition time (TR) of 1500 ms but with increasing echo times (TE) of 6, 12, 18, 24, 30, 36, 42, and 48 ms; total imaging time was 6 min. The stepped unbroken line in the lower part of each image depicts the relative signal intensity at each echo time compared to the minimum (dashed line, 0). If a suitable M_0 (proton density) phantom is included in the RF coil at the time of image acquisition, those signal intensities can be expressed as an absolute value. Less signal is apparent at the longer echo times because it has decayed before it was recorded. The mean T_2 value of cartilage in this joint was automatically calculated to be 23.1 ± 0.5 ms from the decay curve based on a single exponential. In a similar manner, sequential images of the same joint were acquired (data not shown) and processed to calculate T_1 relaxation times; in this case, the TE was kept constant at 6 ms and the TR was decreased.

Magnetization Transfer

Protons within the joint are either freely mobile or bound to relatively immobile polymers. In a magnetization transfer (MT) experiment [42], data from a normal spin-echo sequence is acquired and then the sample is reimaged

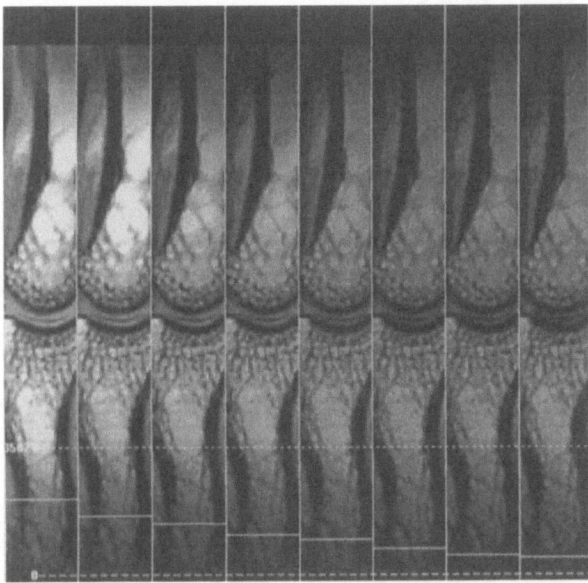

Fig. 1. Magnetic resonance (MR) images acquired during a CPMG (Carr–Purcell–Meiboom–Gill) experiment. The distal interphalangeal (DIP) joint of an asymptomatic volunteer (45-year-old woman) shows decreased signal in the cartilage with increasing echo times (from left to right) during measurement of T_2 relaxation rates. Spin echo: TR (repetition time), 1500 ms; TE (echo time) (from left to right), 6, 12, 18, 24, 30, 36, 42, and 48 ms; FOV (field of view), 3.84 cm with a 256 matrix, slice thickness of 1.5 mm, and in-plane pixel resolution of 150 μm². *Dashed horizontal lines* in lower part of image, minimum (0) signal intensity; *stepped unbroken lines*, relative signal intensity for each echo time

using a weak (0.15-G) source of RF energy 10 kHz off resonance from the frequency of freely mobile water; the signal of water in contact with macromolecules is selectively saturated and suppressed. As energy is transferred from macromolecules to free water, signal is lost until eventually an equilibrium is reached which is characteristic of that tissue. Thus, agarose gels, for example, display marked MT suppression as they have a large polymeric structure and freely exchangeable protons; in contrast, acrylamide gels show no MT suppression because they have no exchangeable protons. Likewise, sodium alginate exhibits no MT suppression even though it forms a fairly viscous gel compared to the same concentration of calcium alginate, which is highly cross linked. Denaturation of polymeric proteins may generate new exchangeable groups (e.g.,—SH) where additional proton cross-relaxation could occur that would contribute to the MT effect [43]. The degree of MT saturation achieved by a suitable polymer is proportional to the concentration of polymer, its affinity with water, and the degree of cross-linking, which decreases lateral mobility [44]. Articular cartilage exhibits very high saturation

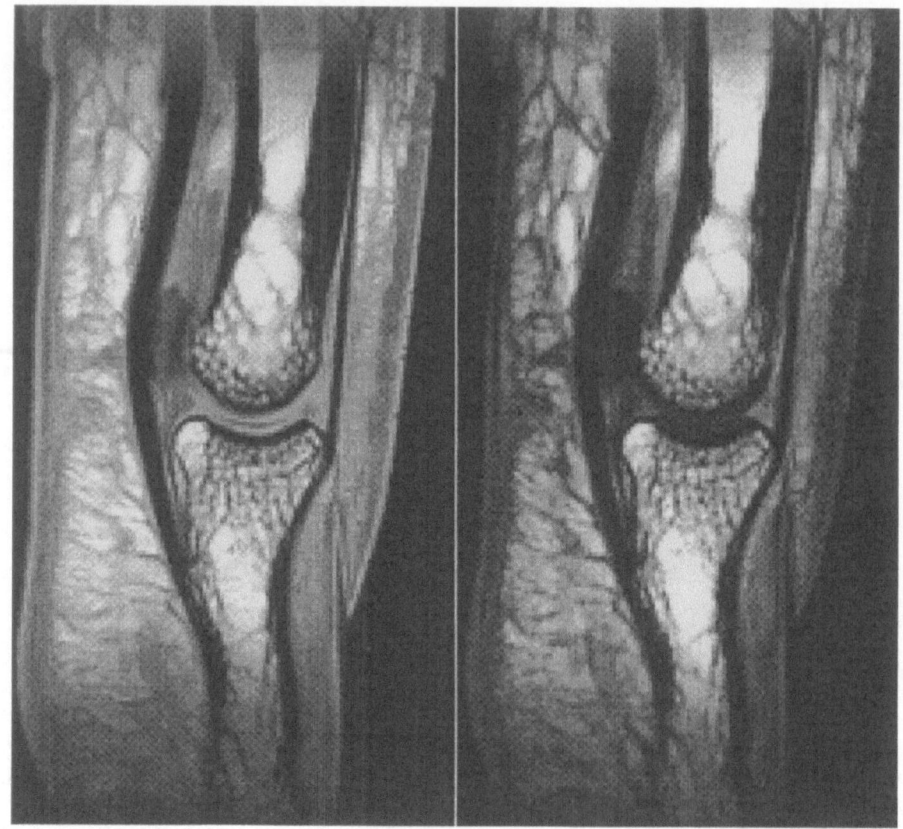

a   b

FIG. 2a,b. MR image of the same DIP joint as in Fig. 1. **a** Spin echo with no magnetization transfer; TR, 1500 ms; TE, 6 ms. **b** Spin echo with magnetization transfer
pre-pulse of 0.15 G, 10 kHz off resonance

of signal, typically more than 80% following an MT sequence (Fig. 2b) compared to a spin-echo image with no MT (Fig. 2a). The mean value for the
cartilage in Fig. 2 was calculated to be 85.1%, or 0.149 as the $Msat/M_0$ ratio of
the signal with and without MT. This effect is thought to be caused in part by
the cross-linked collagen network [45,46], which raises the possibility as to
whether such measurements could be used to identify the initial stages of
cross-link disruption and later loss of collagen from the cartilage during the
progression of OA or, alternatively, to monitor the formation of a new type II
collagen network during repair.

Automatic Report Generation

Following acquisition of the MR data, the image is displayed on the screen and
a region of interest or mask is outlined with a computer-aided tool. The T_1,

T_1sat, T_2, and MT ratio for each pixel within that delineated region is automatically calculated, based on a single exponential decay, and printed. For this study we have chosen to print out a small image of the joint and a histogram plot of the frequency distribution of each parameter. As the distribution is approximately Gaussian, the mean value and standard deviation of the total number of pixels defined by the mask is also given to provide a working MR definition of the quality of cartilage for that specimen. The quantitative information is acquired individually for every pixel of the joint within the field of view. It is therefore possible to calculate mean MR values in the same way for muscle, fat, or any other tissue of interest and compare them with the changes occurring within cartilage during the degenerative process. Alternatively, printouts of each distribution map of T_2, T_1, and MT values or total water content for each joint could be generated to provide spatial information as to where changes occur.

The automated printout of mean cartilage values calculated from qMRI data acquired in vivo from the DIP joint in Fig. 1 is shown in Fig. 3. The histogram plots are for T_1, T_2 (top left and right), Msat/M_0, and T_1sat (bottom

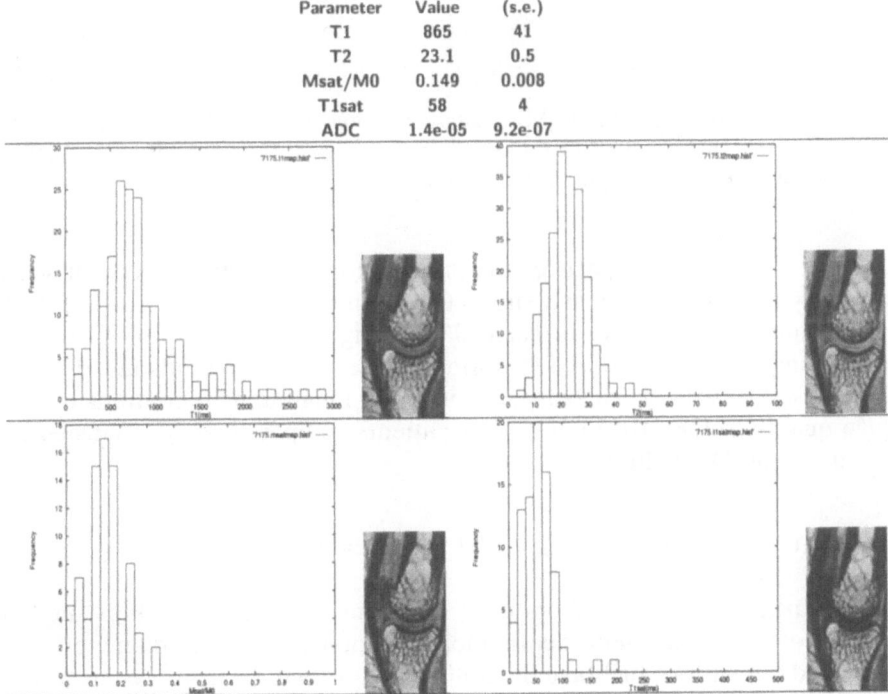

Parameter	Value	(s.e.)
T1	865	41
T2	23.1	0.5
Msat/M0	0.149	0.008
T1sat	58	4
ADC	1.4e-05	9.2e-07

FIG. 3. Automated printout of quantitative MRI (qMRI) data computed from a set of images of asymptomatic cartilage in the DIP joint shown in Fig. 1. Total acquisition time including pilot scan, 35 min

100   J.A. Tyler et al.

Parameter	Value	(s.e.)
T1	1353	106
T2	41.9	1.1
Msat/M0	0.349	0.020
T1sat	44	6
ADC	1.8e-05	1.4e-06

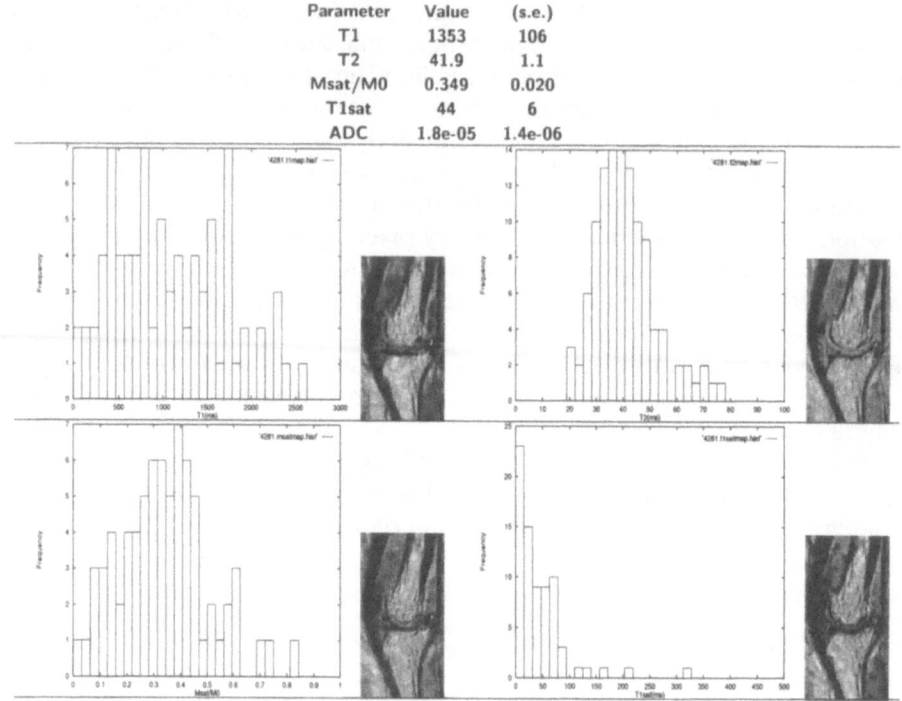

Fig. 4. Automated printout of qMRI data for osteoarthritis (OA) cartilage computed from a set of MR images of DIP joint of an OA patient (64-year-old woman). Total acquisition time including pilot scan, 35 min

left and right). For comparison, the printout for DIP cartilage in the finger of an OA patient (Fig. 4) clearly shows that both the mean and spread of the T_2 values and Msat/M_0 ratio in particular are significantly different in the OA joint compared to those of the normal finger. These methods are presently being used to study both cross-sectional and longitudinal variations in cartilage quality in the DIP joint of OA patients compared to age-matched and younger non-OA volunteers.

Preparation and qMRI of OA Knee Cartilage

Knee cartilage recovered from joint replacement surgery was kept moist to avoid loss of water. Full-depth biopsy samples, 4 mm in diameter, were punched out with an orthopaedic drill from different areas to provide a range of samples with different grades of OA pathology. One sample of such a femoral condyle with some of the punched holes is shown in Fig. 5. The cartilage plugs were immediately placed in a sealed plastic cylinder (4-mm diameter) and examined by qMRI and histology.

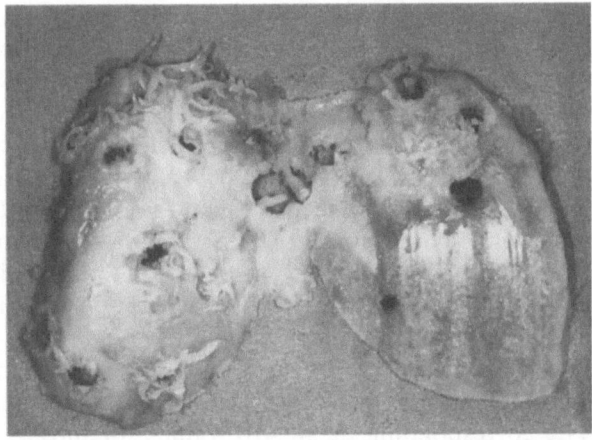

FIG. 5. Part of femoral condyle recovered from OA patient during joint replacement surgery. Full-depth, 4-mm-diameter biopsy plugs were removed from regions of the tissue showing varying stages of cartilage degeneration for qMRI examination and histology

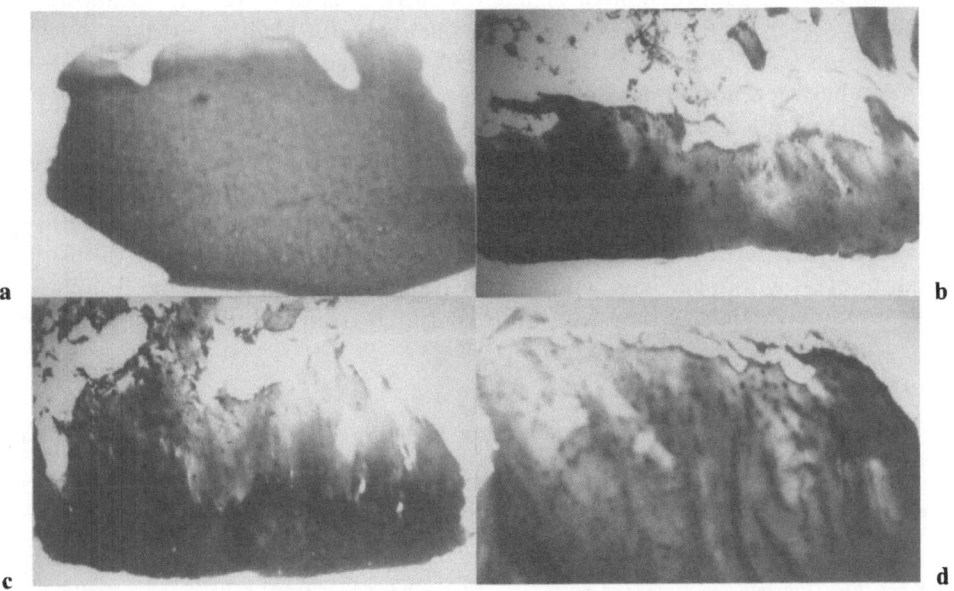

FIG. 6a–d. OA femoral cartilage histology in which 20-μm cryosections of four representative biopsy samples (a–d) were stained with toluidene blue. The MR characteristics of these specimens are shown in Table 1

Quantitative parameters measured were spin-lattice (T_1) relaxation rates (by saturation recovery; TE = 6 ms; TR = 5000, 2500, 1500, 1000, or 500 ms); spin-spin (T_2) relaxation rates (by CPMG, Carr–Purcell–Meiboom–Gill sequence; TR, 1500 ms; TE, 6–48 ms; 8 echoes as in Fig. 1); and magnetization transfer (MT) behavior (with B_1 saturation of 0.15 G off set by 10 Hz and saturation times of 0, 20, 50, 100, 200, and 400 ms) to evaluate T_1sat and Msat/M_0 ratio. Total water content (M_0) and thickness of the cartilage can be calculated from the same data. The method was validated by comparing data acquired from bulk measurements with selected slice data (slice thickness, 1.5 mm; FOV, 3.84 × 1.92 mm) of the appropriate phantom samples; they were found to be the same within experimental error.

After MRI, the specimens were frozen, cryosectioned at 20 μm, and stained with toluidine blue. The histology for four representative specimens is shown in Fig. 6a–d. The corresponding mean MR values for those specimens are listed in Table 1 together with the data acquired from in vivo imaging of the DIP cartilage shown in Figs. 3 and 4. Recent data of quantitative MR parameters obtained from images of healthy femoral cartilage acquired in vivo show values very similar to those for the asymptomatic DIP joint. A systematic and consistent two- to threefold increase in the T_2 relaxation rate and decrease in the degree of suppression of signal with MT was observed, from approximately 23.1 ± 0.5 and 0.149 ± 0.008, respectively, for healthy cartilage to 52.9 ± 0.8 and 0.557 ± 0.082 in degraded OA cartilage. Similar differences were found between normal and OA cartilage from the femoral biopsy specimens imaged ex vivo and the normal and OA DIP cartilage imaged in vivo.

The experiments described here have attempted to relate changes in the composition of cartilage matrix to the change in relaxometry of the cartilage water with respect to the T_1 and T_2 relaxation rates and MT ratio. Other laboratories have, in addition, mapped the spatial distribution of diffusion parameters within cartilage and demonstrated differences with depth [47] or adapted methodology based on the MR signal from sodium imaging, which

TABLE 1. Quantitative magnetic resonance imaging (MRI) values for normal and ostcoarthritis (OA) cartilage

Specimen	T_1 (ms)	T_2 (ms)	Msat/M_0	T_1sat
Knee, OA (Fig. 6a)	833 ± 18	24.1 ± 0.5	0.198 ± 0.005	78 ± 1
Knee, OA (Fig. 6b)	353 ± 6	53.1 ± 0.6	0.492 ± 0.047	152 ± 31
Knee, OA (Fig. 6c)	333 ± 8	52.9 ± 0.8	0.557 ± 0.055	110 ± 16
Knee, OA (Fig. 6d)	593 ± 20	50.9 ± 1.8	0.527 ± 0.082	159 ± 26
DIP, OA	1353 ± 106	41.9 ± 1.1	0.349 ± 0.02	44 ± 6
DIP, normal	865 ± 41	23.1 ± 0.5	0.149 ± 0.008	58 ± 4

DIP, distal interphalangeal.
All data shown are the mean values of all pixels included in the mask outlined on the MR image to define articular cartilage. On average, this was 50 pixels for the knee OA biopsy samples and 160 pixels for the normal DIP cartilage.

may prove promising for assessing changes in the concentration of proteoglycan [48].

Conclusion

A novel method of monitoring cartilage degradation by MRI has been developed and validated. The computer-automated analysis of MR images can monitor statistically significant differences in normal and degraded cartilage in vivo with acquisition times of 6 min and 12 min for the T_2 relaxation rate and MT ratio, respectively. We are confident, therefore, that this methodology can be used to identify and follow progression of cartilage degeneration in vivo in the DIP joint (to a resolution of $150 \mu m^2$) and knee (to a resolution of $600 \mu m^2$) of OA patients and to evaluate novel treatments. Further work is now required to establish whether similar MR protocols can be used to distinguish between fibrous and hyaline cartilage following treatment to induce repair and to validate those measurements by comparison with currently accepted analytical techniques.

Acknowledgments. The authors are indebted to the Arthritis and Rheumatism Council for a Senior Research Fellowship (JAT), the Medical Research Council for a ROPA grant (PJW), and Dr. Herchel Smith for an endowment to the Department of Medicinal Chemistry (LDH). We are also grateful for the enthusiastic sponsorship of this work by Genzyme Tissue Repair. Thanks are also given to Dr. Adrian Carpenter, Cliff Bunch, and Simon Smith for their expert maintenance of the MR scanners.

References

1. Hunziker EB (1992) Articular cartilage structure in humans and experimental animals. In: Kuettner KE, Schleyerbach R, Peyron JG, et al (eds) Articular cartilage and osteoarthritis. Raven Press, New York, pp 183–189
2. Ghadially FN, Thomas I, Oryschak AF, et al (1977) Long term results of superficial defects in articular cartilage: a scanning electron microscope study, J Pathol 121:213–217
3. Charnley J, Cupic Z (1973) The nine and ten year results of low friction arthroplasty of the hip. Clin Orthop 95:9–13
4. Chandler HP, Resnick FT, Wilson RL (1981) Total hip replacement in patients who are under the age of 30 at the time of arthroplasty. A five year follow up study. J Bone Joint Surg 63A:9–12
5. Tyler JA, Hunziker EB (1997) Articular cartilage regeneration. In: Lohmander S, Brandt K, Doherty M (eds) Osteoarthritis. Oxford University Press, Oxford, pp 101–118
6. Bentley G, Greer A (1971) Homotransplantation of isolated epiphyseal and articular cartilage chondrocytes into joint surfaces of rabbits. Nature (Lond) 230:385–388

7. Itay S, Abramovici A, Nevo Z (1987) Use of cultured embryonal chick epiphyseal chondrocytes as grafts for defects in chick articular cartilage. Clin Orthop 220:284–303
8. Grande DA, Pitman MI, Peterson L, et al (1987) The repair of experimentally produced defects in rabbit articular cartilage by autologous chondrocyte transplantation. J Orthop Res 7:208–218
9. Wakitani S, Kimura T, Hirocka A, et al (1989) Repair of rabbit articular surfaces with allograft chondrocytes embedded in collagen gel. J Bone Joint Surg [Br] 71(1):74–80
10. Brittberg M, Lindahl A, Nilsson A, et al (1994) Treatment of deep cartilage defects in the knee with autologous chondrocyte transplantation. N Engl J Med 331(14):889–895
11. Sams AE, Nixon AJ (1995) Chondrocyte-laden collagen scaffolds for resurfacing extensive articular cartilage defects. Osteoarthritis Cartil 3:47–59
12. Benayahu D, Kletter Y, Zipori D, et al (1989) Bone marrow derived stromal cell line expresses osteoblastic phenotype in vitro and osteogenic capacity in vivo. J Cell Physiol 140:1–7
13. Haynesworth SE, Goshima J, Goldberg VM, et al (1992) Characterisation of cells with osteogenic potential from human marrow Bone (NY) 13:81–88
14. Wakitani S, Goto T, Pineda SJ, et al (1994) Mesenchymal cell-based repair of large full-thickness defects of articular cartilage. J Bone Joint Surg 76A:579–592
15. Hunziker EB, Rosenberg LC (1995) Repair of partial thickness articular cartilage defects. Cell recruitment from the synovium. J Bone Joint Surg 78A:721–733
16. Hunziker EB, Shenk RK (1995) A differential treatment protocol for inducing cartilage and bone repair in full-thickness articular cartilage defects. Trans Orthop Res Soc 20:170
17. Johnson LL (1990) The sclerotic lesion: pathology and the clinical response to arthroscopic abrasion arthroplasty. In: Ewing JE (ed) Articular cartilage and knee joint function. Basic science and arthroscopy. Raven Press, New York, pp 319–333
18. Childers ECJ, Ellwood SC (1979) Partial chondrectomy and subchondral bone drilling for chondromalacia. Clin Orthop 144:114–120
19. Insall J (1974) The Pridie debridement operation for osteoarthritis of the knee. Clin Orthop 32-B(3):302–367
20. Matsusue Y, Yamamuro T, Hama H (1993) Case report: arthroscopic multiple osteochondral transplantation to the chondral defect in the knee associated with anterior cruciate ligament disruption. Arthroscopy 9:318–321
21. Bobic V (1996) Arthroscopic osteochondral autograft transplantation in anterior cruciate ligament reconstruction: a preliminary clinical study. Knee Surg Sports Traumatol Arthrosc 3:262–264
22. Edelman RR, Kleefield J, Wentz KU, et al (1990) Basic principles of magnetic resonance imaging. In: Edelman RR, Hesselink JR (eds) Clinical magnetic resonance imaging. Saunders, Philadelphia, pp 3–38
23. Karvonen RL, Negendank WG, Tietge RA, et al (1994) Factors affecting articular cartilage thickness in osteoarthritis and ageing. J Rheumatol 21:1310–1318
24. Peterfy CG, van Dijke SV, Janzen EL, et al (1994) Quantification of articular cartilage in the knee with pulsed saturation transfer subtraction and fast-suppressed MR imaging: optimisation and validation. Radiology 192:485–491

25. Pilch L, Stewart C, Gordon D, et al (1994) Assessment of cartilage volume in femoro-tibial joints with magnetic resonance imaging and 3D computer reconstruction. J Rheumatol 21:2370–2379
26. Eckstein F, Sittek H, Milz S (1995) The potential of magnetic resonance imaging (MRI) for quantifying articular cartilage thickness: a methodological study. Clin Biomech 10:434–440
27. Robson MD, Hodgson RJ, Herrod NJ, et al (1995) A combined analysis and magnetic resonance imaging technique for computerized automatic measurement of cartilage thickness in the distal interphalangeal joint. Magn Reson Imaging 13:709–718
28. Eckstein F, Gavazzeni A, Sittak H (1996) Determination of knee joint cartilage thickness using three-dimensional magnetic resonance chondro-crassometry. Magn Reson Med 36:256–265
29. Kladny B, Bail H, Swonoda C, et al (1996) Cartilage thickness measurement in magnetic resonance imaging. Osteoarthritis Cartil 4:181–186
30. Sittek H, Eckstein F, Gavazzeni A, et al (1996) Assessment of normal patellar cartilage volume and thickness using MRI: an analysis of currently available pulse sequences. Skeletal Radiol 25:55–62
31. Losch A, Eckstein F, Haubner M, et al (1997) A non-invasive technique for assessment of articular cartilage thickness based on MRI. Part 1: method. Development of a computational method. Magn Reson Imaging 15(7):795–804
32. Haubner M, Eckstein F, Schnier M, et al (1997) A non-invasive technique for 3-dimensional assessment of articular cartilage thickness based on MTI. Part 2: Validation using arthrography. Magn Reson Imaging 15(7):805–813
33. Racht MP, Kramer JS, Marcelis S, et al (1993) Abnormalities of articular cartilage in the knee: analysis of available MR techniques. Radiology 187:473–478
34. Disler DG, McCauley TR, Kelman CG (1996) Fat-suppressed three dimensional spoiled gradient-echo MR imaging of hyaline cartilage defects in the knee: comparison with standard MR imaging and arthroscopy. AJR 167:127–132
35. Gahunia HK, Lemaire C, Babyn PS, et al (1995) Osteoarthritis in rhesus macaque knee joint: quantitative magnetic resonance imaging, tissue characterisation of articular cartilage. J Rheumatol 22(9):1747–1755
36. Watson PJ, Carpenter TA, Hall LD, et al (1996) Cartilage swelling and loss in a spontaneous model of osteoarthritis visualised by magnetic resonance imaging. Osteoarthritis Cartil 4:197–207
37. Tyler JA, Watson PJ, Koh W-L, et al (1996) Detection and monitoring of progressive degeneration of osteoarthritic cartilage by MRI. Acta Orthop Scand 66:130–138
38. Wilson D, Paul PK, Roberts ED, et al (1993) Magnetic resonance imaging and morphometric quantitation of cartilage histology after chronic infusion of interleukin 1 in rabbit knees. Proc Soc Exp Biol Med 203(1):30–37
39. Farrar TC, Becker ED (1971) Pulse and Fourier transform NMR: introduction to theory and methods. Academic Press, London
40. Homans SW (1989) A dictionary of concepts in NMR. Clarendon Press, Oxford
41. Callaghan PT (1987) Principles of nuclear magnetism. Oxford University Press, Oxford
42. Wolff SD, Balaban RS (1989) Magnetization transfer contrast (MTC) and tissue water proton relaxation in vivo. Magn Reson Med 10:135–144

43. Grad J, Mendelson D, Hyder F, et al (1991) Applications of nuclear magnetic cross-relaxation spectroscopy to tissues. J Magn Res 17:452–459
44. Tessier J, Potter K, Carpenter TA, et al (1994) Demonstration of the linear dependence of proton magnetisation transfer on polymer concentration in aqueous gels. Magn Reson Chem 32:55–61
45. Kim DK, Ceckler TI, Hascall VC, et al (1993) Analysis of water-macromolecule proton magnetisation transfer in articular cartilage. Magn Reson Med 29:211–215
46. Lesperance LM, Gray ML, Burnstein D (1993) Effect of collagen concentration and structure on MT in hydrated collagen and cartilage. Soc Magn Reson Med 3:1107–1110
47. Xia Y, Farquhar T, Burton-Wurster N, et al (1994) Diffusion and relaxation mapping of cartilage-bone plugs and excised disks using microscopic magnetic resonance imaging. Magn Reson Med 31:273–282
48. Bernstein D, Gray ML, Hartman AL, et al (1993) Diffusion of small solutes in cartilage as measured by nuclear magnetic resonance (NMR) spectroscopy and imaging. J Orthop Res 11:456–478

Gene Delivery to Chondrocytes Using Adenovirus Vector

Toshikazu Kubo[1], Yuji Arai[1], Kappei Kobayashi[2], Jiro Imanishi[2], Masaharu Takigawa[3], and Yasusuke Hirasawa[1]

Summary. The objective of this study was to investigate the effects of adenovirus vector (Ax-)mediated gene transduction of *E. coli* β-galactosidase (LacZ) and transforming growth factor-β1 (TGF-β1) into a human chondrocyte-like cell line (HCS-2/8). The expression of transduced genes and their expression periods were examined by 5-bromo-4-chloroindolyl-β-D-galactoside (X-gal) staining, Northern blotting, ELISA, and Western blotting. To assess the influence of TGF-β1 gene transduction, the expression of mRNAs of type II collagen, proteoglycan core protein, matrix metalloproteinase-3 (MMP-3), and tissue inhibitor of matrix metalloproteinase-1 (TIMP-1) were examined by Northern blotting. Staining with X-gal indicated that the genes were transduced into 99% of the cells. Expression of the transduced genes in the cells was continued for at least 21 days. Transduction of the TGF-β1 gene enhanced mRNA expressions of type II collagen and proteoglycan core protein, but suppressed MMP-3 mRNA expression in the cells. These results indicate Ax is useful in chondrocyte gene therapy, and it could be an efficient mediator of TGF-β1 gene transduction.

Key Words. Gene delivery, Adenovirus vector, Chondrocytes, TGF-β1

Introduction

The number of patients with joint damage, such as rheumatoid arthritis, osteoarthritis, and chondral injury, has been increasing rapidly along with the increase in the elderly population and in numbers of athletes. When damage

---

[1] Department of Orthopaedic Surgery, Kyoto Prefectural University of Medicine, Kawaramachi-Hirokoji, Kamigyo-ku, Kyoto 602, Japan.
[2] Department of Microbiology, Kyoto Prefectural University of Medicine, Kawaramachi-Hirokoji, Kamigyo-ku, Kyoto 602, Japan.
[3] Department of Biochemistry and Molecular Dentistry, Okayama University Dental School, 2-5-1 Shikata-cho, Okayama 700-0914, Japan.

progresses and results in severe destruction of the joint, surgical treatment is often required. Therefore, it is desired to prevent the progress of joint damage by elucidating the pathology of arthritis and by developing effective pharmacological therapies.

Many proteins have recently been reported to protect articular cartilage, and the hope is that they can be used as antiarthritic proteins. However, conventional drug delivery systems, such as oral, intravenous, intramuscular, or intraarticular administration, present difficulties in delivering a drug into specific joints and maintaining long-term therapeutic effects. With these existing administration methods, high dosages and frequent administration of drugs are necessary to achieve a therapeutically effective level.

On the other hand, basic and clinical studies of gene therapy for genetic diseases and malignant diseases have progressed [1,2]. Adenovirus vector (Ax) is a DNA carrier. By using Ax, foreign genes can be transduced easily and efficiently into a target tissue. Moreover, because it uses a recombinant virus without replication capability, Ax is safer than other virus vectors [3–5]. If a genetic code of a certain protein that protects articular cartilage can be transduced into chondrocytes, and if the protein can be expressed locally for a long time, this would be an efficient approach in the treatment of joint diseases.

In this study, we investigated the effects of Ax-mediated gene transduction of the *E. coli* β-galactosidase (LacZ) gene and transforming growth factor-$\beta1$ (TGF-$\beta1$) gene into a human chondrocyte-like cell line. LacZ gene is a marker gene used for evaluating gene transduction efficiency; TGF-$\beta1$ is a multifunctional molecule that plays a central role in embryonic development, tumorigenesis, wound healing, fibrosis, and immunoregulation [6–8]. TGF-$\beta1$ is also reported to promote cartilage repair and is expected to be one of the most effective drugs for joint diseases [9,10]. These characteristics make TGF-$\beta1$ a potential candidate for gene therapy for joint diseases.

We report here the high efficient gene transduction by Ax and demonstrate that the matrix metabolism is stimulated after the transduction of TGF-$\beta1$.

Materials and Methods

Cell Culture

We used an established human chondrocyte-like cell line (HCS-2/8) in this in vitro study [11–13]. HCS-2/8 cells were cultured in Dulbecco's modified Eagle's medium (DMEM; Nissui Pharmaceutical, Tokyo, Japan) supplemented with 10% fetal bovine serum (FBS; Gibco BRL, Gaithersburg, MD, USA), 60μg/ml of kanamycin, and 0.292mg/ml of L-glutamine (Wako BRL, Osaka, Japan). The cells were maintained in a humidified atmosphere of

5% CO_2/95% air environment at 37°C. The medium was changed twice a week.

Adenovirus Vector

We used a adenovirus type 5-based recombinant virus vector that lacks E1A, E1B, and E3 regions and therefore is replication deficient. AxCALacZ, a recombinant virus harboring the *E. coli* β-galactosidase (β-gal) gene (LacZ) under the control of CAG promoter [14], and Ax1w, a control vector harboring no foreign gene expression unit, were generous gifts of Dr. I. Saito (University of Tokyo). The CAG promoter is a potent promoter consisting of cytomegalovirus IE enhancer, chicken β-actin promoter, and rabbit β-globulin polyadenylation signal [14]. Recombinant virus expressing the TGF-β1 gene was constructed as described previously [15]. The TGF-β1 coding sequence, which generates latent TGF-β1, was excised from pHTGF-β2 (obtained from the American Type Culture Collection) by digesting with *Pst*I and *Nco*I, and was inserted into *Pst*I-*Kpn*I-digested pcDL-SRα296 containing SRα promoter [16]. The expression unit was excised from the plasmid and inserted into *Swa*I site of pAx1cw [14], purchased from Riken Gene Bank (Tsukuba, Japan). The recombinant virus clone expressing TGF-β1 was isolated, designated as AxSRTGF, and propagated and titrated as described [17]. Concentrated and purified virus stock was prepared as described previously [17].

Ax-Mediated Gene Transduction

Cells were resuspended to 10% FBS/DMEM and seeded in 60-mm plastic dishes at a density of 3×10^6 cells/4 ml. Two days later, when cells reached to confluent level, the medium was removed and 200 μl of recombinant virus diluted with phosphate-buffered saline (PBS) to contain 7.5×10^8 pfu/ml [multiplicity of infection (MOI) = 50 plaque-forming unit/cell] was added to the cells. In control experiments, cells received Ax1w or PBS. After incubation under humidified atmosphere of 5% CO_2 in air at 37°C for 1 h with occasional agitation, culture medium was added to the cells, and they were cultured until analysis. The day of transduction was defined as day 0.

Histochemical Staining of LacZ-Expressing Cells

Cells were fixed at indicated posttransduction times with AxCALacZ with 1% glutaraldehyde for 15 min at room temperature, rinsed twice with PBS, and then immersed in substrate solution consisting of 0.1 M sodium phosphate buffer, pH 7.5, 10 mM KCl, 1 mM $MgCl_2$, 3 mM $K_3[Fe(CN)_6]$, 3 mM $K_4[Fe(CN)_6]$, 0.1% Triton X-100, 1 mM 5-bromo-4-chloroindolyl-β-D-galactoside (X-gal) for 12 h at 37°C. Efficiency of gene transduction was assessed from the percentage of cells that were stained blue. Experiments were triplicated.

Determination of β-Galactosidase (β-Gal) Activity

AxCALacZ-transduced cells were harvested at indicated times and then soni-cated in o-nitrophenyl-β-D-galactopyranoside (ONPG) assay buffer [10 mM Tris-HCl (pH 7.5), 10 mM KCl, 1 mM MgCl$_2$, 0.1% Triton X-100, and 5 mM 2-mercaptoethanol]. Total protein concentration of the high-speed supernatant was determined by Lowry's method [18]. β-Gal activity was determined using the chromogen ONPG substrate. An aliquot of lysate was incubated with 0.5 mg/ml ONPG at 37°C for 4 min, and the reaction was stopped by add-ing 1 M Na$_2$CO$_3$. Optical density at 450 nm of the reaction product was mea-sured, and β-gal activity was calculated as an increase of A450 per minute per milligram total protein (A450 min^{-1}mg^{-1} protein). Experiments were triplicated.

Northern Blotting and Probe Preparation

Northern blotting was performed according to the previously described method [19]. Total RNA was extracted from the cells at the indicated time by acid guanidium thiocyanate-phenol-chloroform extraction [20]. Total RNA was quantified and analyzed by Northern blotting by using the RNA probes for TGF-β1, type II collagen, proteoglycan core protein, matrix metalloproteinase-3 (MMP-3), and tissue inhibitor of matrix metalloproteinase-1 (TIMP-1) [21–24]. The RNA probes for Northern blot-ting were prepared by transcribing RNA in the presence of digoxigenin-UTP (-uridine triphosphate) (Boehringer-Mannheim Biochemica, Mannheim, Germany) or fluorescein-12-UTP (DuPont NEN, Boston, MA, USA) from the template plasmids generated as follows. The BamHI-NcoI fragment, ex-cised from pHTGFβ-2 (2.14 kbp), was inserted into pBluescript. The reverse transcriptase-polymerase chain reaction (RT-PCR) products of type II col-lagen, proteoglycan core protein, MMP-3, and TIMP-1 were inserted into pCRII (Invitrogen, San Diego, CA, USA). Chemiluminescent detection using Dig luminescent detection kit (Boehringer-Mannheim Biochemica) and Renaissance nucleic acid chemiluminescence reagent kit (DuPont NEN) was performed according to the manufacturer's instructions. Experiments were quadruplicated.

Determination of TGF-β1 Level in Culture Supernatant of AxSRTGF-Transduced Cells

Culture supernatant was collected from control and AxSRTGF-transduced HCS-2/8 cells at day 3, centrifuged, filtered, and then treated with HCl at 4°C for 1h to enable all TGF-β1 molecules to be detectable by active TGF-β1-specific ELISA kit (Amersham Systems, Buckinghamshire, England). The ELISA kit was used according to the manufacturer's instructions. Experiments were triplicated.

Results

In all triplicated or quadruplicated experiments for each test item, almost identical results were obtained. The figures are representative of the repeated experiments.

Evaluation of Ax-Mediated Gene Transduction by Using LacZ Gene

To assess the efficiency of Ax-mediated gene transduction, we transduced the *E. coli* LacZ gene to the cells by using AxCALacZ. Efficiency of gene transduction was estimated as the percentage of cells staining X-gal positive in total cells counted. The LacZ expression was observed in 99% of the cells transduced with 50 MOI of AxCALacZ on day 3 after transduction (Fig. 1). No LacZ expression was observed in control cells under the same staining condition. In addition, there was no evidence of cell death or gross morphological changes as a result of transduction under microscopic examination.

To evaluate the LacZ expression period, we examined the expression at 3, 7, 14, and 21 days after the treatment. The β-gal-positive cell ratio was 99% on

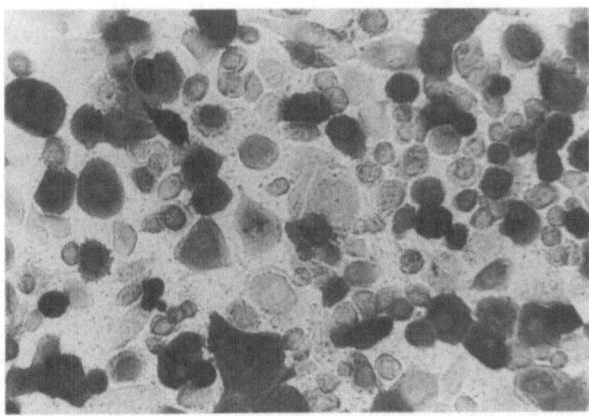

FIG. 1. Photomicrograph of cells transduced with Lac-Z (*E. coli* β-galactosidase). HCS-2/8 cells were treated with AxCALacZ and stained with X-gal on posttransduction day 3. Original magnification, ×200

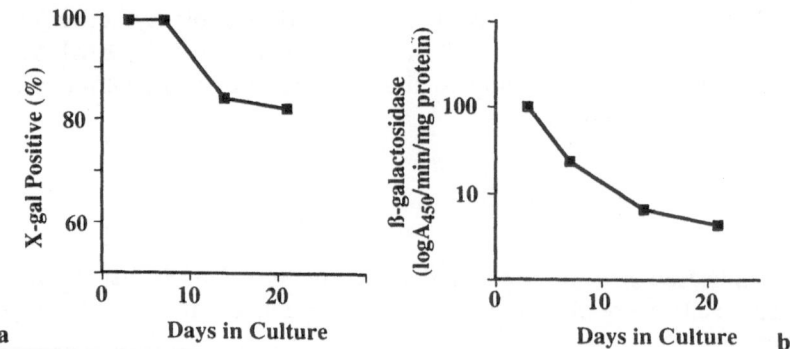

FIG. 2a,b. Durability of LacZ expression in LacZ-transduced cells. **a** Chronological change in the percentage of LacZ-positive cells. HCS-2/8 cells were treated with AxCALacZ, stained with X-gal on posttransduction days 3, 7, 14, and 21, and the percentage of LacZ-positive cells determined. **b** Chronological change in β-gal activity. HCS-2/8 cells were treated with AxCALacZ, and β-gal activity was determined on posttransduction days 3, 7, 14, and 21

post-transduction day 3 and thereafter decreased; 99%, 84%, and 82% on posttransduction days 7, 14, and 21, respectively (Fig. 2a). The β-gal activity was maintained at posttransduction day 21, even though total β-gal activity in transduced cells gradually decreased during the study period (Fig. 2b). No β-gal activity was detected in the control cells under the identical assay condition (data not shown).

Expression and Effect of Transduced TGF-β1 Gene

Expression of transduced TGF-β1 was confirmed by Northern blotting and ELISA. In the control cells, endogenous TGF-β1 mRNA was detected as a 2.5-kilobase (kb) band. When cells were treated with AxSRTGF-encoded TGF-β1 gene, both endogenous and exogenous TGF-β1 mRNA (2.0 kb) were detected (Fig. 3a; TGF). Expression of the exogenous TGF-β1 gene was observed to continue for at least 21 days (Fig. 3b). As expected from the result of Northern analysis, cells secreted a significant amount of TGF-β1. Transduction of TGF-β1 gene resulted in a threefold increase (control cells, 0.760 $\pm$ 0.058 ng/ml, mean$\pm$SD; TGF-β1 transduced cells, 2.352 $\pm$ 0.213 ng/ml) in secreted TGF-β1 level.

We then examined the expression of proteins that are related to cartilage metabolism. Messenger RNAs for type II collagen, proteoglycan core protein, MMP-3, and TIMP-1 were readily detectable in the cells (Fig. 4). Ax-mediated transduction of the TGF-β1 gene elevated the expression of type II collagen and proteoglycan core protein mRNA, and downregulated the expression of MMP-3 mRNA (Fig. 4a–c), but did not affect TIMP-1 mRNA expression (Fig. 4d).

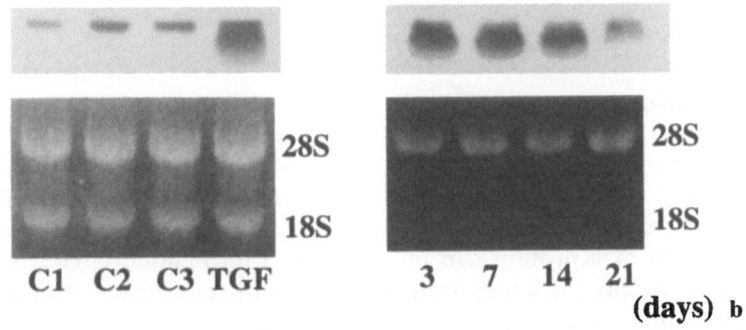

FIG. 3a,b. Northern blot analysis for transduced transforming growth factor beta-1 (TGF-β1) gene expression. **a** RNA samples from untreated cells (*C1*), PBS-treated cells (*C2*), Ax1w-treated cells (*C3*), and AxSRTGF-treated cells (*TGF*) were analyzed. Transduced TGF-β1 gene expression was detected in AxSRTGF-treated cells. Ethidium bromide staining (*lower panel*) confirmed that an equal amount of RNA was analyzed. **b** HCS-2/8 cells were treated with AxSRTGF, and RNA was extracted on posttransduction days 3, 7, 14, and 21. Transduced TGF-β1 mRNA (2.0 kb) was detected throughout the experimental period. Ethidium bromide staining (*lower panel*) confirmed that an equal amount of RNA was analyzed

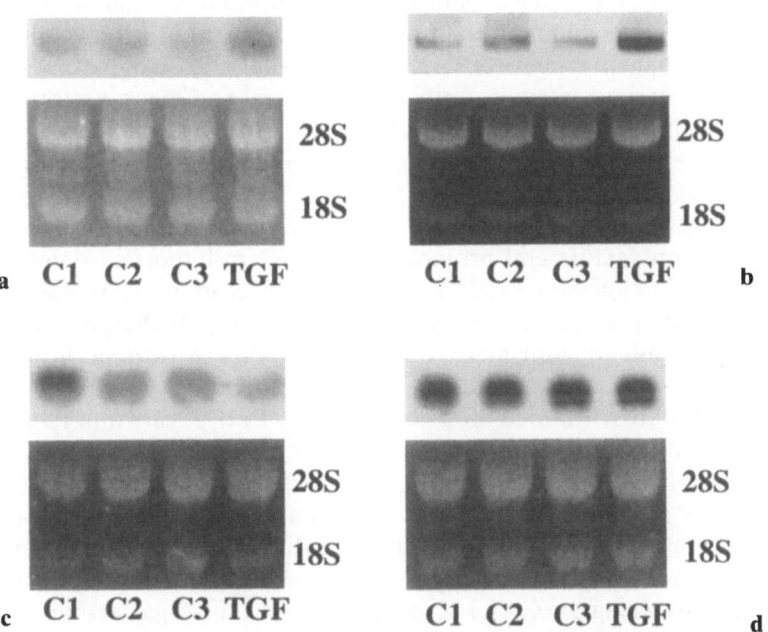

FIG. 4a–d. Effects of TGF-β1 gene transduction on the expression of cartilage matrix-related genes. RNA samples from untreated cells (*C1*), PBS-treated cells (*C2*), Ax1w-treated cells (*C3*), and AxSRTGF-treated cells (*TGF*) were analyzed. Northern blots were performed with RNA probe for type II collagen (**a**), proteoglycan core protein (**b**), matrix metalloprotem (MMP-3) (**c**), or tissue inhibitor of matrix metalloproteinase-1 (TIMP-1) (**d**). Ethidium bromide staining (*lower panel* of each set) confirmed that an equal amount of RNA was analyzed

113

Discussion

Many proteins that have antiarthritic potential are expected to be new drugs for arthritis. However, traditional drug delivery methods cannot target specific joints and cannot maintain effective concentrations of drugs for a long time. If gene coding of a protein can be transduced into chondrocytes, and can be expressed locally for a long time, this would be an efficient strategy in treatment for joint diseases.

Since the first gene therapy for adenosine deaminase (ADA) deficiency was performed in 1990, some experiments on gene therapy have been conducted, and basic and clinical experiments of gene therapy for many diseases, such as genetic diseases [1], cancer [2], and AIDS [25] have progressed. Experiments of gene therapy for joint diseases have also been performed, and transduction to the synovium has been conducted [26–32]. However, gene transduction to articular chondrocytes has not been well studied. If we can transduce chondroprotective genes into the chondrocytes of cartilage, this treatment would be an efficient therapy for joint diseases.

In this study, efficiency of gene transduction was investigated by using HCS-2/8. HCS-2/8 cells maintain their phenotype throughout a long culture period, produce collagen type II, IX, XI, and cartilage proteoglycans (aggrecan), respond to various vitamins and growth factors, and express protooncogenes similar to those of normal chondrocytes [11–13]. For these reasons, the HCS-2/8 cell line is a good model of human normal chondrocytes and is useful to evaluate the success rate of gene transduction. In this study, using this cell line, we demonstrated Ax is an effective mean to transduce TGF-β1 gene.

Expression vectors and promoter elements are important determinants of gene transduction and expression. Various vectors such as naked plasmid DNA, retrovirus vector [33], adenovirus vector [34], herpes simplex virus vector [35], adeno-associated virus vector [36], and cationic liposomes [37] with various promoters are used in gene transduction. Previous studies have shown that retroviral-mediated gene delivery to the synovium requires surgical removal of the tissue [26–32], but Ax mediates expression of foreign transgenes by direct in vivo methods in a variety of terminally differentiated cells, such as neurons, glia cells, pulmonary epithelium, hepatocytes, and skeletal muscle [34,38–40]. In most cases, the efficiency of gene transduction was high, and long-term transgene expression was observed. In this study, experiments using AxCALacZ demonstrated that β-gal activity was maintained at posttransduction day 21, even though total β-gal activity in transduced cells gradually decreased during the study period. Possible factors for the decreased levels are the decreased number of vectors resulting from their disruption and dilution of cDNA level by cell growth. Even though terminal proteins are connected to both ends of the adenovirus vector to protect cDNA from DNase, vectors are not perfectly free from destruction. On the other hand, HCS-2/8 grows quite slowly even in the culture period; therefore, the cDNA levels of cells could be diluted in the later culture period. If there is no cell growth, β-galactosidase levels might be higher than our findings. In addition, Ax has more features; that is, Ax easily propagates without integrating into the host genome, and Ax does not affect host cell replication [4,5]. Therefore, Ax is regarded as an appropriate vector for gene transduction into chondrocytes.

TGF-β1, which is one of the major growth factors, is reported to increase articular cartilage proteoglycan synthesis and to suppress proteoglycan degradation [9,10]. Therefore, TGF-β1 is considered to accelerate cartilage repair. However, to obtain efficacy in actual treatment, frequent and repeated intraarticular injection is required [41]. In our study, the TGF-β1 gene was efficiently transduced by using Ax, and its expression continued for at least 21 days. Expression of the transduced TGF-β1 gene enhanced expression of mRNAs of type II collagen and proteoglycan core protein, which are major components of articular cartilage. We used the TGF-β1 gene that encodes latent TGF-β1, which is necessary to maintain the three-dimensional structure of TGF-β when it is released from a cell. The latent TGF-β1 generated from this gene may be activated when it is secreted to outside the cell, and it then changes to an active form. On the other hand, expression of transduced TGF-β1 gene suppressed the expression of MMP-3 mRNA, which can degrade proteoglycan. These results indicated that Ax-mediated transduction of TGF-β1 gene can improve the tissue repair capability in cartilage metabolism. On the other hand, frequent, large-dose direct intraarticular injection of TGF-β1 is reported to induce such unwanted effects as synovium inflammation and osteophytes [41]. Concerning these problems, gene transduction has an advantage: by changing the promoter area of the gene, a specific gene can be expressed in the target tissue. By using a promoter for a specific collagen, such as type II or type XI, it is possible to limit TGF-β1 expression to the cartilage tissue and to reduce the severity of unwanted effects on other tissues.

In this study, we used vectors to control the expression of various genes. If Ax is directly injected into a healthy joint in vivo, the permeability of Ax will be a matter of concern because cartilage has a matrix that may prohibit the deep distribution of Ax. However, in joints with osteoarthritis or traumatic cartilage injury, the cartilage matrix is usually degenerated and swollen; therefore, it is possible for Ax to enter the cells in a deep area. In addition, mechanical effects in vivo, such as joint motion and weight-bearing, would contribute to the distribution of Ax. We are at present conducting an in vivo study using Ax containing such genes.

In conclusion, gene delivery using Ax could be an attractive method for gene therapies for joint diseases.

Acknowledgments. We thank Dr. Y. Kanegae and I. Saito for the gift of Ax1w and AxCAlacZ. This work was supported by a grant-in-aid for scientific research (no. 05454411) from the Ministry of Education of Japan.

References

1. Blaese RM (1990) The ADA human gene therapy clinical protocol. Hum Gene Ther 1:327–362
2. Rosenberg SA (1992) Gene therapy for cancer (clinical conference). JAMA 268:2416–2419
3. Roemer K, Friedmann T (1992) Concepts and strategies for human gene therapy. Eur J Biochem 208:211–225
4. Graham FL, Ludvik P (1991) Manipulation of adenovirus vectors. In: Murray EJ, Walker JM (eds) Methods in molecular biology, vol 7. Gene transfer and expression protocols. Humana, Clifton, NJ, pp 109–127
5. Kozarsky KF, Wilson JM (1993) Gene therapy: adenovirus vectors. Curr Opin Genet Dev 3:499–503
6. Kehrl JH, Wakefield LM, Roberts AB, et al (1986) Production of transforming growth factor beta by human T lymphocytes and its potential role in the regulation of T cell growth. J Exp Med 163:1037–1050
7. Espevik T, Figari IS, Shalaby MR, et al (1987) Inhibition of cytokine production by cyclosporin A and transforming growth factor beta. J Exp Med 166:571–576
8. Mule JJ, Schwarz SL, Roberts AB, Sporn MB, Rosenberg SA (1988) Transforming growth factor-beta inhibits the *in vitro* generation of lymphokine-activated killer cells and cytotoxic T cells. Cancer Immunol Immunother 26:95–100
9. Morales TI, Roberts AB (1988) Transforming growth factor-β regulates the metabolism of proteoglycans in bovine cartilage organ cultures. J Biol Chem 263:12828–12831
10. Redini F, Galera P, Mauviel A, et al (1988) Transforming growth factor-β stimulates collagen and glycosaminoglycan biosynthesis in cultured rabbit articular chondrocytes. FEBS Lett 234:172–176
11. Takigawa M, Tajima K, Pan H-O, et al (1989) Establishment of a clonal human chondrosarcoma cell line with cartilage phenotypes. Cancer Res 49:3996–4002
12. Enomoto MI, Takigawa M (1992) Regulation of tumor-derived and immortalized chondrocytes. In: Adolphe M (ed) Biological regulation of the chondrocytes. CRC Press, Boca Raton, pp 321–328
13. Zhu JD, Pan HO, Suzuki F, Takigawa M (1994) Proto-oncogene expression in a human chondrosarcoma cell line: HCS-2/8. Jpn J Cancer Res 85:364–371
14. Kanegae Y, Gwang L, Sato Y, et al (1995) Efficient gene activation in mammalian cells by using recombinant adenovirus expressing site-specific Cre recombinase. Nucl Acids Res 23:3816–3821
15. Miyake S, Makimura M, Kanegae Y, et al (1996) Efficient generation of recombinant adenoviruses using adenovirus DNA-terminal protein complex and a cosmid bearing the full-length virus genome. Proc Natl Acad Sci USA 93:1320–1324
16. Takebe Y, Seiki M, Fujisawa J, et al (1988) SRα Promoter: an efficient and versatile mammalian cDNA expression system composed of the simian virus 40 early promoter and the R-U5 segment of human T-cell leukemia virus type 1 long terminal repeat. Mol Cell Biol 8:466–472
17. Kanegae Y, Makimura M, Saito I (1994) A simple and efficient method for purification of infectious recombinant adenovirus. Jpn J Med Sci Biol 47:157–166
18. Lowry OH, Rosenbrough NJ, Farr AL, Randall RJ (1951) Protein measurement with the folin phenol reagent. J Biol Chem 193:265–275

19. Kobayashi K, Ohgitani E, Tanaka Y, Kita M, Imanishi J (1994) Herpes simplex virus-induced expression of 70 kD heat shock protein (HSP70) requires early protein synthesis but not viral DNA replication. Microbiol Immunol 38:321–325

20. Chomczynski P, Sacchi N (1987) Single-step method of isolation by acid guanidium thiocyanate-phenol-chloroform extraction. Anal Biochem 162:156–159

21. Su MW, Lee B, Ramirez F, Machado M, Horton W (1989) Nucleotide sequence of the full length cDNA encoding for human type II procollagen. Nucl Acids Res 17:9473

22. Doege KJ, Sasaki M, Kimura T, Yamada Y (1991) Complete coding sequence and deduced primary structure of the human cartilage large aggregating proteoglycan, aggrecan: human-specific repeats, and additional alternatively spliced forms. J Biol Chem 266:894–902

23. Whitham SE, Murphy G, Angel P, et al (1986) Comparison of human stromelysin and collagenase by cloning and sequence analysis. Biochem J 240:913–916

24. Onisto M, Garbisa S, Caenazzo C, et al (1993) Reverse transcription-polymerase chain reaction phenotyping of metalloproteinases and inhibitors involved in tumor matrix invasion. Diagn Mol Pathol 2:74–80

25. Anderson WF (1992) Human gene therapy. Science 256:808–813

26. Bandara G, Robbins PD, Georgescu HI, Mueller GM, Glorioso JC, Evans CH (1992) Gene transfer to synoviocytes. DNA Cell Biol 11:227–231

27. Roessler BJ, Allen ED, Wilson JM, Hartman JW, Davidson BL (1993) Adenoviral-mediated gene transfer to rabbit synovium in vivo. J Clin Invest 92:1085–1092

28. Makarov SS, Olsen JC, Johnston WN, et al (1995) Retrovirus mediated in vivo synovium in bacterial cell wall-induced arthritis in rats. Gene Ther 2:424–428

29. Bandara G, Mueller GM, Galea-Lauri J, et al (1993) Intraarticular expression of biologically active interleukin 1-receptor-antagonist protein by ex vivo gene transfer. Proc Natl Acad Sci USA 90:10764–10768

30. Roessler BJ, Hartman JW, Vallance DK, Latta JM, Janich SL, Davidson BL (1995) Inhibition of interleukin-1-induced effects in synoviocytes transduced with the human IL-1 receptor antagonist cDNA using an adenoviral vector. Hum Gene Ther 6:307–316

31. Makarov SS, Olsen JC, Johnston WN, et al (1996) Suppression of experimental arthritis by gene transfer of interleukin 1 receptor antagonist cDNA. Proc Natl Acad Sci USA 93:402–406

32. Hung GL, Galea-Lauri J, Mueller GM, et al (1994) Suppression of intra-articular response to interleukin-1 receptor antagonist gene to synovium. Gene Ther 1:64–69

33. Miller AD (1992) Human gene therapy comes of age. Nature (Lond) 357:455–460

34. Rosenfeld MA, Yoshimura K, Trapnell BC, et al (1992) In vivo transfer of the human cystic fibrosis transmembrane conductance regulator gene to the airway epithelium. Cell 68:143–155

35. Glorioso JC, DeLuca NA, Goins WF, Fink DJ (1994) Development of herpes simlpex virus vectors for gene transfer to the central nervous system. In: Wolff JA (ed) Gene therapeutics. Methods and applications of direct gene transfer. Birkhauser, Boston, pp 281–302

36. Kotin RM (1994) Prospects for the use of adeno-associated virus as a vector for human gene therapy. Hum Gene Ther 5:793–801

37. Singhal A, Huang L (1994) Gene transfer in mammalians cells using liposomes as carriers. In: Wolff JA (ed) Gene therapeutics. Methods and applications of direct gene transfer. Birkhauser, Boston, pp 118–142
38. Le Gal La Salle G, Robert JJ, Berrard S, et al (1993) An adenovirus vector for gene transfer into neurons and glia in the brain. Science 259:988–990
39. Ragot T, Vincent N, Chafiy P, et al (1993) Efficient adenovirus-mediated transfer of a human minidystrophin gene to skeletal muscle of mdx mice. Nature (Lond) 361:647–650
40. Morsy MA, Alford EL, Bett A, Graham FL, Caskey CC (1993) Efficient adenoviral-mediated ornithin transcarbamylase expression in deficient mouse and human hepatocytes. J Clin Invest 92:1580–1586
41. Van Beuningen HM, Van der Kraan PM, Arntz OJ, Van den Berg WB (1994) Transforming growth factor-$\beta 1$ stimulates articular chondrocyte proteoglycan synthesis and induces osteophyte formation in the murine knee joint. Lab Invest 71:279–290

C. New Cartilage Markers

The Recently Discovered Collagenase-3: A Key Role in Osteoarthritis

JOHANNE MARTEL PELLETIER[1] and JEAN-PIERRE PELLETIER[2]

Summary. Osteoarthritis (OA) is a progressive degenerative joint disease characterized by a gradual loss of cartilage, with synovitis as a secondary phenomenon. Although the etiology of OA remains to be determined, the progression of this disease can generally be divided into different stages in which proteolytic breakdown of the cartilage matrix occurs at an early point. Current knowledge indicates an important involvement of the metalloprotease (MMP) family in the catabolic process of this degenerative process. As the high tensile strength of the cartilage is for the most part provided by type II collagen, the breakdown of the collagen network must be a highly regulated event. The MMP members accounting for this macromolecular degradation are the collagenases. Three such enzymes are found in human articular cartilage: collagenase-1 (MMP-1), collagenase-2 (MMP-2), and the recently discovered collagenase-3 (MMP-13). In this chapter, we have summarized data from our laboratory which suggests that, in addition to collagenase-1, collagenase-3 is a key contributing factor in cartilage collagen degradation during the OA process. The different collagenases likely have distinct yet complementary roles.

Key Words. Collagenase-3, Osteoarthritis, Cartilage, Chondrocytes, Collagenase-1

Introduction

The dominant feature in osteoarthritis (OA) is a loss of cartilage. At the clinical stage of the disease, however, changes caused by OA involve not only the cartilage but also the synovial membrane, where an inflammatory reaction

[1]University of Montréal and Osteoarthritis Research Unit, Centre hospitalier de l'Université de Montéal, Campus Notre-Dame, 1560 Rue Sherbrooke, Montréal, Québec, H2L 4M1 Canada.
[2]Rheumatic Disease Unit, University of Montréal and Osteoarthritis Research Unit, Centre hospitalier de l'Université de Montéal, Campus Notre-Dame, 1560 Rue Sherbrooke, Montréal, Québec, H2L 4M1 Canada.

is often seen, and the subchondral bone, where significant bone remodeling occurs [1].

In the cartilage matrix, collagen is particularly important because its breakdown results in loss of the tissue's structural integrity. The high tensile strength provided by type II collagen in cartilage is a key factor in the biomechanical function of this tissue [2]. Because of this importance, as well as the poor inherent healing capacity of the tissue, the initial and specific cleavage of type II collagen must be a highly regulated event. A prominent hypothesis attributes such cartilage matrix breakdown to the proteolytic enzymes secreted by the chondrocytes.

Much attention is currently focused on determining the protease responsible for the initiation of matrix digestion. Current knowledge indicates an important involvement of the metalloproteases (MMP) [1,3–5]. The enzyme class responsible for collagen type II degradation in pathological tissue is the collagenase. It had been thought that the collagenase responsible for collagen breakdown was collagenase-1 (MMP-1). However, and despite the fact that the level of collagenolytic activity in cartilage increases with the severity of the disease, in situ production and synthesis of collagenase-1 is generally low [6,7], suggesting that other enzymes are responsible for collagen turnover. In the last few years other collagenases, or enzymes having collagenase activity, have been identified in human cartilage: the neutrophil collagenase, or collagenase-2 (MMP-8) [8], collagenase-3 (MMP-13) [9,10], and an enzyme of a different class of MMP, the membrane-bound MMP, named MT-MMP, in which the type 1 (MT1-MMP) shows collagenase activity [11]. However, their exact role in human OA is not yet clear [12].

Of note, it has recently been shown that collagenase-3 has a high level of homology with rat and mouse collagenase-1 (86%) and only 46% homology with human collagenase-1 [13]. Homology has also been found, but to a lesser extent, with stromelysin-1 (MMP-3), as well as neutrophil collagenase (MMP-8).

Studies from our laboratory have contributed significantly to the understanding of the role of collagenase-3 in the pathophysiology of OA. In this chapter, we summarize some of our findings suggesting that, in addition to collagenase-1, collagenase-3 is involved in the degradation of cartilage collagen matrix during the OA process and that these two enzymes possibly have different functions in this disease.

Collagenase-3 Promoter

We recently cloned and sequenced the 5'-flanking region of collagenase-3. Analysis of the sequence revealed the presence of consensus sequences as potential binding sites for several transcription factors: TATA and CCAAT-binding proteins, AP-1 and PEA-3, as well as three core motifs of hormone-response elements (HRE/) [14]. Comparison of the human collagenase-3 promoter sequence with that of rodent or human collagenase-1 showed, as for the open reading frame [13], a strong homology between human collagenase-3 promoter and mouse collagenase-1 but very little with the human collagenase-1 promoter [14–17]. These findings are represented by the vertical bars in Fig. 1.

```
-338  TTATTACCTG   AAAAACTCAG   AGTAGCTGTT   TTCCCTACAA   AAGGAAGACA   ACATTTTTGT   M   Coll-1
       |  | |        ||       ||    |  |||     |  |  |      || | |    | ||||||||
-349  ATTATTCGAA   GAAGCAAAAG   TAGATACGTT   CTTACAGAAG   GCAAAAAAAA   AAATTTTTGC   H   Coll-3
         ||           | |         ||          | | |         |       |  | ||||
-344  GCACTTTATG   ACCATCAGAA   CCAGCCTTTT   TCAAAAAGAC   CATGGAG--T   AC-TCTTTGA   H   Coll-1


-278  CCAGTGAAGT   GAAAAAT--A   CTAGCTG-CT   GCTTCTCCCC   ACTA-TATCC   ATGAAA-ATG   M   Coll-1
      ||||||||     ||||||  |    ||| ||  ||   ||||||  |||   || | |||||   || ||| |||
-289  TAAGTGAAGT   AAAAAATGTA   CTA-CTCTCT   GCTTCTTCCC   AC-AGTATCC   AT-AAATATG   H   Coll-3
       ||| |        || ||   |      ||||        |          | |          || |
-287  CCTGTGTATA   TAACAAG--A   ACCTTTCTC-   AAATAGGAAA   GAAATGAATT   GGAGAAAA--   H   Coll-1


-223  CTGAGGCTGT   TTATTTTGCC   AGATGAGTTT   TGATATTCCC   CCACTGAAAG   TAGAGATGC-   M   Coll-1
      ||||||| ||   |||||||||||   ||||| ||||   ||| | |||     ||||||     ||||||||
-232  CTGAGGCCGT   TTATTTTGCC   AGATGGGTTT   TGAGA--CCC   TG-CTGAAAC   AAGAGATGCT   H   Coll-3
        | ||       |||    |||    |||  | |      |    | |    ACA-CATCTT   || | |
-232  ---CCACTGT   TTA-CATGGC   AGA--GTGTG   TCTCCTTGC   ACA-CATCTT   GTTTGAAGTT   H   Coll-1


                               AML-1      AML-1
-164  CTTCATTT-T   CCATTTCCCT   CAGATTCTGC   CACAACCAC   ACTT---AGG   ---AAGAAAA   M   Coll-1
      || ||||| |    ||||||||    || ||||| |   |||||||||   ||  |||       |||||||
-175  CT-CATTTAT   --ATTTCCCT   CAAATTCTAC   CACAACCAC   ACTCGGGAGG   GAAAAGAAAA   H   Coll-3
       |||          |          ||| |  ||    | ||  |      ||||          |
-179  AATCATGACA   TTGC-AACAC · CAAGTGATTC   C-AAATAATC   TGCTAGGAG-   -----TCACC   H   Coll-1


                                            PEA-3
-111  AAAAAATA-CC   ATGTAAGCAT   GTTTACCTTC   GCCTCACTAG   GAAGTT-AAC   ACAC-ACCCC   M   Coll-1
       |   |  ||   |  ||||||||   |||||||||||   |  |||||   |||||  ||    ||  |  | ||
-118  AG---TCGCC   ACGTAAGCAT   GTTTACCTTC   AAGTGACTAG   GAAGTGGAA-   AC-CTATCC-   H   Coll-3
       |          |  ||          |  |   |      | ||||        || |     |
-127  ATTTCTAA-T   GATTGCCTAG   TCTATTCATA   GCTAATCAAG   AGGATGTTAT   AAA-------   H   Coll-1


            AP-1
-54   A-AAGTGGTG   ACTCATCACT   AT-CATG---   ----------   --------CT   ATAAAATAGA   M   Coll-1
      |  ||||| ||   ||||| || |    | ||| | ||                            |||||   |
-64   ATAAGTGATG   ACTCACCA-T   -TGCAGGC--   ----------   --------CT   ATAAAAGTAA   H   Coll-3
       |          || |  |||  |     | |||                        ||    ||| |   |
-75   ----GCA-TG   AGTCAG-ACA   CCTCTGGCTT   TCTGGAAGGG   CAAGGACTCT   ATATATACAG   H   Coll-1


-17   AGATGCTTGC   CCTGGGA                                                      M   Coll-1
      || |  |       || |
-26   AGGTAATCTC   TGCGGAAAGA   CAACAG                                          H   Coll-3
      |||| |  ||    |  ||
-21   AGGGAGCTTC   CTAGCTGGGA   T                                               H   Coll-1
```

FIG. 1. Sequence comparison and alignment of the proximal promoter regions of human collagenase-3 (*H Coll-3*) [14,15], mouse collagenase-1 (*M Coll-1*) [17], and human collagenase-1 (*H Coll-1*) [16] genes. The TATA box and consensus binding sites for the transcription factors AP-1, PEA-3, and AML-1 (family of proteins related to osteoblast-specific factor-2) are boxes. *Vertical lines* indicate conserved nucleotides between the sequences

Collagenase-3 mRNA Distribution in Human Tissue

Investigation by other authors [10] of the expression of collagenase-3, collagenase-1, and stromelysin-1 mRNA using the reverse transcription-DNA amplification (RT-PCR) method in various normal human tissues (i.e., heart, kidney, liver, lung, skeletal muscle, small intestine, spleen, testis, thymus, and articular chondrocytes) has revealed that collagenase-3 is expressed only in chondrocytes. Collagenase-1 has been identified in articular chondrocytes and the small intestine, and stromelysin-1 in brain, kidney, skeletal muscle, small intestine, testis, and articular chondrocytes.

Further experiments performed in our laboratory [9] using various samples of chondrocytes from primary culture, and synovial fibroblasts stimulated or not with interleukin-1β (IL-1β), have revealed that, although both collagenase-1 and stromelysin-1 are expressed by chondrocytes and synovial fibroblasts, collagenase-3 is expressed in chondrocytes but virtually not at all in synovial fibroblasts. Together, these data suggest that collagenase-3 is expressed very selectively in normal tissue but is present in human articular cartilage.

Collagenase-3 Expression and Synthesis in OA Chondrocytes

To document whether this new collagenase is involved in the pathophysiology of OA, we conducted further investigations [9]. Northern blot analysis using mRNA from human OA chondrocytes has revealed bands corresponding to 3.0 and 2.5 kb in all specimens examined, with some variation in amount among different individuals. For some specimens, a third band corresponding to 2.2 kb was also detected. A statistically significant increase in expression (mRNA) of the enzyme of the two major bands was found when OA values (3.0 kb, 0.66 $\pm$ 0.14; 2.5 kb, 0.76 $\pm$ 0.15) were compared to normal (3.0 kb, 0.26 $\pm$ 0.07; $P < .05$; 2.5 kb, 0.38 $\pm$ 0.08, $P < .03$).

Further data have demonstrated that not only the mRNA of collagenase-3 but also its synthesis are enhanced in OA [9]. Results from Western blot analysis have revealed that approximately 9.5 times more collagenase-3 protein is found in OA samples than in normal ones.

Digestion of Types I and II Collagen by Collagenase-3

Further investigations were carried out to examine the activity level of collagenase-3 on type I and II collagen [9]. Collagens were incubated with aminophenylmercuric acid (APMA)-activated collagenase-3 or collagenase-1 and the products examined by electrophoresis. Results showed that both collagenases cleave type I and type II collagen at a typical locus (Fig. 2). Degradation products were analyzed, and the collagen cleavage rate activity of

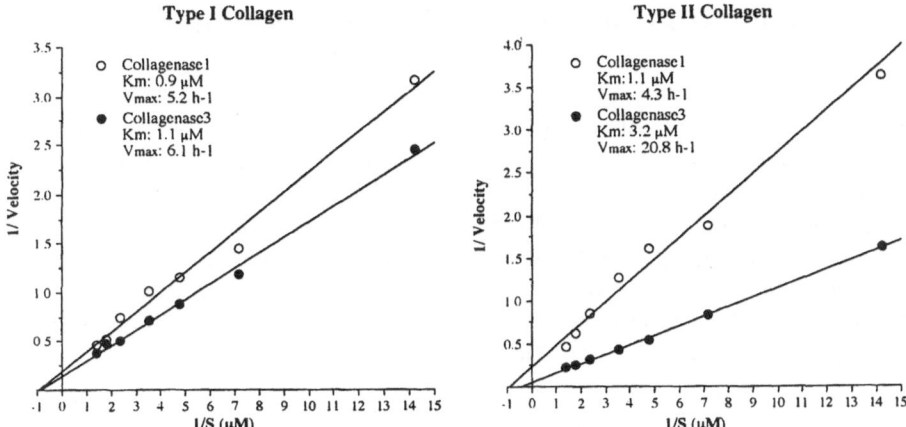

FIG. 2. Lineweaver–Burk plots of the cleavage rates of collagenase-1 and collagenase-3 on soluble type I and type II collagens. The collagens were incubated for 3 h at 25°C in the presence of aminophenylmercuric acid (APMA) (1.5 mM) -activated collagenase-1 or collagenase-3. The catalytic velocity (V_{max}) is expressed as the number of collagen molecules degraded per molecule of collagenase per hour and the K_m in molarity. Reproduced from results published in The Journal of Clinical Investigation, 1996, vol. 97, pp 2011–2019

both collagenases, as well as values for K_m and the catalytic velocity (V_{max}) were determined. Collagenase-3 degraded type II collagen more readily (by about fivefold) than collagenase-1; K_m, 3.2 μM vs. 1.1 μM; V_{max}, 20.8 h^{-1} vs. 4.3 h^{-1}. Collagenase-3 also cleaves the type I collagen (K_m, 1.1 μM; V_{max}, 6.1 h^{-1}); however, the cleavage rate is similar to that of collagenase-1 (K_m, 0.9 μM; V_{max}, 5.2 h^{-1}).

Stimulation of Collagenase-3 Production by Proinflammatory Cytokines

We also looked at whether collagenase-3 production can be modulated by the proinflammatory cytokines interleukin-1-beta (IL-1β) and tumour necrosis factor-alpha (TNF-α) [9]. Dose–response experiments revealed that both IL-1β and TNF-α (0–100 units/ml) exhibit a dose-dependent increase in the mRNA expression of collagenase-3. IL-1β stimulated simultaneously and proportionally the three collagenase-3 transcripts. Compared to IL-1β, TNF-α induction produced a lower level of collagenase-3 mRNA expression, and only the two higher collagenase-3 transcripts (3.0 and 2.5 kb) were detected.

We performed similar dose–response experiments for protein synthesis using Western blotting [9], and findings were consistent with the mRNA results in that the synthesis of collagenase-3 could be modulated by these cytokines, an effect that increased in a dose-dependent manner.

Topographical Localization of Collagenase-3 in OA Cartilage

To clarify the role of collagenase-3 in cartilage degradation, we thought that information regarding the in situ distribution of the enzyme in human articular cartilage under both normal and arthritic conditions would be extremely valuable. For this purpose, we employed immunohistochemical analysis utilizing a specific antibody against collagenase-3 [18]. In normal cartilage (Fig. 3A), the collagenase-3 level is very low, while in OA cartilage (Fig. 3B), there is a dramatic enhancement in the number of chondrocytes staining positive throughout the entire cartilage thickness.

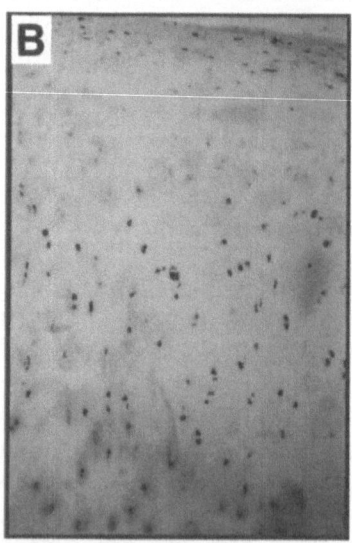

FIG. 3A,B. Representative sections of collagenase-3 immunostaining of human (**A**) normal articular cartilage and (**B**) osteoarthritic cartilage (original magnification, ×63)

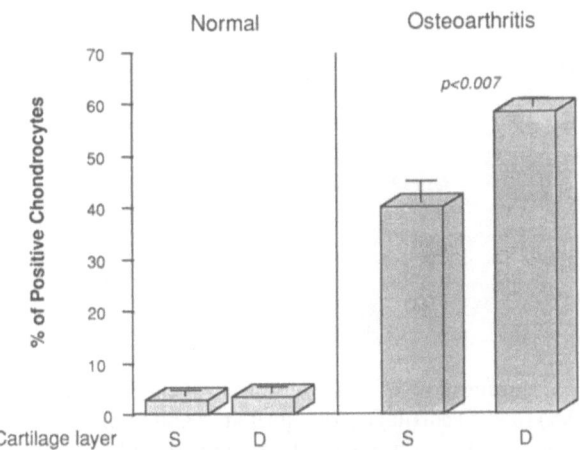

FIG. 4. Cell score of chondrocytes staining positive for collagenase-3 of human articular cartilage from normal ($n = 8$) or osteoarthritis ($n = 10$) patients. After processing for immunohistochemistry, the total number of chondrocytes and the total number of positive chondrocytes were counted separately at $\times 40$ magnification from each of the following two zones: the superficial and upper intermediate layers (S), and the lower intermediate and deep layers (D). Results were expressed as the percentage of positive chondrocytes. Student's t-test was used for comparison between the S and D layers. (Modified from [18], with permission)

In each specimen, the percentage of chondrocytes staining positive for collagenase-3 from each cartilage section was determined by morphometric analysis. Cartilage sections were divided into two zones: the superficial zone, which corresponds to the superficial and upper intermediate layers, and the deep zone, comprising the lower intermediate and deep layers. Results from normal cartilage showed no difference between these two cartilage zones (Fig. 4). However, in OA specimens, there was a statistically significant difference between the superficial and deep cartilage zones, with a greater percentage of chondrocytes staining positive in the deeper zones.

Experiments were also carried out to assess the amount of collagenase-3 in fibrillated and nonfibrillated cartilage from normal and OA tissue. For this experiment, proteins were extracted directly from each cartilage sample and processed for Western immunoblotting. Results confirmed the previous immunohistochemistry data of the secreted collagenase-3 (Fig. 5), where a higher amount of this enzyme was found in OA than in normal tissue. In this study, however, data also revealed no major differences in the amount of collagenase-3 when comparing the fibrillated and nonfibrillated areas of cartilage from both normal and OA specimens.

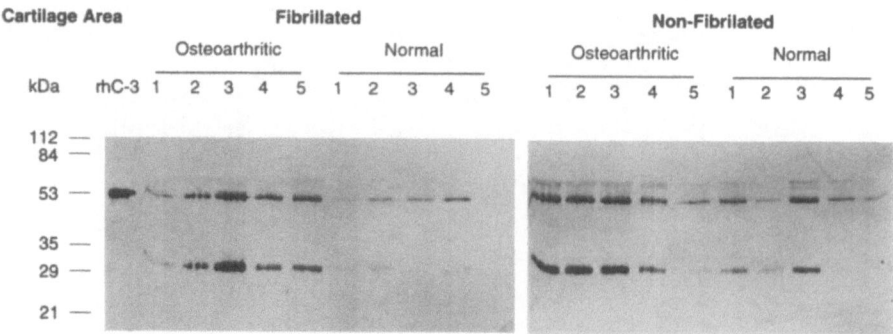

FIG. 5. Western immunoblot of collagenase-3 of human normal ($n = 5$) and osteoarthritis (OA) ($n = 5$) cartilage from fibrillated and nonfibrillated areas. No major difference was noted in the protein level between the fibrillated and nonfibrillated areas for either normal or OA cartilage. Of note is a smaller band that possibly represents a collagenase-3 degradation product

Correlations of Collagenase-3 and Collagenase-1 Versus Severity of Histological Lesions in OA Cartilage

To further investigate the correlation of collagenase-3 and collagenase-1 as regards the severity of histological lesions in cartilage of early OA, we studied the in situ distribution of these collagenases using the canine experimental model of OA [19]. The OA model is created on dogs by sectioning the anterior cruciate ligament of the right stifle joint with a stab wound, and lesions are generally well established by 12 weeks [20,21].

In this experiment, the dogs were killed at staggered intervals following surgery (4, 8, or 12 weeks) [19]. A fourth group of unoperated (normal) dogs was included in the study as control. Immunohistochemical analysis was performed as for human cartilage, using a specific antibody for either collagenase-3 or collagenase-1. The immunohistological cartilage pattern of collagenase-3 was consistent with that previously observed in human OA cartilage in which positive staining was observed throughout the cartilage, but predominantly in the lower intermediate and deep layers (Fig. 6). It is interesting to note that chondrocytes staining for collagenase-1 were detected mostly in the superficial and upper intermediate layers (Fig. 6).

Cell score comparison between the time of surgery and the development of histological lesions in the femoral condyles and tibial plateaus (Fig. 6A) indicated that, for collagenase-3, the elevation is consistently higher in chondrocytes from both superficial and deep layers, with a statistical difference found at 8 and 12 weeks in the deep layers compared to the superficial. This increase reached its zenith at 8 weeks. For collagenase-1 (Fig. 6B), cell score increased steadily up to the 12th week in the superficial layers. In the deep layers, no change was observed following the first histological modifications (i.e., at 4 weeks after surgery).

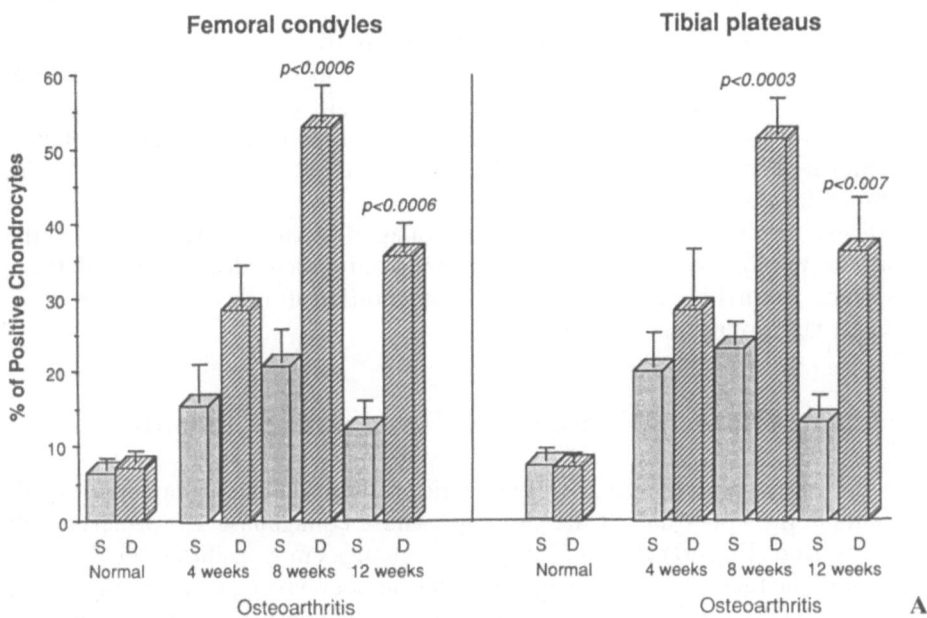

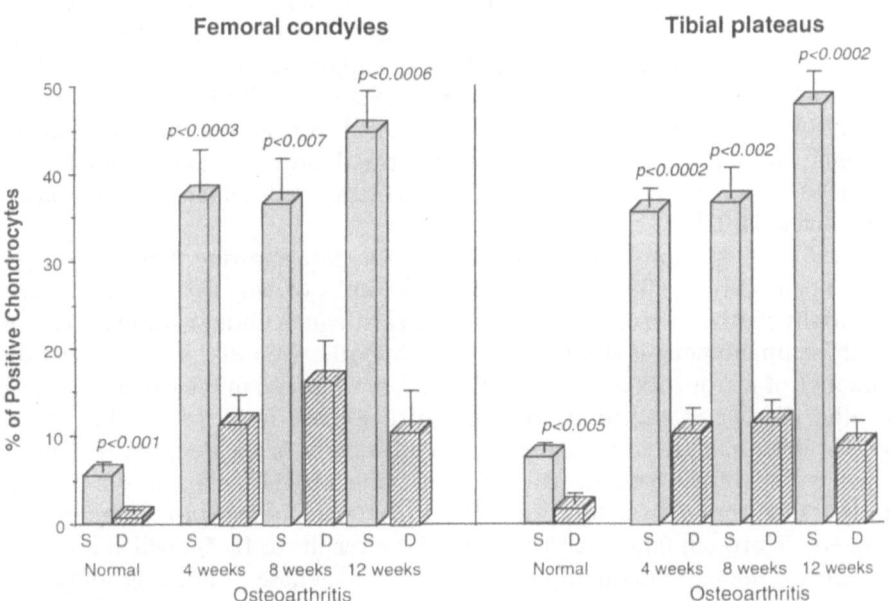

FIG. 6A,B. Cell score for chondrocytes staining positive for (**A**) collagenase-3 or (**B**) collagenase-1 of articular cartilage from normal ($n = 4$) or osteoarthritis dogs following the Pond–Nuki model at 4 ($n = 4$), 8 ($n = 4$), and 12 ($n = 4$) weeks post surgery. For further details, see legend of Fig. 4. (Modified from [19], with permission)

We further [19] correlated cell score with histological grading using the Mankin scale [22]. Results for both collagenase-1 and collagenase-3 showed a correlation of the second order for both superficial and deep layers, and a strong correlation for collagenase-3 was found in the deep layers (femoral condyles, $r = .65, P < .0004$; tibial plateaus, $r = .46, P < .004$]. In contrast, the strongest correlation for collagenase-1 was found in the superficial layers (femoral condyles, $r = .69, P < .0001$; tibial plateau, $r = .65, P < .0003$), with a much lower correlation in the deep layers.

These results suggest that both these collagenases are likely involved in the pathophysiology of OA. The different topographical distribution of these enzymes in cartilage suggests they may have different roles in the breakdown of cartilage collagen.

Factors That Can Upregulate Collagenase-3 Synthesis

In the early stage of OA, disorganization of the collagen network initially occurs in the upper half of the cartilage, where collagenase-1 is preferentially synthesized (Fig. 6B) [1,6,19,23,24]. These changes may facilitate the diffusion of catabolic factors from the superficial to the deep layers, which in turn could upregulate the synthesis of enzymes such as collagenase-3 in the deep layers of cartilage.

In a study performed on the OA experimental model [24], it was shown that the increase in collagenase-1 chondrocyte score in the superficial layers coincided with the presence of IL-1β in this pathological cartilage. Indeed, immunohistochemical analysis of dog OA cartilage stained with IL-1β revealed that this cytokine is found mostly in the superficial layers and in the matrix at the lesional areas [24]. This result also confirmed previous data from human cartilage where IL-1β was found in OA cartilage predominantly at the superficial layers [1,23].

These findings, however, do not explain the data showing that the collagenase-3 cell score reached a maximum at 8 weeks or why this enzyme is preferentially synthesized in the deep layers of cartilage. Although the exact reason for these phenomena is still unknown, we hypothesized that it may reflect the influence of factors other than IL-1 that are synthesized in the cartilage and/or in other tissues in the joint. We therefore looked for a factor that would specifically stimulate collagenase-3 in chondrocytes of the deep layers, and/or which would diffuse from the subchondral bone into the cartilage. We chose to study transforming growth factor-β (TGF-β), which belongs to the bone morphogenetic protein family, and compared the results to IL-1β, which is able to upregulate the expression and synthesis of collagenase-3. For this study [18], human cartilage was incubated in the presence or absence of IL-1β or TGF-β and processed for immunohistochemistry using the collagenase-3 antibody.

Data showed that both IL-1β and TGF-β increase the production of collagenase-3 in normal cartilage (Fig. 7). IL-1β stimulates chondrocytes in both the

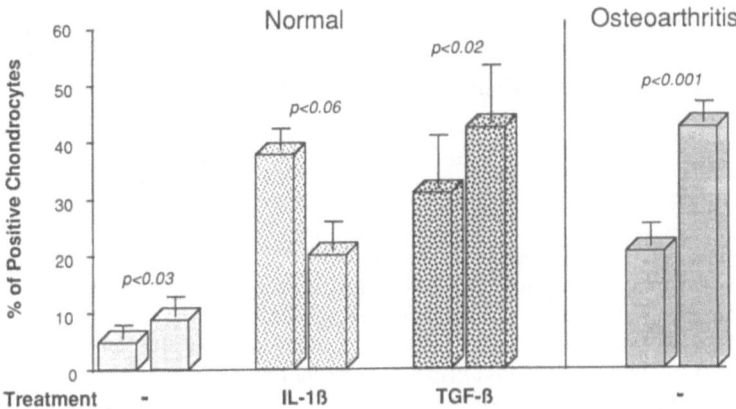

FIG. 7. Cell score of chondrocytes staining positive for collagenase-3 of human normal ($n = 5$) and osteoarthritis ($n = 7$) cartilage explants incubated for 72h at 37°C in the absence ($-$) or presence of IL-1β (100 units/ml) or transforming growth factor-beta (TGF-β) (150ng/ml) and processed for immunohistochemistry. For further details, see legend of Fig. 4. (Modified from [18], with permission)

superficial and deep zones, with a predominant increase observed in the superficial layers. Interestingly, TGF-β also stimulates collagenase-3 production, but to a greater extent on chondrocytes from the deeper layers, therefore mimicking the in vivo pattern observed in OA cartilage (Figs. 5 and 7).

The results of this study indicate that TGF-β may be an alternative or complementary factor to the action of IL-1β in upregulating collagenase-3 synthesis in OA cartilage.

Conclusion

In summary, our data present several lines of evidence supporting the involvement of collagenase-3 in the pathophysiology of OA. The greater correlation coefficient found for collagenase-3 compared to collagenase-1 in the deep layers of cartilage, combined with the high capacity of collagenase-3 to cleave type II collagen, makes this enzyme an excellent candidate for involvement in the degradation of the collagen network in cartilage and is likely responsible for the progression of lesions in this disease.

The different localization of collagenase-1 and collagenase-3 in pathological cartilage may indicate a different function allocated to these collagenases in the diseased tissue. Because collagenase-3 is not found in most normal tissue, but is present in cartilage and involved in OA pathophysiology, and as collagenase-1 is found in all articular tissues, future therapeutic treatment of this disease may well incorporate the use of compounds that specifically inhibit collagenase-3.

Acknowledgments. The authors thank the researchers, research assistants, students, and secretarial staff of the laboratories of Drs. Johanne Martel-Pelletier and Jean-Pierre Pelletier for their invaluable contribution to these studies on collagenase-3.

References

1. Pelletier JP, Martel-Pelletier J, Howell DS (1997) Etiopathogenesis of osteoarthritis. In: Koopman WJ (ed) Arthritis and allied conditions. A textbook of rheumatology, 13th edn. Williams & Wilkins, Baltimore, pp 1969–1984
2. Pelletier JP, Martel-Pelletier J (1993) Articular cartilage. In: Schumacher HR Jr, Klippel J, Koopman WJ (eds) Primer on the rheumatic diseases, 10th edn. Arthritis Foundation, Atlanta, pp 8–11
3. Dean DD, Martel-Pelletier J, Pelletier JP, et al (1989) Evidence for metalloproteinase and metalloproteinase inhibitor imbalance in human osteoarthritic cartilage. J Clin Invest 84:678–685
4. Martel-Pelletier J, McCollum R, Fujimoto N, et al (1994) Excess of metalloproteases over tissue inhibitor of metalloprotease may contribute to cartilage degradation in osteoarthritis and rheumatoid arthritis. Lab Invest 70:807–815
5. Pelletier JP, Martel-Pelletier J, Howell DS, et al (1983) Collagenase and collagenolytic activity in human osteoarthritic artilage. Arthritis Rheum 26:63–68
6. Nguyen Q, Mort JS, Roughley PJ (1992) Preferential mRNA expression of prostromelysin relative to procollagenase and in situ localization in human articular cartilage. J Clin Invest 89:1189–1197
7. Mort JS, Dodge GR, Roughley RJ, et al (1993) Direct evidence for active metalloproteinases mediating matrix degradation in interleukin 1-stimulated human articular cartilage. Matrix 13:95–102
8. Cole AA, Chubinskaya S, Schumacher BL, et al (1996) Chondrocyte matrix metalloproteinase-8. Human articular chondroctyes express neutrophil collagenase. J Biol Chem 271:11023–11026
9. Reboul P, Pelletier JP, Tardif G, et al (1996) The new collagenase, collagenase-3, is expressed and synthesized by human chondrocytes but not by synoviocytes: a role in osteoarthritis. J Clin Invest 97:2011–2019
10. Mitchell PG, Magna HA, Reeves LM, et al (1996) Cloning, expression, and type II collagenolytic activity of matrix metalloproteinase-13 from human osteoarthritic cartilage. J Clin Invest 97:761–768
11. Ohuchi E, Imai K, Fujii Y, et al (1997) Membrane type 1 matrix metalloproteinase digests interstitial collagens and other extracellular matrix macromolecules. J Biol Chem 272:2446–2451
12. Martel-Pelletier J, Pelletier JP (1996) Wanted—the collagenase responsible for the destruction of the collagen network in human cartilage. Br J Rheumatol 35:818–820
13. Freije JM, Diez-Itza I, Balbin M, et al (1994) Molecular cloning and expression of collagenase-3, a novel human matrix metalloproteinase produced by breast carcinomas. J Biol Chem 269:16766–16773

14. Tardif G, Pelletier JP, Dupuis M, et al (1997) Cloning, sequencing and characterization of the 5'-flanking region of the human collagenase-3 gene. Biochem J 323:13–16
15. Pendas AM, Balbin M, Llano E, et al (1997) Structural analysis and promoter characterization of the human collagenase-3 gene (MMP-13). Genomics 40:222–233
16. Angel P, Baumann I, Stein B, et al (1987) 12-O-Tetradecanoly-phorbol-13-acetate induction of the human collagenase gene is mediated by an inducible enhancer element located in the 5'-flanking region. Mol Cell Biol 7:2256–2266
17. Schorpp M, Mattei M-G, Herr I, et al (1995) Structural organization and chromosomal localization of the mouse collagenase type I gene. Biochem J 308:211–217
18. Moldovan F, Pelletier J, Hambor J, et al (1997) Collagenase-3 (MMP-13) is preferentially localized *in situ* in the deeper layer of human arthritic cartilage. *In vitro* mimicking effect by TGF-β. Arthritis Rheum 40:1653–1661
19. Fernandes JC, Martel-Pelletier J, Lascau-Coman V, et al (1998) Collagenase-1 and collagenase-3 synthesis in early experimental osteoarthritic canine cartilage. An immunohistochemical study. J Rheumatol 8:1585–1594
20. Adams ME, Pelletier JP (1990) Canine anterior cruciate ligament transection model of osteoarthritis. In: Greenwald RA, Diamond HS (eds) Animal models for the rheumatic diseases, vol 2. CRC Press, Boca Raton, pp 57–81
21. Pelletier JP, Di Battista JA, Raynauld JP, et al (1995) The *in vivo* effects of intraarticular corticosteroid injections on cartilage lesions, stromelysin, interleukin-1 and oncogene protein synthesis in experimental osteoarthritis. Lab Invest 72:578–586
22. Mankin HJ, Dorfman H, Lippiello L, et al (1971) Biochemical and metabolic abnormalities in articular cartilage from osteoarthritic human hips. II. Correlation of morphology with biochemical and metabolic data. J Bone Joint Surg [Am] 53:523–537
23. Pelletier JP, Martel-Pelletier J (1989) Evidence for the involvement of interleukin 1 in human osteoarthritic cartilage degradation: protective effect of NSAID. J Rheumatol 16:19–27
24. Pelletier JP, Faure MP, Di Battista JA, et al (1993) Coordinate synthesis of stromelysin, interleukin-1, and oncogene proteins in experimental osteoartrits. An immunohistochemical study. Am J Pathol 142:95–105

Calpain and Its Role in Arthritis

KATSUJI SHIMIZU

Summary. Calpain, originally considered to be an intracellular proteinase, was demonstrated to be present extracellularly in various biological events including enchondral bone formation and arthritides. The proteoglycan-degrading proteolytic activities of calpain were demonstrated in vitro and in osteoarthritic synovial fluid. These data plus some recent reports of other investigators suggest that the calpain-calpastatin system may play an important role in the metabolism of the extracellular matrix and especially in cartilage degradation in arthritides, although the pathways of externalization of these intracellular proteinase remain unclarified. In this chapter, the roles of calpain in matrix degradation and in arthritides are reviewed.

Key Words. Calpain, Matrix proteinase, Arthritis, Proteoglycan, Degradation

Introduction

Calpain, also called calcium-activated neutral proteinase (CANP), is a Ca^{2+}-dependent neutral cystein proteinase that is widely distributed among animal species. Two forms of calpain are now known to exist, and they differ in their Ca^{2+} requirements for activation: μ-calpain, or calpain I, requires low concentrations (micromolar), and m-calpain, or calpain II, requires high concentrations (millimolar). A natural specific inhibitor of calpain, which is called calpastatin, is also present (Table 1). Calpain, originally considered to be an intracellular proteinase, was recently demonstrated to be present extracellularly in the hypertrophic zone of the growth cartilage of the rat [1], in fracture healing of the rat [2], and in rat growth plate chondrocyte cultures [3]. Consequently, calpain was also demonstrated in synovial fluids of osteoarthritic

Department of Orthopaedic Surgery, Gifu University School of Medicine, 40 Tsukasamachi, Gifu 500-8705, Japan.

TABLE 1. Calpain and calpastatin

Protease (80 kDa + 30 kDa)		Inhibitor (14 kDa)n
μ-Calpain (calpain I)	m-Calpain (calpain II)	Calpastatin
Low Ca^{2+} requirement ($\sim 2\mu M$)	High Ca^{2+} requirement ($\sim 200\mu M$)	Not Ca^{2+} binding

TABLE 2. Evidence of calpain as a matrix proteinase

Enchondral bone formation	
Growth cartilage (rat)	[1]
Growth cartilage chondrocyte culture (rat)	[3]
Experimental fracture callus (rat)	[2]
Arthritis	
Synovial fluids of osteoarthritis (human)	[4,7]
Synovial fluids of rheumatoid arthritis (human)	[7,14]
Synovial cell culture (human)	[7,15]
Collagen-induced arthritis (mouse)	[8.9]
Substrate	
Cartilage proteoglycan (aggrecan)	[4,5]

patients with extracellular proteolytic activity on proteoglycan (aggrecan) [4]. Calpains degrade proteoglycan aggregate as well as monomers very rapidly in vitro [5,6] and are considered to degrade the matrix proteoglycan of cartilage in osteoarthritis, in rheumatoid arthritis [7], and in murine collagen-induced arthritis (CIA) [8,9]. Thus, calpain may have pivotal roles in cartilage degradation of arthritides (Table 2). In this chapter, the general concept of calpain as a matrix proteinase is illustrated by highlighting several important topics on its roles in arthritides.

Calpain

The occurrence of Ca^{2+}-dependent neutral protease in rat brain was first described by Guroff in the National Institutes of Health, (United States), as early as 1964 [10]. Meyer and others at Seattle, WA, then also described a kinase-activating factor in skeletal muscle [11], which later turned out to be a Ca^{2+} protease [12]. In the 1970s, a large number of studies were done on this protease in various tissues and cells and their important roles in intracellular proteolysis discussed. In 1981, these proteinases were named calpain by Murachi on the basis of the implication that *cal* stands for calcium, while the ending *-pain* conforms to thiol proteinases including papain [13].

Calpain in Growth Cartilage of Rats

We began the study of calpain in growth cartilage of rats as it may be related to the calcification process, because its activity is highly dependent on calcium ions. In the calcifying zone of growth cartilage, several matrix proteinases such as collagenase and stromelysin are known to exist, and they are thought to degrade cartilage matrix and facilitate conversion of cartilage to bone. Immunohistochemical staining of growth cartilage of rats revealed a positive staining of m-calpain in hypertrophic chondrocytes and no staining in the chondrocytes of the resting zone.

Higher magnification of the immunohistochemistry showed an intracellular staining of hypertrophic chondrocytes, but at the same time, a vague staining of calpain in the cartilage matrix could be seen in spite of deep staining with methyl green. We then repeated the same immunohistochemistry, but with a very light counterstaining with methyl green (Fig. 1). In this picture an intracellular proteinase, calpain, was first demonstrated in the extracellular matrix. Subsequently, calpain was demonstrated in an experimental fracture callus in rats [2] and pelleted growth chondrocyte culture from rat epiphyseal cartilage [3], and is thought to be functioning as a matrix proteinase promoting enchondral bone formation through proteoglycan degradation.

Proteoglycan-Degrading Activity of Calpain

We then studied the ability of calpain to degrade cartilage proteoglycan (aggrecan), as it was the most important substrate in the growth cartilage as well as type II collagen. m-Calpain was extracted from the kidney of swine, and proteoglycan monomer (A1 D1 fraction), proteoglycan aggregate (A1 fraction), and link protein were prepared from the articular cartilage of swine as substrates. These substrates were examined for changes in molecular size with the combined use of Sepharose-2B gel filtration chromatography, sucrose density gradient ultracentrifugation, and agarose polyacrylamide gel electrophoresis after incubation with m-calpain.

The findings are summarized as follows. (1) Decrease of molecular size was observed in proteoglycan monomers, proteoglycan aggregates, and link proteins at neutral pH and calcium dependently with a trace amount of the enzyme. (2) An inhibitory study confirmed that the above-mentioned effects were produced by calpain. (3) Besides such decrease of molecular size of proteoglycan monomers, effects were observed on the molecular functions of preteoglycan, including loss of the ability to reaggregate with hyaluronic acid [4,5].

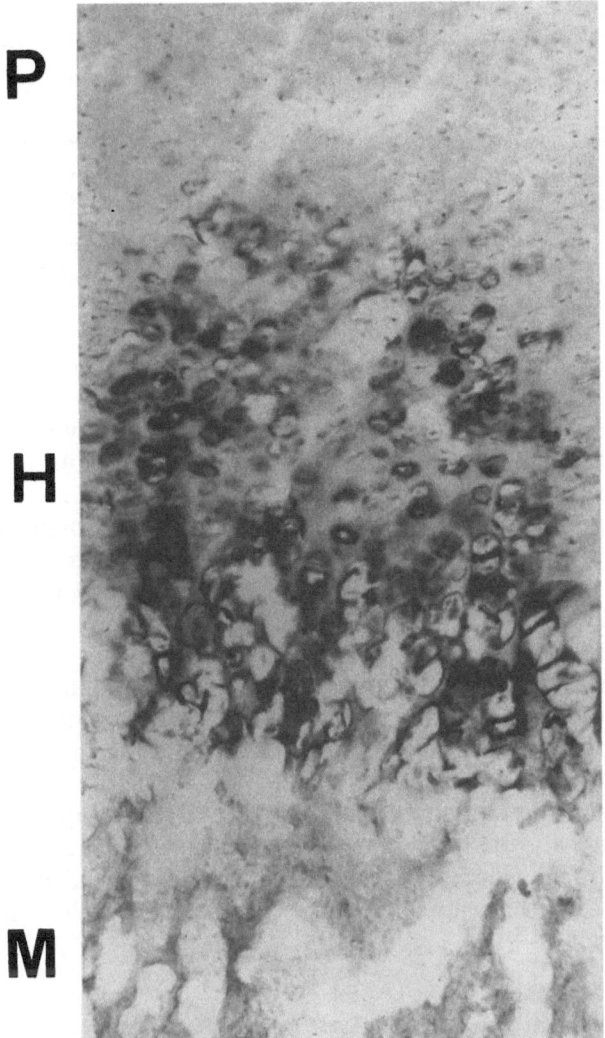

FIG. 1. Extracellular presence of calpain in hypertrophic zone (*H*) of growth cartilage. Immunohistochemical staining with DAB (diaminobenzide stain) of growth cartilage of the proximal tibia from day 3 newborn Wistar rat. *P*, proliferative zone; *M*, metaphysis. ×100

Calpain and Calpastatin of Synovial Fluids of Osteoarthritis

Once calpain was found to have a strong effect on degradation of cartilage proteoglycan, our interest focused on whether calpain and calpastatin are present in synovial fluids. If calpain activity can be demonstrated in synovial fluids, (1) the matrix of articular cartilage, which consists mostly of proteoglycan, would come in contact with calpain, thus possibly causing calpain to take part in degradation of articular cartilage, and (2) an extracellular presence of calpain would be proved.

Synovial fluid of osteoarthritis (OA) was selected for the material to start with in proving the extracellular presence of calpain in synovial fluid, because the synovial fluid obtained from subjects with rheumatoid arthritis, which is rich in cellularity, may well be contaminated by cellular fragments and would not be proper for this purpose. The cellularity of the synovial fluid of osteoarthritis is known to be very low. We nevertheless examined the activity of the synovial fluid, which had been further processed by filtration so as to prevent contamination by calpain and calpastatin from cellular component.

By passing a linear gradient of sodium chloride through the synovial fluids absorbed to DEAE-cellulose, peaks of caseinolytic activity were observed at 150 and 300 mM. The inhibitor study and immunoblotting using monospecific antiserum proved these peak fractions to be μ-calpain and m-calpain, respectively. With the use of peak fractions of μ-calpain and m-calpain obtained from the synovial fluids by DEAE-cellulose chromatography, cartilage proteoglycan-degrading activity was assayed: this activity was proved to be subjected to nearly 100% inhibition by E64 (a cysteine proteinase inhibitor) and calpastatin (a specific inhibitor of calpain).

Calpastatin was observed as a heat-stable calpain inhibitor at a 120-mM sodium chloride concentration of DEAE-cellulose chromatography of synovial fluids, and was identified by immunoblotting using anticalpain antibody. Quantitative assay on synovial fluid samples used in the current study could be carried out, and the quantity of inhibitor activity was superior to the total quantity of activity of the two calpains; therefore, in the total activity of synovial fluids, the inhibitor was dominant. Calpain and calpastatin were found to be present in synovial fluids of osteoarthritis while remaining active extracellularly.

Calpain in Rheumatoid Arthritis

A study published by Fukui et al. [14] found calpain and calpastatin to be present in synovial fluids of rheumatoid arthritis. Subsequently, synovial tissues from rheumatoid arthritis (RA) and osteoarthritis (OA) were stained immunohistochemically using anticalpain antibody. Calpain immunoreactivity was demonstrated in synovial lining cells, endothelial cells, and interstitial fibroblasts. Immunoblotting of synovial tissues, synovial fluid, cultured synovial fibroblast, and culture medium showed a specific band of calpain.

Calpain activity was assayed in synovial fluids of RA and OA, and the results showed both the degrading activity of calpain and the inhibitory activity of calpastatin; total degrading activity was higher than inhibitory activity

[7]. Because the balance of the calpain/calpastatin system is inclined toward degradation or inhibition at the cartilage in osteoarthritis and rheumatoid arthritis, the matrix of articular cartilage consisting mostly of proteoglycan would be in contact with the proteoglycan-degrading, activity-possessing calpain. Therefore, it is highly possible that calpain is involved in degeneration of articular cartilage in such diseases.

In synovial cell culture from rheumatoid arthritis, calpain was secreted by synovial fibroblasts (synovial B cells) and not by synovial macrophages (synovial A cells) [15]. An autoantibody that reacts with calpastatin has been identified in systemic rheumatic diseases including rheumatoid arthritis [16]. The presence of anticalpastatin antibodies in patients may increase the enzymatic activity of calpain that mediates cartilage degradation or inflammation and may participate in the pathogenic mechanisms of arthritis.

Calpain in Collagen-Induced Arthritis of Mice

Type II collagen-induced arthritis (CIA) in mice is an experimental model for inflammatory arthritis, and provides reproducible in vivo conditions similar to those in human rheumatoid arthritis. m-Calpain was detected in murine CIA [8]. The appearance of calpain in CIA correlated with both a histological grade of arthritis and an acute phase of cartilage destruction. Further development of the disease showed continual presence of m-calpain but with reduced intensity. Intraarticular inflammatory cells (mainly polymorphonuclear leucocytes, synovial lining cells, and sublining fibroblasts) were found to be the most positively stained, but extracellular localization of m-calpain on the surface of cartilage and synovium and in the articular cartilage matrix and chondrocyte lacunae was also observed. In knee joint lavage obtained at the most intensive stage of acute arthritis, m-calpain was detected by immunoelectrophoretic blotting [9]. These findings suggest that m-calpain may act at an early phase of CIA as a matrix proteinase and may take part in the destruction of articular cartilage or activate other destructive enzymes.

So far, two types of matrix proteinases are known: proteinases that are secreted outside the cell through the Golgi body, such as collagenase, and lysosomal enzymes (a typical example is cathepsin D). These proteinases, secreted from the inside to the outside of the cell, are known in general to have signal peptides that determine the transportation pathway between intracellular compartments. Calpain is not a lysosomal enzyme, and signal peptide is not contained either in calpain or in calpastatin [17–22]. Also known is the presence of proteins such as interleukin 1, which has no signal peptide, yet exerts its effects after moving outside the cell [23]. The pathway that interleukin 1 takes to come out of the cell without the help of a signal peptide remains unsolved. Yet it is believed that during its movement from the cell, the molecular size of interleukin 1 simultaneously decreases [23]. It is unknown whether calpain and interleukin 1 share a common mechanism of secretion.

Calpains have been generally known as intracellular proteinases, and catalyze selective but limited proteolytic modification of proteins. Findings from the current study suggest that calpain occurs with extracellular activity and has an extracellular role of proteoglycan-degrading activity. Some previous studies have demonstrated extracellular localization of calpain in the skeletal muscle after sciatic denervation or starvation of rats using immunogold electron microscopy [24]. Although the pathway which calpain takes to move out of the cell is not yet known, it would be encouraging to carry out further studies on calpain because of its provision of such properties of matrix proteinase that it possesses enzyme activity outside the cell and can degrade matrix proteoglycan.

References

1. Shimizu K, Hamamoto T, Hamakubo T, et al (1991) Immunohistochemical and biochemical demonstration of calcium-dependent cystein proteinase (calpain) in calcifying cartilage of rats. J Orthop Res 9:26–36
2. Nakagawa Y, Shimizu K, Hamamoto T, et al (1994) Calcium-dependent neutral proteinase (calpain) in fracture healing of rats. J Orthop Res 12:58–69
3. Yasuda T, Shimizu K, Nakagawa Y, et al (1995) m-Calpain in rat growth plate chondrocyte cultures: its involvement in the matrix mineralization process. Dev Biol 170:159–168
4. Suzuki K, Shimizu K, Hamamoto T, et al (1990) Biochemical demonstration of calpains and calpastatin in osteoarthritic synovial fluid. Arthritis Rheum 33:728–732
5. Suzuki K, Shimizu K, Hamamoto T, et al (1992) Characterization of proteoglycan degradation by calpain. Biochem J 285:857–862
6. Suzuki K, Shimizu K, Sandy JD (1994) Aggrecan degradation by calpain. In: Abstracts, 40th annual meeting, Orthopaedic Research Society, February 21–24, New Orleans, LA, USA
7. Yamamoto S, Shimizu K, Shimizu K, et al (1992) Calcium-dependent cysteine proteinase (calpain) in human arthritic synovial joints. Arthritis Rheum 35:1309–1317
8. Fujimori Y, Shimizu K, Suzuki K, et al (1994) Immunohistochemical demonstration of calcium-dependent cysteine proteinase (calpain) in collagen-induced arthritis in mice. Z Rheumatol 53:72–75
9. Szomor Z, Shimizu K, Fujimori Y, et al (1995) Appearance of calpain correlates with arthritis and cartilage destruction in collagen-induced arthritic knee joints of mice. Ann Rheum Dis 54:477–483
10. Guroff G (1964) A neutral, calcium-activated proteinase from the soluble fraction of rat brain. J Biol Chem 239:149–155
11. Meyer WL, Fisher EH, Krebs EG (1964) Activation of skeletal muscle phosphorylase b kinase by Ca^{2+}. Biochemistry 3:1033–1039
12. Huston RB, Krebs EG (1968) Activation of skeletal muscle phosphorylase kinase by Ca^{2+}. II. Identification of the kinase activating factor as a proteolytic enzyme. Biochemistry 7:2116–2122

13. Murachi T (1983) Calpain and calpastatin. Trends Biochem Sci 8:167–169
14. Fukui I, Tanaka K, Murachi T (1989) Extracellular appearance of calpain and calpastatin in the synovial fluid of the knee joint. Biochem Biophys Res Commun 162:559–566
15. Yamamoto S, Shimizu K, Niibayashi H, et al (1994) Immunocytochemical demonstration of calpain in synovial cells in human arthritic synovial joints. Biomed Res 15:77–88
16. Mimori T, Suganuma K, Tanami Y, et al (1995) Autoantibodies to calpastatin (an endogenous inhibitor for calcium-dependent neutral protease, calpain) in systemic rheumatic diseases. Proc Natl Acad Sci USA 92:7267–7271
17. Suzuki K, Ohno S, Imajoh S, et al (1985) Identification and distribution of mRNA for calcium-activated neutral protease (CANP). Biochem Res 6:323–327
18. Sakihama T, Kakidani H, Zenita K, et al (1985) A putative Ca-binding protein: structure of the light subunit of porcine calpain elucidated by molecular cloning and protein sequence analysis. Proc Natl Acad Sci USA 82:6075–6079
19. Suzuki K, Hayashi H, Hayashi T, et al (1983) Amino acid sequence around the active site cysteine residue of calcium-activated neutral protease (CANP). FEBS Lett 152:67–70
20. Emori Y, Kawasaki H, Sugihara H, et al (1986) Isolation and sequence analyses of cDNA clones for the large subunits of two isozymes of rabbit calcium-dependent protease. J Biol Chem 261:9465–9471
21. Emori Y, Kawasaki H, Sugihara H, et al (1986) Isolation and sequence analysis of cDNA clones for the small subunit of rabbit calcium-dependent protease. J Biol Chem 261:9472–9476
22. Ohno S, Emori Y, Imajoh S, et al (1984) Evolutionary origin of a calcium-dependent protease by fusion of genes for a thiol protease and a calcium-binding protein? Nature (Lond) 312:566–570
23. Oppenheim JJ, Kovacs EJ, Matsushima K (1986) There is more than one interleukin 1. Immunol Today 7:45–56
24. Kumamoto T, Kleese WC, Cong JY, et al (1987) Localization in electron micrographs of the Ca^{2+}-dependent proteinases and their inhibitor in normal, starved, and denervated rat skeletal muscle. J Cell Biol 105:280

Immunohistochemical Localization of Cartilage-Specific and Non-Cartilage-Specific Proteoglycans in Experimental Osteoarthritic Articular Cartilage in Rats

Hiroshi Satsuma, Chiaki Hamanishi, Makoto Hashima, and Seisuke Tanaka

Summary. To demonstrate the localization of cartilage-specific or abnormal proteoglycans in normal and osteoarthritic joints, chondroitin-4-sulfate, keratan sulfate, and dermatan sulfate were examined immunohistochemically using monoclonal antibodies in control and mechanically induced osteoarthritic rat knee joints. Chondroitin-4-sulfate (CS-4) was observed both pericellularly and intracellularly, and keratan sulfate (KS) was observed mainly pericellularly, in normal cartilage. In early osteoarthritic joints, these immunohistochemical reactions were enhanced. In contrast, dermatan sulfate (DS) was not observed in control cartilage but appeared only in osteoarthritic knees intracellularly and extracellularly. Increased production of cartilage-specific proteoglycans is suspected to be a protective reaction of mechanically stressed chondrocytes, although it was not clear whether production of abnormal small proteoglycan DS represented a chondroprotective reaction or initiated destructive changes of the articular cartilage.

Key Words. Osteoarthritis, Experimental osteoarthritis, Chondroitin sulfate, Keratan sulfate, Dermatan sulfate, Immunohistochemistry

Introduction

Osteoarthritis is a chronic, degenerative, and proliferative joint disease, and several biochemical or biomechanical causative factors have been reported [1–5]. Several metabolic changes of the chondrocytes in relation to proteoglycan (PG) synthesis [6–9] have also been demonstrated, mainly biochemically, and chondrocytes have been thought to be activated and to produce increased amounts of primitive PGs [10,11]. Immunohistochemical observations of altered cartilage, however, have not been carried out using

Department of Orthopaedic Surgery, Kinki University School of Medicine, 377-2 Ohno-Higashi, Osaka-Sayama, Osaka 589-8511, Japan

142

reproducible experimental osteoarthritis models and monoclonal antibodies. In this study, we introduced experimental osteoarthritis in rat knee joints and observed the localization of cartilage-specific or abnormal PGs immunohistochemically.

Materials and Methods

Preparation of Osteoarthritis in Rat Model

The right knees of 15 male Wistar rats weighing 150–200 g were opened under anesthesia induced by intraperitoneal injection of pentobarbital (40 mg/kg). Under a surgical microscope, the anterior and posterior cruciate ligaments and the medial collateral ligament were dissected out. Skin incision and capsulotomy were performed on the left knee as a sham-operated control. The rats were fed and kept in their cages under standard conditions.

Preparation of Tissue Sections

At 2, 4, and 6 weeks after the operation, five rats at each timepoint were anesthetized and perfused through the left ventricle with 30 ml of 0.9% NaCl, followed by 200 ml of the fixative containing 4% paraformaldehyde and 0.2% picric acid in 0.1 M phosphate buffer at a flow rate of 120 ml/min. Both knee joints were dissected out. Twenty articular cartilage blocks were trimmed out together with the thin subchondral bone layer from the lateral and medial femoral condyles in each rabbit, immersed for 2 days in a fixative containing 4% paraformaldehyde and 0.2% picric acid, and washed for 1 day with 30% sucrose in 0.1 M phosphate buffer, decalcified with 5% EDTA solution for 1 week, and kept in 30% sucrose in 0.1 M phosphate buffer. The 20 chondroosseous blocks from each rat were then frozen and sectioned consecutively frontally at a thickness of 10–15 μm using a cryostat.

Immunohistochemical Staining

The consecutive sections were preincubated in chondroitinase avidin-biotm-peroxidase complex (ABC) solution (Seikagaku-Kogyo, Osaka, Japan) for 1 h at 37°C, and 0.3% H_2O_2 and 5% normal rabbit serum in phosphate-buffered salme (PBS) containing 0.03% Triton X-100 (PBS-T) for 20 min to block the endogenous peroxidase activity and nonspecific antibody-binding sites. The consecutive sections were subsequently incubated with primary monoclonal antibodies to chondroitin 4-sulfate (2-B-6), keratan sulfate (5-D-4), and dermatan sulfate (6-B-6) (Seikagaku-Kogyo, Osaka, Japan) at appropriate concentrations in PBS-T containing 5% normal rabbit serum for 18 h at 4°C. After washing with PBS-T, the sections were incubated for an additional 4 h with rabbit antimouse IgG, then for 1.5 h with mouse peroxidase-antiperoxidase (PAP) complex (Zymed, San Francisco, CA, USA). After three rinses, the preparations were developed with 0.02% 3,3'-diaminobenzidine (Sigma), 0.2% nickel ammonium sulfate, and 0.005% H_2O_2 in 50mM Tris-HCL buffer (pH 7.4). The sections were stained also with hematoxylin-eosin, or with safranine-O, then observed and photographed under a Zeiss light microscope.

Results

HE and Safranine-O Staining

Sham-Operated Control Joints

The articular cartilage had a smooth surface, and normal tangential, transitional, and radial layers of chondrocytes. Normal safranine-O staining was observed in the pericellular and extracellular matrix.

Osteoarthritic Joints

At 2 weeks after operation, fibrillation and hypocellularity in the tangential layer and clonal expansion of the chondrocytes in the transitional layer were observed. The columnar appearance in the radial layer seemed to be intact. The matrices were less stained with safranine-O than were the controls. At 6 weeks after operation, the tangential and half of the transitional layers were worn away, and marked clonal expansion or cluster formation of the chondrocytes was observed in the residual transitional and radial layers. The columnar appearance of the radial layer had almost entirely disappeared. The tidemark was partially doubled, and the width of the calcified cartilage layer was decreased. Vascular buds traversed the tidemark in some portions.

Immunohistological Findings

Chondroitin-4-Sulfate

Sham-Operated Control Joints (Fig. 1a)

Immunoreactivity was strongly observed in the cytosol of the chondrocytes in the tangential layer. No immunoreactivity was observed in the calcified layer.

Osteoarthritic Cartilage

At 2 weeks after operation (Fig. 1b), strong immunoreactivity was observed in the superficial layer and, in the cytosol and matrices in the tangential and transitional layers. Chondrocytes were immunoreactive in the calcified layer. At 6 weeks after operation (Fig. 1c), immunoreactivity was observed in the cytosol and matrix in the residual layers. Chondrocytes were immunoreactive in the calcified layer.

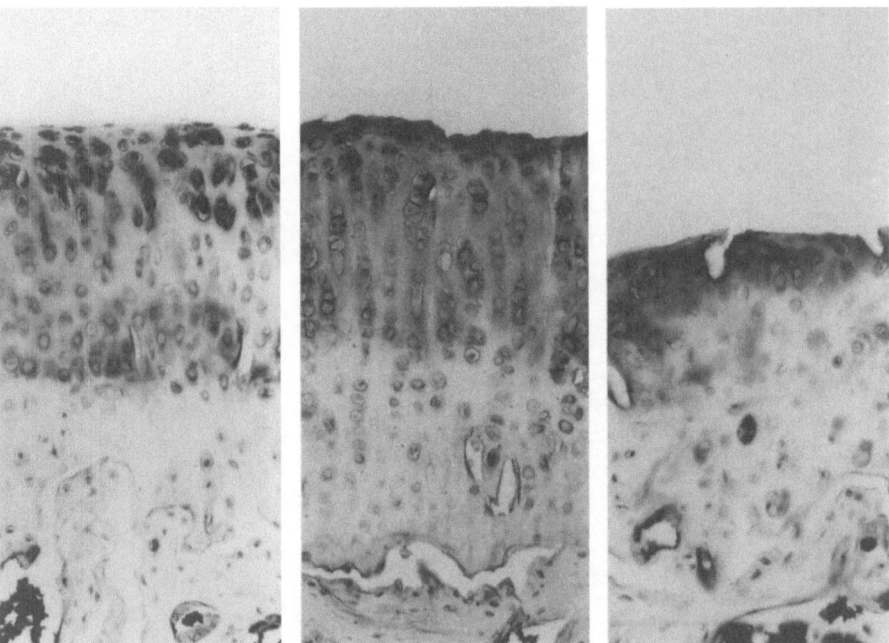

a,b   c

Fig. 1a–c. Immunohistochemical staining using monoclonal antibody to chondroitin-4-sulfate. **a** In sham-operated control joints, the cytosol of the chondrocytes was immunoreactive. In osteoarthritic cartilage at 2 weeks after operation (**b**), the cytosol and matrices were immunoreactive; at 6 weeks after operation (**c**), the cytosol and matrix in the residual layers also were immunoreactive

Keratan Sulfate

Sham-Operated Control Joints (Fig. 2a)

Immunoreactivity was observed in the pericellular and extracellular matrices from the tangential to the radial layer, while the cytosol was stained weakly.

Osteoarthritic Cartilage

At 2 weeks after operation (Fig. 2b), immunoreactivity was enhanced in the matrices in the tangential and transitional layers and in the upper half of the radial layer. At 6 weeks after operation (Fig. 2c), immunoreactivity was observed in the matrix in the residual transitional and radial layers.

Dermatan Sulfate

Sham-operated Control Joints (Fig. 3a)

No immunoreactivity was observed in articular cartilage.

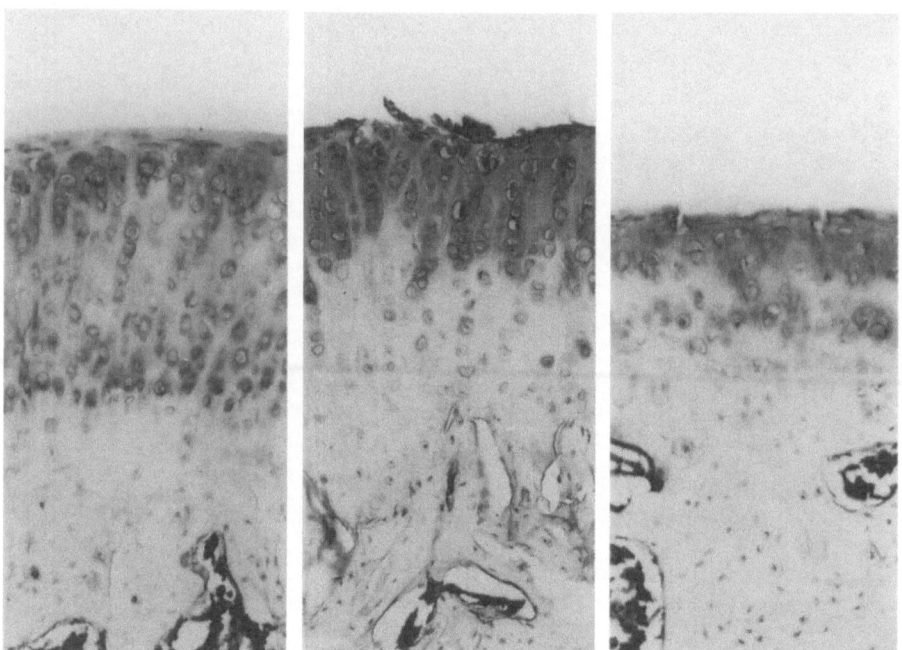

a,b   c

Fig. 2a–c. Immunohistochemical staining using monoclonal antibody to keratan sulfate. **a** In sham-operated control joints, the pericellular and extracellular matrices were immunoreactive. In osteoarthritic cartilage at 2 weeks after operation (**b**), immunoreactivity was enhanced in the matrices; at 6 weeks after operation (**c**), the matrix in the residual layer was immunoreactive

Osteoarthritic Cartilage

At 2 weeks after operation (Fig. 3b), immunoreactivity was observed mainly in the extracellular matrices in the transitional and upper part of the radial layers. At 4 weeks after operation (Fig. 3c), immunoreactivity was observed on the joint surface, in the pericellular and extracellular matrices in the residual transitional and radial layers. At 6 weeks after the operation, the matrix in the residual transitional radial layer was positively stained.

Discussion

Although many kinds of animals have been used to produce osteoarthritis, no study has used rat joints to produce a reproducible osteoarthritic model. Rats have several advantages as an experimental animal because of their genetic homogeneity and versatility with regard to the availability of many kinds of monoclonal antibodies and cDNA probes.

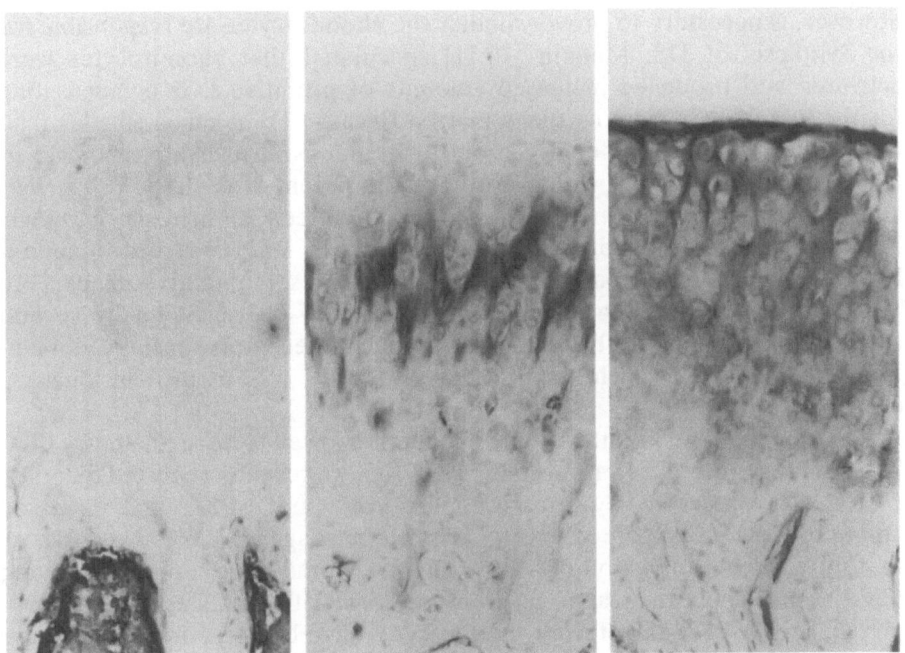

a,b   c

FIG. 3a–c. Immunohistochemical staining using monoclonal antibody to dermatan sulfate. **a** In sham-operated control joints, no immunoreactivity was observed in the articular cartilage. In osteoarthritic cartilage at 2 weeks after operation, the extracellular matrices were immunoreactive; at 4 weeks after operation (**c**), the pericellular and extracellular matrices were immunoreactive

The histological findings of osteoarthritis induced by multiple ligamentous dissection in this study were reproducible and similar to those in man. In osteoarthritis, several metabolic changes such as disturbed GAG synthesis [6,7] and decrease in synthesis of CS [8] or KS [9] have been reported in chondrocytes. In this study, the localizations of these PGs were determined immunohistochemically under normal conditions and in osteoarthritis. In normal cartilage, CS-4 was observed both intracellularly and pericellularly, and KS was observed mainly pericellularly in tangential and radial layers. In osteoarthritic cartilage, increased staining of both CS-4 and KS was observed pericellularly at 2 weeks in all layers, and CS-4 was observed even in the calcified layer at 6 weeks when the tangential layer was worn away.

Dermatan sulfate (DS) is a major component of the extracellular matrix of mesenchymal tissue in the limb bud before chondrogenesis [12] and has also been detected biochemically in epiphyseal cartilage [13], aged articular cartilage [14], and reparative cartilage tissue [15]. In this study, DS was detected histologically for the first time in the pericellular matrix of the chondrocytes in osteoarthritic cartilage using a monoclonal antibody. Further elucidation, however, is necessary to prove whether the chondrocytes are responsible for the synthesis of DS. Mankin [10,11] speculated that chondrocytes were activated and produced increased amounts of primitive PGs compensating for the loss of PGs from cartilage matrix. Because DS is much smaller than the cartilage-specific proteoglycan and does not bind to hyaluronic acid to form large aggregates, it would not have the potent viscoelastic properties, and replacement by DS may have deleterious effects on articular cartilage. Recently, altered chondroitin sulfate synthesis was observed immuno-histochemically in osteoarthritic joints in canines [16] and humans [17]. The synthesis of PGs has been demonstrated to be regulated by several cytokines and hormones through certain specific receptors on the cell membrane, signals from which are transduced by Ca^{2+} [18] or protein kinase-C (PKC) [19].

The production of keratan sulfate has been reported to be regulated by PKC [20]. Among more than ten subspecies of PKC, we recently reported that only ε-PKC was observed in normal chondrocytes, and α-PKC and increased amounts of ε-PKC appeared in osteoarthritic cartilage [21]. We also observed that intraarticular injection of a PKC agonist, tetradecanoyl-phorbol-acetate (TPA), protected the cartilage from osteoarthritic changes almost completely [22]. α-PKC-transfected chondrocytes have been reported to produce increased amounts of PGs [23] in vitro. Increased production of cartilage-specific CS-4 and KS are suspected to be protective reactions of mechanically stressed chondrocytes. The appearance of DS, however, does not merely represent a chondroprotective reaction as suggested by Mankin et al. because of its poor viscoelastic properties, and could be deleterious for the articular cartilage.

Acknowledgment. This work was supported by a grant-in-aid for scientific research (no. 07671630) from the Ministry of Education, Science, Sports and Culture, Japan.

References

1. Ehrlich MG, Houle PA, Vigliani G, Mankin HJ (1978) Correlation between articular cartilage collagenase activity and osteoarthritis. Arthritis Rheum 21:761–766
2. Dean DD, Pelletier JM, Pelletier JP, Howell DS, Woessner JF Jr (1989) Evidence for metalloproteinase and metalloproteinase inhibitor imbalance in human osteoarthritic cartilage. J Clin Invest 84:678–685
3. Heine J (1926) Uber die Arthritis deformans. Virchows Arch 260:521–663
4. Pelletier JM, Pelletier JP, Cloutier JM, Howell DS, Mnaymneh LG, Woessner JF (1984) Neutral proteases capable of proteoglycan digesting activity in osteoarthritic and normal human articular cartilage. Arthritis Rheum 27:305–312
5. Chrisman OD (1969) Biochemical aspects of degenerative joint disease. Clin Orthop 64:77–86

6. Mathews MB, Glagov S (1966) Acid mucopolysaccharide patterns in aging human cartilage. J Clin Invest 45:1103–1111
7. Matthews BF (1953) Composition of articular cartilage in osteoarthritis. Br Med J 19:660–661
8. Bollet A, Nance J (1966) Biochemical finding in normal and osteoarthritic articular cartilage. II. Chondroitin sulfate concentration and chain length, water, and ash content. J Clin Invest 45:1170–1177
9. Benmaman JD, Ludowieg JJ, Anderson CE (1969) Glucosamine and galactosamine distribution in human articular cartilage: relationship to age and degenerative joint disease. Clin Biochem 2:461–464
10. Mankin HJ, Lippiello L (1971) The glycosaminoglycans of normal and arthritic cartilage. J Clin Invest 50:1772–1779
11. Mankin HJ, Dorfman H, Lippiello L, Zarins A (1971) Biochemical and metabolic abnormalities in articular cartilage from osteo-arthritic human hips. II. Correlation of morphology with biochemical and metabolic data. J Bone Joint Surg 53A:523–537
12. Goetinck PF, Pennypacker JP, Royal PD (1974) Proteochondroitin sulfate synthesis and chondrogenic expression. Exp Cell Res 87:241–248
13. Rosenberg LC, Tang LH, Choi H, et al (1983) Isolation, characterization and immunofluorescent localization of a dermatan sulfate containing proteoglycan from bovine fetal epiphyseal cartilage. In: Kelley RO, Goetinck PF, Maccabe JA (eds) Limb development and regeneration, part B. Liss, New York, pp 67–84
14. Rosenberg LC, Choi H, Johnson T, Pal S, Poole AR, Tang L (1985) Structure and properties of cartilage-specific proteoglycans and dermatan sulfate proteoglycans present in the extracellular matris of articular cartilages. In: Hirohata K, Matsubara T (eds) Cartilage in health and disease. Medical View, Tokyo, pp 103–112
15. Furukawa T, Eyre DR, Koide S, Glimcher M (1980) Biochemical studies on repair cartilage resurfacing experimental defects in the rabbit knee. J Bone Joint Surg 62A:79–80
16. Visco DM, Johnstone B, Hill MA, Jolly G, Caterson B (1993) Immunohistochemical analysis of 3-B-3($-$) and 7-D-4 epitope expression in canine osteoarthritis. Arthritis Rheum 36:1718–1725
17. Slater RR Jr, Bayliss MT, Lachiewicz PF, Visco DM, Caterson B (1995) Monoclonal antibodies that detect biochemical markers of arthritis in humans. Arthritis Rheum 38:655–659
18. Eilam Y, Beit-Or A, Nevo Z (1985) Decrease in cytosolic free Ca^{2+} and enhanced proteoglycan synthesis induced by cartilage derived growth factors in cultured chondrocytes. Biochem Biophys Res Commun 132:770–779
19. Arner EC, Pratta MA (1991) Modulation of interleukin-1-induced alterations in cartilage proteoglycan metabolism by activation of protein kinase C. Arthritis Rheum 34:1006–1013
20. Fukuda K, Yamasaki H, Nagata Y, et al (1991) Histamine H1-receptor-mediated keratan sulfate production in rabbit chondrocytes: involvement of protein kinase C. Am J Physiol 261C:413–416
21. Satsuma H, Saito N, Hamanishi C, Hashima M, Tanaka S (1996) Alpha and epsilon isozymes of protein kinase C in the chondrocytes in normal and early osteoarthritic articular cartilage. Calcif Tissue Int 58:192–194

22. Hamanishi C, Hashima M, Satsuma H, Tanaka S (1996) Protein kinase C-activator inhibits progression of osteoarthritis induced in rabbit knee joints. J Lab Clin Med 127:540–544
23. Kimura T, Hujioka H, Matsubara T, Itoh T (1994) The role of protein kinase C in glycosaminoglycan synthesis by cultured bovine articular chondrocytes (In Japanese). Clin Rheumatol 5:240–246

D. Promising Treatments 1

Results of a Phase II Rheumatoid Arthritis Clinical Trial Using T-Cell Receptor Peptides

S.W. Brostoff[1], D.J. Carlo[1], J.P. Diveley[1], E.E. Morgan[1],
C.J. Nardo[1], S.P. Richieri[1], T.C. Adamson[2], Z. Fronek[2],
L.H. Calabrese[3], J.M. Cash[3], J.A. Markenson[4], J. Bathon[5],
A.K. Matsumoto[5], E.L. Matteson[6], K.M. Uramoto[6], C.M. Weyand[6],
V. Strand[7], L.W. Heck[8], W.J. Koopman[8], and L.W. Moreland[8]

Summary. Restricted T-cell receptor gene use has been found in animal models of autoimmune disease. This observation has resulted in the successful use of T-cell receptor peptide therapy in animal studies. Initial phase I studies in patients with rheumatoid arthritis (RA) indicated that this therapy was safe and well tolerated. A double-blind, placebo-controlled, multicenter phase II rheumatoid arthritis clinical trial was undertaken using IR501 therapeutic vaccine, which consists of a combination of three peptides derived from T-cell receptors (Vβ3, Vβ14, Vβ17) in incomplete Freund's adjuvant (IFA). These T-cell receptors were previously reported to be restricted in RA patients. A total of 99 patients received either 90μg (31 patients) or 300μg (35 patients) of IR501 therapeutic vaccine or IFA alone (33 patients) as a control. IR501 therapeutic vaccine was administered as a 1.0-ml intramuscular injection at weeks 0, 4, 8, and 20. Patients were followed for 32 weeks. The results of the trial indicated that the treatment was safe, with none of the patients discontinuing the trial because of treatment-related adverse events. No significant adverse events attributable to the study drug were observed. Patients in both dose groups treated with IR501 therapeutic vaccine showed improvement in disease condition. Most importantly, the 90-μg dose group showed a statistically significant improvement when compared to control patients after the

[1] Immune Response Corporation, 5935 Darwin Court, Carlsbad, CA 92008, U.S.A.
[2] Sharp Rees-Stealy, 2001 Fourth Avenue, San Diego, CA 92101, U.S.A.
[3] Cleveland Clinic, 9500 Euclid Avenue, Cleveland, OH 44195, U.S.A.
[4] Cornell University Medical College, 535 East 70th Street, New York, NY 10021, U.S.A.
[5] Johns Hopkins University, 5501 Hopkins Bayview Circle, Baltimore, MD 21224, U.S.A.
[6] Mayo Clinic, 200 First Street SW, Rochester, MN 55905, U.S.A.
[7] Stanford University, San Francisco, CA 94131, U.S.A.
[8] University of Alabama, 068 Spain Rehabilitation Center, 1717 Sixth Avenue South, Birmingham, AL 35294-0006, U.S.A.

third and fourth injections. More than 50% of the treated patients showed improvement compared to 19% of controls, as measured in accordance with the American College of Rheumatology definition for clinical response (ACR 20 criteria).

Key Words. T-cell receptor peptide vaccine, Phase II rheumatoid arthritis trial, Vβ3, Vβ14, and Vβ17 T-cell receptors, Rheumatoid arthritis

Introduction

The immune system must be able to distinguish self from nonself. When inappropriate reactions to self (autoreactivity) result in pathological tissue damage, an autoimmune disease occurs. Rheumatoid arthritis, along with multiple sclerosis and psoriasis, is one of the major autoimmune diseases in which this tissue damage is caused by autoreactive T cells. Because T cells are responsible for pathological tissue damage in these diseases, these T cells can be considered pathogens. With this consideration, therapies can be developed to treat T-cell-mediated autoimmune disease using strategies similar to those used to control other pathogens, such as bacteria or viruses. Perhaps the most successful strategy developed to control pathogens has been the use of vaccines made from attenuated, killed, or subunits of the pathogen.

Early studies by Cohen and co-workers indicated that in experimental autoimmune encephalomyelitis (EAE), an animal model of T-cell-mediated autoimmune disease, an attenuated form of the pathogenic T cell could be used to protect animals from EAE [1]. Although this approach is currently being tested in human clinical trials, its shortcoming is the need to use this approach as an autologous T-cell immunization. Because of the outbred nature of the human population, it would have to be administered in an individualized manner (i.e., T cells removed from an individual, attenuated, and reinfused back into that individual) because of transplantation antigen differences. We have used a different approach in treating T-cell-mediated disease by employing a subunit vaccine of the pathogenic T cell as a practical alternative to the whole killed or attenuated T-cell approach. The subunit of the T cell that distinguishes one T cell from another, and therefore, distinguishes the pathogenic T cells from normal T cells, is the T-cell receptor (TCR), which is the portion of the T cell that recognizes and binds to tissue antigens. The T-cell receptor (Fig. 1) consists of two amino acid chains called the α- and β-chains, each composed of gene elements (V, D, J, C) that are rearranged during development in such a way as to leave each β-chain with a single V, D, J, and C and each α-chain with a single V, J, and C. Thus, each T cell has one specific combination of these elements of the millions of different possible combinations or specificities.

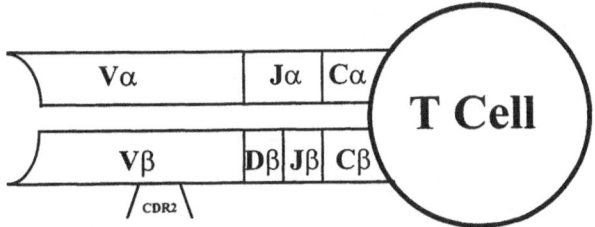

FIG. 1. T-cell receptor structure showing the various gene elements (V, D, J, C) that comprise the α- and β-chains. The CDR2 or second (complementarity-determining) hypervariable region is indicated

Animal Studies

Studies in animal models of T-cell-mediated autoimmune disease indicated that the pathogenic T cells use a limited number of T-cell receptor gene elements [2–5]. Using the EAE model, we extended the strategy used by Cohen and co-workers [1] by using synthetic peptides comprising amino acid sequences from the gene elements found to be conserved on encephalitogenic T cells as subunit vaccines to treat EAE. Vβ peptides from complementarity-determining region (CDR)2 were among those used [6,7]. Figure 1 is a representation of the α- and β-chains of the T-cell receptor with the location of the CDR2 region indicated.

The results of experiments in EAE using CDR2 peptides are shown in Fig. 2. In these experiments, Lewis rats were injected with T-cell receptor peptides in complete Freund's adjuvant and were challenged 30 days later with myelin basic protein in complete Freund's adjuvant. The disease course was graded on a 3-point scale, and the animals were followed until they recovered. Lewis rats generally spontaneously recover from disease within a week after the most severe clinical signs (usually paralysis, grade 3) have occurred. A significant impact on the disease was demonstrated; the severity and duration of the clinical signs were reduced.

The animal studies using T-cell receptor peptides to treat EAE [6–9] suggest that this approach can be used to treat human T-cell-mediated autoimmune disease. In human diseases in which the majority of pathogenic T cells use a limited number of Vβ gene elements, one can hope to downregulate a population of cells that contain the pathogenic T cells by targeting these specific gene elements. In contrast to other strategies that broadly target T cells, this kind of immunotherapeutic approach should be specific without compromising the immune system because it will affect only the pathogenic T cells, while sparing the rest of the T cells which are needed to protect against other diseases and infections. This approach may also be helpful in treating B-cell-mediated disease to the extent that T-cell help is needed and, in fact, any

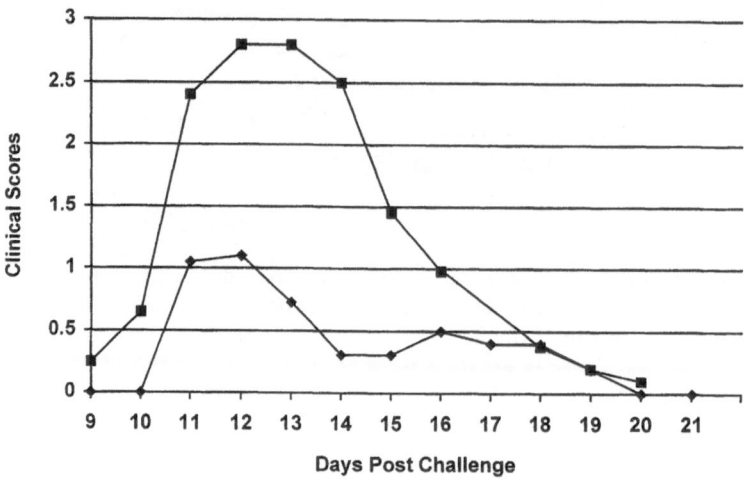

FIG. 2. The effect of CDR2 T-cell receptor peptide vaccination on the course of experimental autoimmune encephalomyelitis (EAE) in the Lewis rat. Rats were graded on a 3-point scale as follows: (1) loss of motor control of the tail, (2) hindleg weakness, and (3) hindleg paralysis. Controls are denoted by *squares*; CDR2 peptide-treated animals are denoted by *diamonds*. Clinical scores are graded for each day after challenge with myelin basic protein in complete Freund's adjuvant. (See [7] for more details)

T-cell-mediated pathology involving oligoclonal T-cell populations, such as T-cell lymphoma.

Human Application

To apply T-cell receptor peptide immunization therapy to human autoimmune disease, restriction in T-cell receptor gene use must be a feature of the disease. Therefore, our basic strategy has been to try to identify T cells involved in human autoimmune disease and analyze their T-cell receptor gene use. This strategy is depicted in Fig. 3 for rheumatoid arthritis. We obtained synovial tissue from rheumatoid arthritis patients undergoing joint replacement surgery and, using magnetic beads coated with antibody, we isolated IL-2 receptor-positive (IL-2R+) T cells infiltrating these tissues. Previous animal studies [10] have indicated that most of the T cells infiltrating target tissues in EAE were not involved in the disease. Rather, it was the small percent of activated (IL-2R+) T cells that correlated with disease activity [10]. This observation led us to focus on the small population of infiltrating IL-2R+ T cells for analysis of the T cells involved in rheumatoid arthritis. Our analysis of infiltrating T cells in rheumatoid arthritis [11] indicated an over representation of three Vβ gene families: Vβ17, Vβ14, and Vβ3. Sequence analysis of infiltrat-

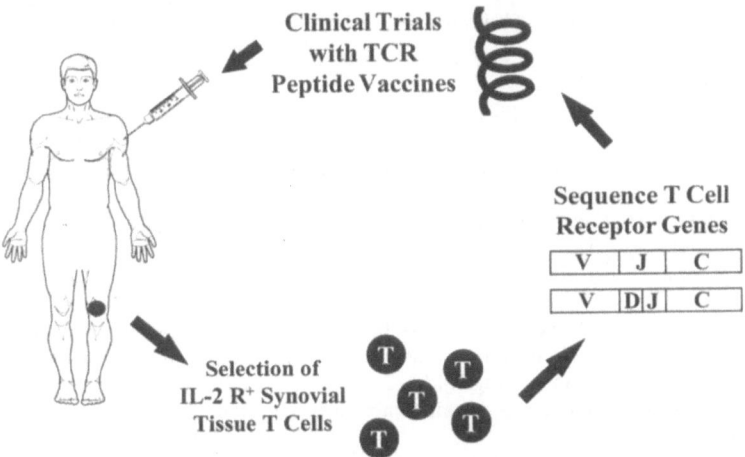

FIG. 3. Strategy for determining which T-cell receptor (*TCR*) peptides to use in clinical trials. T cells infiltrating synovial tissue were removed and fractionated. IL-2 receptor positive (IL-2 R+) T cells were analyzed for T-cell receptor gene use. T-cell receptors that displayed elevated expression and evidence of clonality were identified. (See [11] for details on analysis of T-cell receptors from synovial tissue of rheumatoid arthritis patients)

ing IL-2R+ T cells bearing these Vβs indicated a clonal expansion in situ had occurred because many of these T cells were either clonal or oligoclonal [11]. Of significant interest is the fact that these three Vβ gene families are quite homologous to each other. Other workers in the field have subsequently made similar observations regarding the Vβ genes associated with rheumatoid arthritis [12–18].

Phase I Trials

We completed three phase I trials in rheumatoid arthritis using the T-cell receptor peptide technology, one of which recently has been published [19]. These early trials all indicated that the therapy was safe and well tolerated. We recently completed a double-blind, placebo-controlled, multicenter phase II trial using IR501 therapeutic vaccine, which consists of a combination of three peptides derived from T-cell receptors (Vβ3, Vβ14, and Vβ17) in incomplete Freund's adjuvant. A total of 99 patients received either 90μg (31 patients) or 300μg (35 patients) of IR501 therapeutic vaccine or IFA alone (33 patients) as a control (Moreland et al., in manuscript). IR501 Therapeutic Vaccine or control was administered as a 1.0-ml, intramuscular injection at weeks 0, 4, 8, and 20. Patients were followed for 32 weeks. The inclusion and exclusion criteria are included in Table 1. The trial was performed at six clinical sites: Cleveland Clinic Foundation, Cornell University, Johns Hopkins University,

TABLE 1. Inclusion and exclusion criteria for patients in the IR501 therapeutic vaccine phase II trial

Inclusion criteria
Diagnosis of rheumatoid arthritis (RA) by American College of Rheumatology (ACR) criteria
Moderate to severe rheumatoid arthritis (stage II or III) as defined by ACR functional criteria
Active RA ($\geq$9 tender and $\geq$6 swollen joints)
18–70 years of age
Exclusion criteria
Medications
Variable doses of hydroxychloroquine/sulfasalazine; prednisone >10 mg/day; oral gold >6 mg/day; or >1 gold injection/months for 2 months before study entry
Cytotoxic or investigational drugs within 2 months before study entry
Investigational immunotherapy within 6 months before study entry
Medical conditions
Severe extraarticular manifestations of rheumatoid arthritis, such as vasculitis or Felty's syndrome
Other rheumatic illness (e.g., systemic lupus erythematosus, overlap syndrome)
Active substance or alcohol abuse
Pregnant or lactating women
Abnormal clinical laboratory results and/or known to be HIV positive
Cancer within past 5 years
Active systemic infection

Mayo Clinic and Foundation, Sharp Rees-Stealy Medical Groups, and the University of Alabama, Birmingham (all U.S.A.).

The patient demographics for the study were quite similar for all dose groups. The mean age of the patients in the trial was 51.5 years (range, 21–73); 77% were women and 23% were men. The mean disease duration was 10.9 years (range, 0.4–40). The mean number of tender joints was 28.6 (range, 9–63) and that of swollen joints 21.0 (range, 3.5–40.5).

Discussion

The results of the trial indicated that the treatment was safe and well tolerated, and none of the patients discontinued the trial because of treatment-related adverse events. No significant adverse events attributable to the study drug were observed. No differences in the incidence or character of adverse events between treated and control patients were observed, and there were no clinically significant or meaningful changes in physical examinations, vital signs, or laboratory parameters.

During the course of the study, we observed increases in in vitro proliferative responses to Vβ peptide over time in all dose groups. No host antibody response to the administered peptides was detected in any dose group. No skin reactivity to administered peptides was observed, and there were no decreases

TABLE 2. ACR 20 criteria for defining a "Responder"

A 20% or greater improvement in
  tender joint count, and
  swollen joint count

AND
A 20% decrease or more in three of these five criteria:
  Modified health assessment questionnaire (MHAQ)
  Visual analog scale of pain (VAS)
  Patient global assessment
  Physician global assessment
  Erythrocyte sedimentation rate (ESR) or C-reactive protein (CRP) levels

in peripheral Vβ17, Vβ14 or Vβ13 TCR-positive T cells. Based on animal studies and previous phase I studies, no antibody responses to the administered peptides and no decreases in circulating levels of peripheral Vβ17-, Vβ14-, and Vβ3-positive T cells were expected. There was no indication of generalized immunosuppression as a result of this treatment.

Using the American College of Rheumatology definition for clinical response (ACR 20), patients in both dose groups showed improvement in disease condition during the course of this trial. In the American College of Rheumatology definition for clinical response (Table 2), a responder is defined by 20% or greater improvement in *both* tender joint count and swollen joint count, accompanied by 20% or greater decrease in three of the following five criteria: (1) Modified Health Assessment Questionnaire (MHAQ), (2) Visual Analog Scale of Pain (VAS), (3) Patient Global Assessment, (4) Physician Global Assessment, and (5) erythrocyte sedimentation rate (ESR) or C-reactive protein (CRP) levels.

Statistical Analysis

Statistical analyses were used to evaluate efficacy using the ACR 20 criteria. Perhaps the analysis reflecting the best assessment of efficacy was the one performed using patients who completed the trial per protocol without using prohibited or rescue medications. The resulting total of 59 patients was approximately equally divided between the three dose groups as follows: IFA control (21 patients), 90 μg (18 patients), and 300 μg (20 patients). In this per protocol analysis (Fig. 4), the 90-μg dose group showed a statistically significant improvement when compared to control patients after the third and fourth injections, according to the ACR 20 criteria. After the third injection at week 20, 56% of the treated patients improved using this criteria, compared to 19% in the control group. The difference between treated and control patients was statistically significant at this timepoint. After the fourth injection at week 24, 50% of the treated patients in this dose group showed improvement, compared to 19% of controls. The difference between treated and control

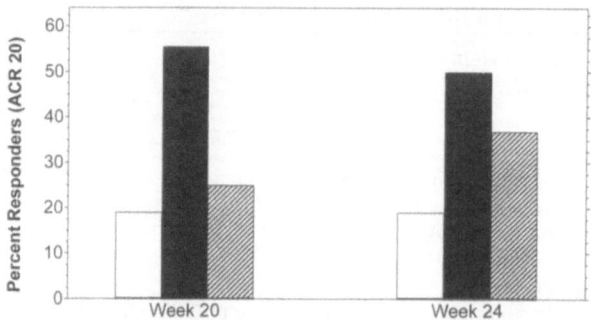

FIG. 4. Per protocol analysis using the American College of Rheumatology (ACR) 20 criteria, at weeks 20 and 24 of patients completing the trial per protocol. Weeks 20 and 24 were after the third and fourth injection, respectively, of IR501 therapeutic vaccine. Controls, *unshaded*; 90-μg dose group, *black*; 300-μg dose group, *hatched*

patients was statistically significant at this timepoint as well. The 300-μg dose group had favorable trends, with 25% of the patients showing improvement after the third injection at week 20 and 37% after the fourth injection at week 24, compared to a 19% improvement in the control group. The 19% improvement in the control group in this study using this analysis is similar to the placebo effect found in other rheumatoid arthritis clinical trials.

The most conservative analysis used in evaluating efficacy of the treatment was the intent-to-treat analysis using all the patients enrolled. In this analysis, all patients were *nonresponders* if they discontinued the treatment or took prohibited or rescue medications before the completion of the trial, whether or not they had improved earlier in the study. Using this analysis (Fig. 5), there was a statistically significant improvement in the 90-μg treated group compared to controls at the 20-week timepoint and trends toward improvement in both the 90-μg and 300-μg dose groups at week 24. This analysis underestimates the treatment effect because patients would not be considered as responders even if they exit early with a 20% improvement and effectively lowers the percent responders. This is illustrated by the fact that the response noted in the control group (about 10%) is below the placebo effect usually found in rheumatoid arthritis clinical trials. Nevertheless, more than 30% of the patients in the 90-μg dose group showed improvement using the most conservative analysis.

Conclusion

In conclusion, IR501 therapeutic vaccine was found to be safe and was well tolerated after multiple intramuscular injections. Although the trial was not powered to show statistical significance, the product demonstrated efficacy in

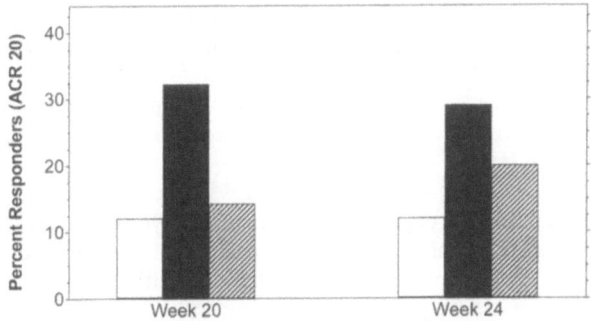

FIG. 5. Intent-to-treat analysis, using the ACR 20 criteria, of all patients enrolled in the trial. Patients who discontinued or who used rescue or prohibited medication were retained in the analysis as nonresponders. Weeks 20 and 24 were after the third and fourth injection, respectively, of IR501 therapeutic vaccine. Controls, *unshaded*; 90-μg dose group, *black*; 300-μg dose group, *hatched*

patients with rheumatoid arthritis by the ACR 20 criteria. According to the design of the trial, there was less than a 30% ($1 - \beta = 0.28$) chance of detecting a statistically significant difference ($\alpha = .05$) between the control and each treatment group. The observation that the 90-μg dose group showed a statistically significant treatment effect in the most conservative analysis warrants additional studies to confirm the usefulness of this therapy as a treatment for rheumatoid arthritis.

References

1. Ben-Nun A, Wekerle H, Cohen IR, et al (1981) Vaccination against autoimmune encephalomyelitis with T-lymphocyte line cells reactive against myelin basic protein. Nature (Lond) 292:60–61
2. Acha-Orbea H, Mitchell DJ, Timmermann L, et al (1988) Limited heterogeneity of T cell receptors from lymphocytes mediating autoimmune encephalomyelitis allows specific immune intervention. Cell 54:263–273
3. Urban JL, Kumar V, Kono DH, et al (1988) Restricted use of T cell receptor V genes in murine autoimmune encephalomyelitis raises possibilites for antibody therapy. Cell 54:577–592
4. Burns FR, Li X, Shen N, et al (1989) Both rat and mouse T cell receptors specific for the encephalitogenic determinants of myelin basic protein use similar Vα or Vβ chain genes even though the major histocompatibility complex and encephalitogenic determinants being recognized are different. J Exp Med 169:27–39
5. Chluba J, Steeg C, Becker A, et al (1989) T cell receptor β chain usage in myelin basic protein-specific rat T lymphocytes. Eur J Immunol 19:279–284
6. Howell MD, Winters ST, Olee T, et al (1989) Vaccination against experimental allergic encephalomyelitis with T cell receptor peptides. Science 246:668–670

7. Brostoff SW (1993) Vaccination with T-cell receptor peptides. In: Bach J-F (ed) Monoclonal antibodies and peptide therapy in autoimmune diseases. Dekker, New York, pp 203–218
8. Vandenbark AA, Hashim G, Offner H (1989) Immunization with a synthetic T-cell receptor V-region peptide protects against experimental autoimmune encephalomyelitis. Nature (Lond) 341:541–544
9. Offner H, Hashim GA, Vandenbark AA (1991) T cell receptor peptide therapy triggers autoregulation of experimental encephalomyelitis. Science 251:430–432
10. Sedgwick J, Brostoff S, Mason D (1987) Experimental allergic encephalomyelitis in the absence of a classical delayed-type hypersensitivity reaction. J Exp Med 165:1058–1075
11. Howell MD, Dively JP, Lundeen KA, et al (1991) Limited T cell receptor β-chain heterogeneity among IL-2R+ synovial T cells suggests a role for superantigen in rheumatoid arthritis. Proc Natl Acad Sci USA 88:10921–10925
12. Alam A, Lulé J, Coppin H, et al (1995) T-cell receptor variable region of the β-chain gene use in peripheral blood and multiple synovial membranes during rheumatoid arthritis. Hum Immunol 42:331–339
13. Williams WV, Kieber-Emmons T, Fang Q, et al (1993) Conserved motifs in rheumatoid arthritis synovial tissue T-cell receptor β chains. DNA Cell Biol 12:425–434
14. Zagon G, Tumang JR, Li Y, et al (1994) Increased frequency of Vβ17-positive T cells in patients with rheumatoid arthritis. Arthritis Rheum 37:1431–1440
15. Kim SY, Lee EY, Kim YI, et al (1995). T cell receptor Vβ gene usage in rheumatoid arthritis of Korean patients. FASEB J 9:A525
16. Goronzy JJ, Bartz-Bazzanella P, Hu W, et al (1994) Dominant clonotypes in the repertoire of peripheral CD4+ T cells in rheumatoid arthritis. J Clin Invest 94:2068–2076
17. Grom AA, Thompson SD, Luyrink L, et al (1993) Dominant T-cell-receptor β chain variable region Vβ14+ clones in juvenile rheumatoid arthritis. Proc Natl Acad Sci USA 90:11104–11108
18. Paliard X, West SG, Lafferty JA, et al (1991) Evidence for the effects of a superantigen in rheumatoid arthritis. Science 253:325–329
19. Moreland LW, Heck LW Jr, Koopman WJ, et al (1996) Vβ17 T cell receptor peptide vaccination in rheumatoid arthritis: results of phase I dose escalation study. J Rheumatol 23:1353–1362

Chondroprotective Activity of a Matrix Metalloprotease Inhibitor, CGS 27023A, in Animal Models of Osteoarthritis

ELIZABETH O'BYRNE[1], VINCENT BLANCUZZI[1], HEM SINGH[1], LAWRENCE J. MACPHERSON[1], DAVID T. PARKER[1], and E. DONALD ROBERTS[2]

Summary. Breakdown of articular cartilage is a primary feature of osteoarthritis (OA) that leads to loss of joint function. Cartilage degradation involves a progressive loss of proteoglycan matrix and chondrocytes, surface fraying, and erosion. Matrix metalloproteases (MMPs) have been implicated in the destruction of cartilage in OA. CGS 27023A is an orally active inhibitor of stromelysin (MMP-3) and collagenase (MMP-1). CGS 27023A was used to evaluate the effects of an MMP inhibitor on the development of cartilage pathology in a surgical model of OA in rabbits and naturally occurring OA in guinea pigs. Focal OA lesions were produced in rabbits by partial lateral meniscectomy (MNX). Rabbits given CGS 27023A at 100 mg/kg in food for 8 weeks following MNX had a lower mean score for cartilage pathology ($P < .005$) than controls. Spontaneous OA occurs naturally in the knees of guinea pigs, starting during the first 6 months of age and progressing during the next year. By 12 months of age, articular cartilage degeneration including loss of proteoglycan and chondrocytes and surface fibrillation were observed in the medial tibia of the majority of untreated guinea pigs. Guinea pigs administered CGS 27023A in food from 6 months to 12 months of age had reduced histology scores for cartilage lesions ($P < .05$). These observations support the hypothesis that an MMP inhibitor would ameliorate cartilage destruction by protecting the collagen framework and proteoglycan matrix in OA patients.

Key Words. Matrix metalloprotease inhibitor, Cartilage degradation, Animal models

[1] Novartis Institute for Biomedical Research, 556 Morris Avenue, Summit, NJ 07901, U.S.A.
[2] Tulane Regional Primate Research Center, 18703 Three Rivers Road, Covington, LA 70433, U.S.A.

163

Introduction

Osteoarthritis (OA) is a degenerative joint disease that results in the destruction of articular cartilage. Cartilage pathology can be scored for progressive changes in the extracellular matrix [1]. Signs of matrix deterioration include loss of proteoglycan, surface fibrillation, and fissures. Early chondrocyte responses involve hyperplasia and cloning, which appears to be an attempt to repair. Eventually, cell death leads to hypocellular cartilage in later stages of the disease [1]. Cartilage erosion results in loss of the ability to distribute load and in joint dysfunction. Currently available therapies relieve painful symptoms but do little to halt the tissue destruction. Our goal is to develop new drugs to control the underlying processes leading to joint degeneration.

Matrix metalloproteases (MMPs) are a family of zinc endopeptidases that include collagenases 1, 2, and 3 (MMP 1, 8, and 13), stromelysins 1 and 2 (MMP 3 and 10), and gelatinases A and B (MMP 2 and 9) [2]. MMPs can destroy the structural proteins of cartilage such as collagen and proteoglycan [3]. MMPs have been implicated in cartilage degeneration in clinical OA in humans [4–16]. Also, MMPs are elevated in osteoarthritic cartilage. Thus we hypothesized that inhibition of MMPs would reduce cartilage destruction in OA. The evaluation of MMP inhibitors in animal models of OA may predict clinical efficacy in OA patients.

We utilized a surgical partial lateral meniscectomy (MNX) model of OA in rabbits [17–20]. In this model, focal osteoarthritic cartilage lesions develop when the biomechanics of the rabbit knee are altered by severing the fibular collateral and sesamoid ligaments and removing a section of the meniscus. MMPs are elevated in the cartilage lesions in the rabbit MNX model of OA [21–22].

Osteoarthritic changes in both guinea pigs and humans begin in the medial compartment of the knee [23–30]. Early lesions of focal chondrocyte death and proteoglycan depletion become progressively more severe with age [25]. Matrix metalloproteases (MMPs) have been implicated in cartilage degeneration in aging guinea pigs [31,32].

CGS 27023A is a nonpeptidic, potent, and orally active inhibitor of collagenase (MMP-1), 72K gelatinase (MMP-2), and stromelysin (MMP-3) [33]. The purpose of these experiments was to determine whether inhibition of MMPs by treatment with a broad-spectrum MMP inhibitor would retard the development of cartilage degeneration in these animal models of secondary and spontaneous OA. CGS 27023A was given in food at 100 mg/kg per day from week 1 through week 8 after MNX to rabbits [34] and from 6 months to 12 months of age to guinea pigs [35]. To assess the effects of the MMP inhibitor on development of OA, histological sections of articular cartilage were scored for pathological changes. We demonstrate a reduction in cartilage pathology in CGS 27023A-treated meniscectomized rabbits and aging guinea pigs.

Materials and Methods

In Vitro and In Vivo Inhibition of MMP

CGS 27023A, a nonpeptidic sulfonamide-based hydroxamic acid (Fig. 1), was assayed for inhibition of stromelysin-1 (MMP-3), collagenase-1 (MMP-1), 72-kDa gelatinase (MMP-2), and 92-kDa gelatinase (MMP-9) using synthetic substrates [36,37]. Oral activity was determined using a rabbit model of stromelysin-induced cartilage degradation (Fig. 2) [38]. For evaluation in this acute model of MMP-induced cartilage degradation, test compounds were suspended in a cornstarch vehicle at the concentration to provide the specified dose in 5 ml/kg body weight orally (p.o.) by gavage. Rabbits were restrained (Nalgene polycarbonate restraining cage; Fisher Scientific), and the drug was gavaged through a syringe attached to a tube (Robinson urethral catheter, Seamless Hospital Products, Dart, Wallingford, CT, USA) inserted 24–25 cm through a hollow mouthpiece into the stomach. At various times following dosing, 40 units recombinant human stromelysin-1 (rhSLN) in 0.1 ml was injected into both knees by inserting a 26-gauge 0.5-inch needle through the suprapatellar ligament into the joint space.

FIG. 1. Chemical structure of CGS 27023A, an orally active inhibitor of matrix metalloproteases

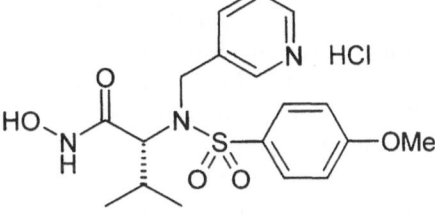

Stromelysin Intra-articular Injection Rabbit Model

- Administer Test Compound
- Inject Stromelysin into Knees
- Collect synovial lavages
- Measure Proteoglycan fragments released

Oral Activity and Duration of Action

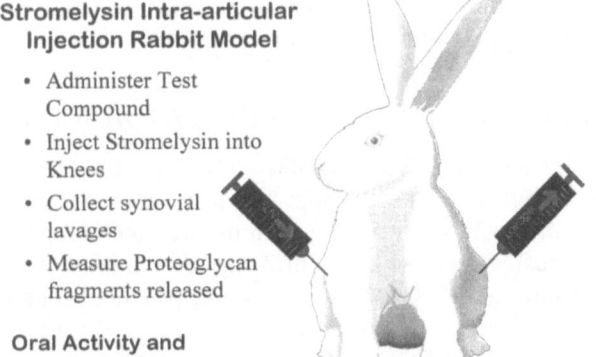

FIG. 2. Diagram of the model of acute matrix metalloprotease-(MMP-) induced cartilage matrix degradation in rabbits

Two hours after injection of rhSLN, the joints were lavaged to collect synovial fluid. To lavage the knee, 1 ml isotonic saline was injected into the joint space through the suprapatellar ligament. The knee was then flexed ten times, then opened, and the lavage was withdrawn with a syringe and a 20-gauge 1-in. needle. The joint lavage was centrifuged at 13 600 × g for 20 min to remove cells [39]. This cell-free joint lavage was analyzed for proteoglycan released into the synovial fluid. The cell-free synovial fluid was first treated with *Streptomyces* hyaluronidase (5 U/ml) for 1 h at 56°C to reduce viscosity. Sulfated glycosaminoglycan (S-GAG) was measured by a modification [40] of the 1,9-dimethylmethylene blue dye binding assay [41]. Keratan sulfate (KS) was quantitated by an enzyme-linked immunosorbent assay (ELISA) [42].

Oral Administration of MMP Inhibitor in Food

CGS 27023A was administered to male New Zealand White rabbits, HAR:PF/CF(NZW)BRSPF (4.0–5.0 kg), in NIH-09 cereal-based rabbit diet formulated to be free of Fe, Mg, Mn, Zn, Cr, Cu, and Co (Dyets, Bethlehem, PA, USA [#620057]). Rabbits were fed 40 g chow per kilogram of body weight per day. Rabbits were weighed weekly, and daily food rations were weighed into labeled ziplock bags. Control rabbits were fed 40 g/kg NIH 09 diet without the drug. The efficacy and stability of CGS 27023A as dosed in food was determined in the intraarticular injection of the rhSLN model [38]. In the rabbit MNX model of OA, CGS 27023A was administered at 100 mg/kg per day in Dyets #670057 containing 100 mg CGS 27023A per 40 g of pellets from week 1 through week 8 post surgery [34].

For the spontaneous model of OA in guinea pigs, CGS 27023A was milled into NIH-34M cereal-based guinea pig diet formulated to be free of Fe, Mg, Mn, Zn, Cr, Cu, and Co (Dyets, #653000). The concentration of CGS 27023A, 4.3 g/kg chow, was calculated to deliver 100 mg/kg to guinea pigs weighing up to 1.5 kg with a consumption of 35 g chow per day. Treatment was started in male Hartley guinea pigs at 6 months of age [9].

Surgical Induction of Experimental OA in Rabbits

Adult male New Zealand White rabbits, HAR:PF/CF(NZW)BRSPF (4.0–5.0 kg) were acclimated in the vivarium 1 month before surgery [26,27]. Only rabbits more than 4 kg in body weight with mature skeletal growth were used. Rabbits were anesthetized with an intramuscular injection of 1 ml/kg body weight of a 1:1 mixture of Rompun (20 mg/ml xylazine; Miles Animal Health Products, Shawnee Mission, KS, USA) and Ketaset (100 mg/ml ketamine; Fort Dodge Laboratories, Fort Dodge, IA, USA).

In the surgical preparation room, the hair was shaved from the knee. The skin in the surgical area and surrounding area were swabbed with betadine, then rinsed with 70% alcohol. All surgery was performed under aseptic conditions in the surgical suite. The right knee was flexed to allow the surgeon to locate the joint space between the femur and tibia. The knee was opened laterally by making a vertical incision approximately 1 cm below the groove to expose the fibular collateral ligament horizontal to the incision. The fibular collateral ligament was severed and a section approximately 3 mm thick was removed (Fig. 3). Severing the fibular collateral ligament exposed the thicker sesamoid ligament running vertical to it. A forceps was placed under the sesamoid ligament to lift it and remove a 3- to 4-mm section using a #10 scalpel blade.

Removal of the sesamoid ligament exposed the lateral meniscus. A toothed forceps was used to firmly grasp the lateral meniscus to sever a 3- to 4-mm section using a #11 scalpel blade (see Fig. 2). The capsule was sutured with 2.0 chromic gut (#6-123H; Ethicon, Somerville, NJ, USA) and the skin closed with 2.0 silk (#679H; Ethicon). Following surgery, each animal received an intramuscular injection of 1 ml Durapen (combined penicillin G benzathine and penicillin G procaine, 300 000 units/ml; Vedco, St. Joseph, MO, U.S.A.). An analgesic, buprenorphine (0.33 ml of 0.3 mg/ml buprenorphine HCl, Buprenex; Reckitt & Colman Pharmaceuticals, Richmond, VA, USA) was administered subcutaneously during recovery on the day of surgery and twice the following day. An Elizabethan collar (#412 SAF-T Shield 12 in.; Ejay International, Glendora, CA, USA) was placed around the neck of each rabbit to prevent chewing of the surgical site. Ten days after surgery, rabbits were anesthetized with 0.5 ml/kg 1:1 mixture of Rompun and Ketaset to remove external sutures.

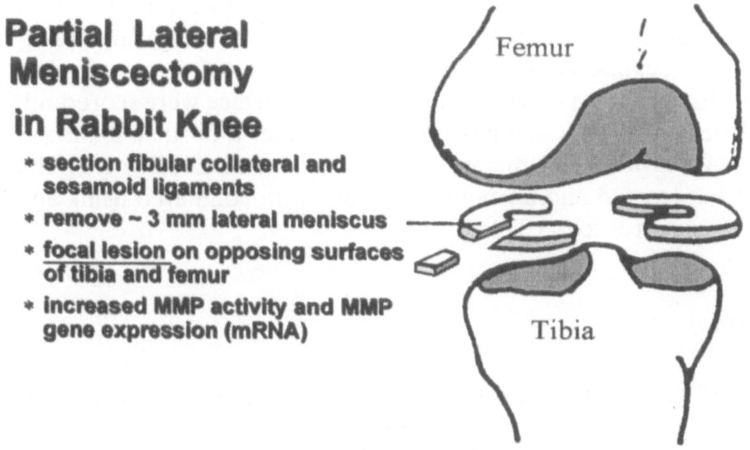

Partial Lateral Meniscectomy in Rabbit Knee

* section fibular collateral and sesamoid ligaments
* remove ~ 3 mm lateral meniscus
* focal lesion on opposing surfaces of tibia and femur
* increased MMP activity and MMP gene expression (mRNA)

Femur

Tibia

FIG. 3. Diagram of partial lateral meniscectomy (MNX) surgery showing removal of a section of the lateral meniscus

Spontaneous OA in Guinea Pigs

Male Hartley guinea pigs were acclimated in the vivarium for 3 months until they were 6 months old, at which time they were utilized for the study. To evaluate cartilage histology at the onset of treatment, ten guinea pigs were necropsied at 6 months of age. Six-month-old guinea pigs were assigned to groups fed ad libitum control chow or chow containing the test compound. At 12 months of age, knee joints were processed for histological staining and scoring.

Histological Scoring of Cartilage Pathology

In the rabbit study, at 8 weeks after partial lateral meniscectomy, knees were fixed in 10% neutral-buffered formalin. Guinea pig knees were immediately fixed in Streck tissue fixative (Streck, Omaha, NE, USA). All fixed tissues were sent to Tulane Regional Primate Research Center for processing. Fixed tissues were demineralized using a 20% solution of formic acid, neutralized in 5% ammonium hydroxide, and washed in running tap water. The articular cartilage was stained with safranin O/fast green with hematoxylin counterstain for histological scoring. Slides were numbered and evaluated by a veterinary pathologist (E.D. Roberts).

Rabbit articular cartilage was graded for changes in chondrocyte pathology on the following scale: 1, normal; 2, minimal changes in chondrocyte organization, palisades; 3, chondrocyte cloning; 4, moderate loss of safranin O staining, with loss of cellularity and focal areas of chondrocyte hyperplasia; and 5, hypocellular cartilage depleted of Safranin O stain with fissures and erosions.

Guinea pig tissues collected from a complete cross section of the knee joint, which included both weight-bearing portions of the femur and tibia, were processed in paraffin, sectioned at 6 nm and stained with safranin O-fast green with hematoxylin counterstain. Degenerative joint changes including reduced chondrocyte cellularity, loss of matrix safranin O staining, osteophyte formation, and fissuring and fraying of the frictional surface were scored subjectively to grade lesion severity using the following scale: 1, normal; 2, mild; 3, moderate; and 4, marked. Results are reported as mean $\pm$ SEM (n). Histological scores from treated and untreated animals were compared using an unpaired t-test (Microsoft Excel 5.0).

Results

CGS 27023A inhibits the MMPs that can degrade the structural proteins of articular cartilage. The K_i of CGS 27023A for inhibition of stromelysin-1 (MMP-3), collagenase-1 (MMP-1), 72-kDa gelatinase (MMP-2), and 92-kDa gelatinase (MMP-9) were 43 nM, 33 nM, 20 nM, and 8 nM, respectively.

In rabbits, CGS 27023A at 50 and 100 mg/kg in food blocked the increase in synovial fluid proteoglycan following in vivo injection of recombinant human MMP-3 into the knee. Feeding chow providing 100 mg CGS 27023A/40 g of pellets per kilogram of body weight per day was selected to block MMP-mediated damage to proteoglycan and collagen in the knee for 24 h/day in the OA model. Rabbits were given food containing CGS 27023A for 8 weeks after MNX surgery. Cartilage pathology scores at 8 weeks post MNX surgery ranged from 4.0 ± 0.4 (7) in untreated rabbits to 1.8 ± 0.5 (5), $P < .05$, in CGS 27023A-treated rabbits (Fig. 4). Inhibition of MMPs ameliorated the loss of matrix and chondrocytes.

In a pilot experiment in 3-month-old guinea pigs, CGS 27023A at 4.3 g/kg diet fed ad libitum for 1 week produced plasma levels of 400–440 nM. Before starting treatment at 6 months of age, tibial cartilage from the knees of ten randomly selected control guinea pigs was evaluated histologically. The mean lesion score was $1.40 + 0.68$ ($n = 20$) in 6-month-old guinea pigs. By 12 months of age, articular cartilage degeneration including loss of proteoglycan, surface fibrillation, and loss of chondrocytes was observed in the medial tibia of the majority of untreated guinea pigs. The mean lesion score was 2.95 ± 0.67 ($n = 20$) in untreated guinea pigs (Fig. 5). Treatment with CGS 27023A lowered the mean lesion score to 2.16 ± 0.16 ($n = 12$) in CGS 27023A-fed guinea pigs, $P < .05$ (Fig. 5). Treatment with an MMP inhibitor retarded cartilage degradation in this model of spontaneous OA.

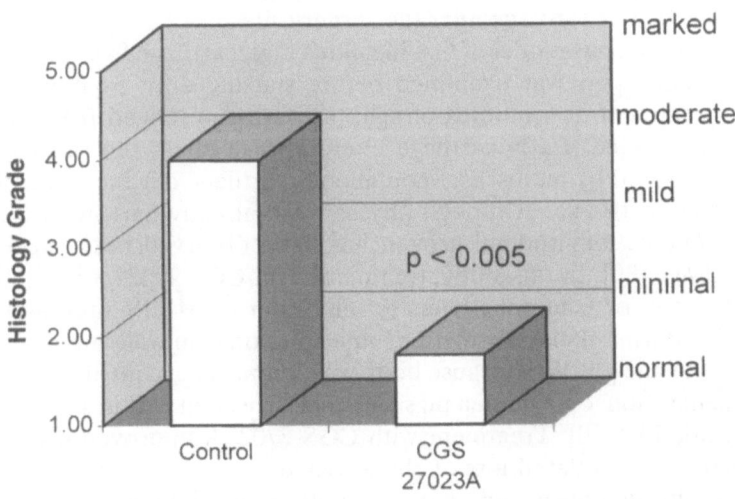

Fig. 4. Histology grades for cartilage lesions in lateral femoral condyle 8 weeks after MNX in control rabbits and CGS 27023A-treated rabbits. OA, osteoarthritis

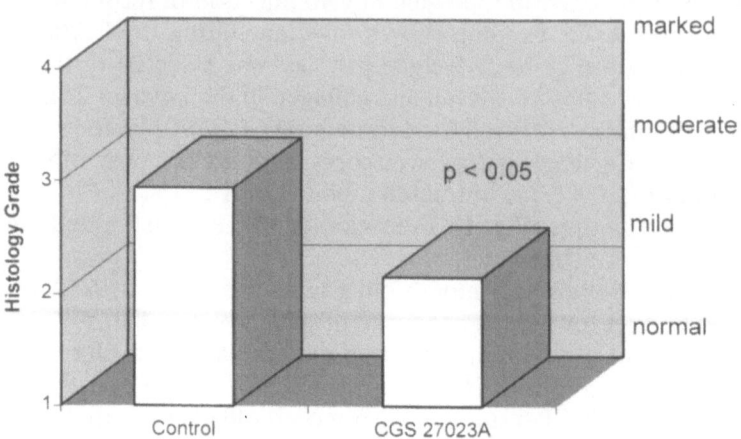

Fig. 5. Histology grades for cartilage lesions in medial tibial condyle of 12-month-old control guinea pigs and animals given CGS 27023A in food from age 6 months to age 12 months

Discussion

By 8 weeks following MNX to induce OA in rabbits, focal, full-thickness cartilage lesions develop. Treatment with the MMP inhibitor, CGS 27023A, reduced loss of proteoglycan stain, chondrocytes, surface fibrillation, and fraying of the articular cartilage near the surgery site.

In the spontaneous model of OA in guinea pigs, cartilage from ten randomly selected guinea pigs was examined before starting drug treatment. At the onset of treatment at 6 months of age, the cartilage ranged from normal to mildly degenerated. Early cartilage alterations occur in the medial tibia in areas not covered by meniscus. Spontaneous cartilage degeneration develops progressively with age. Although physes were already narrow at 6 months, slow continuous longitudinal growth has been observed between 6 and 12 months of age [30]. In this study, treatment with CGS 27023A was not begun before the age of 6 months because inhibition of MMPs may interfere in remodeling during skeletal growth. Guinea pigs do gain weight between 6 and 12 months of age [29,30]. Because body weight may be a contributing factor in joint degeneration, only guinea pigs with a body weight within 1 SD of normal were included [29,30]. Treatment with CGS 27023A improved histology and prevented the age-related loss of chondrocytes.

Our results demonstrated that an orally active inhibitor of MMPs can significantly retard cartilage destruction in a surgical model of OA in rabbits and a naturally occurring OA in guinea pigs and suggest that such an agent is likely to impede the course of OA in human patients. In this report, we have described experiments demonstrating a key role for the MMP family of enzymes in the destruction of the articular cartilage in two animal models of OA.

References

1. Mankin HJ, Dorfman H, Lipiello L, et al (1971) Biochemical and metabolic abnormalities in articular cartilage from osteoarthritic human hips. II. Correlation of morphology with biochemical and metabolic data. J Bone Joint Surg [Am] 53A:523–537
2. Birkedal-Hansen H, Moore WGI, Boden MK (1993) Matrix metalloproteases: a review. Crit Rev Oral Biol Med 4:197–250
3. Docherty AJP, Murphy G (1990) The tissue metalloprotease family and the inhibitor TIMP: a study using cDNAs and recombinant proteins. Ann Rheum Dis 49:469–479
4. Sapolsky AI, Keiser H, Howell DS, et al (1976) Metalloproteases of human articular cartilage that digest cartilage proteoglycan at neutral pH. J Clin Invest 58:1030–1041
5. Ehrlich MG, Mankin HJ, Jones H, et al (1977) Collagenase and collagenase inhibitors in osteoarthritic and normal human cartilage. J Clin Invest 59:226–233
6. Dean DD, Azzo W, Martel-Pellitier J, et al (1987) Levels of metalloproteases and tissue inhibitors of metalloproteases in human osteoarthritic cartilage. J Rheumatol 14S:43–44.
7. Pelletier J-P, Martel-Pelletier J, Howell DS, et al (1983) Collagenase and collagenolytic activity in human osteoarthritic cartilage. Arthritis Rheum 26:63–68
8. Martel-Pelletier J, Pelletier J-P, Cloutier J-M, et al (1984) Neutral proteases capable of proteoglycan digesting activity in osteoarthritic and normal human articular cartilage. Arthritis Rheum 27:305–312
9. Martel-Pelletier J, Pelletier J-P, Malemud CJ (1988) Activation of neutral metalloprotease in human osteoarthritic knee cartilage: evidence of degradation in the core protein of sulfated proteoglycan. Ann Rheum Dis 47:801–808
10. Dean DD, Martel-Pelletier J, Pelletier J-P, et al (1989) Evidence for metalloprotease and metalloprotease inhibitor (TIMP) imbalance in human osteoarthritic cartilage. J Clin Invest 84:678–685
11. Gunja-Smith Z, Nagase H, Woessner JF (1989) Purification of the neutral proteoglycan-degrading metalloprotease from human articular cartilage tissue and its identification as stromelysin matrix metalloprotease-3. Biochem J 258:115–119
12. Okada Y, Shinmei M, Tanaka O, et al (1992) Localization of matrix metalloprotease 3 (stromelysin) in osteoarthritic cartilage and synovium. Lab Invest 66:680–690
13. Dodge GR, Poole AR (1989) Immunohistochemical detection and immunochemical analysis of type II collagen degradation in human normal, rheumatoid and osteoarthritic articular cartilages and in explants of bovine articular cartilages cultured with interleukin-1. J Clin Invest 83:647–661
14. Martel-Pelletier J, McCollum R, Fujimoto N, et al (1994) Excess of metalloproteases over tissue inhibitor of metalloprotease may contribute to cartilage degradation in osteoarthritis and rheumatoid arthritis. Lab Invest 70:807–815

15. Hollander AP, Heathfield TF, Webber C, et al (1994) Increased damage to type II collagen in osteoarthritic articular cartilage detected by a new immunoassay. J Clin Invest 93:1722–1732

16. Hollander AP, Pidoux I, Reiner A, et al (1995) Damage to type II collagen in aging and osteoarthritis starts at the articular surfaces, originates around chondrocytes, and extends into the cartilage with progressive degeneration. J Clin Invest 96:2859–2869

17. Moskowitz R, Davis W, Sammarco J, et al (1973) Experimentally induced degenerative joint lesions following partial meniscectomy in the rabbit. Arthritis Rheum 16:397–405

18. Moskowitz RW, Goldberg VM (1987) Studies of osteophyte pathogenesis in experimentally induced osteoarthritis. J Rheumatol 14:311–320

19. Colombo C, Butler M, O'Byrne E, et al (1983) A new model of osteoarthritis in rabbits. I. Development of knee joint pathology following partial lateral meniscectomy and section of the fibular collateral and sesamoid ligaments. Arthritis Rheum 26:875–886

20. Colombo C (1988) Partial lateral meniscectomy with section of fibular collateral and sesamoid ligaments in the rabbit. In: Greenwald RA, Diamond HS, (eds) Handbook of animal models for the rheumatic diseases, vol 2. CRC Press, Boca Raton, pp 27–55

21. Mehraban F, Riera H, Fuo SY, et al (1993) Cartilage metalloprotease genes are up-regulated in experimental osteoarthritis and in isolated osteoarthritic chondrocytes in culture. Trans Orthop Res Soc 18:682

22. Mehraban F, Riera H, Fuo SY, et al (1994) Prostromelysin and procollagenase are differentially up-regulated in chondrocytes from the knees of rabbits with experimental osteoarthritis. Arthritis Rheum 37:1189–1197

23. Bendele AM, White SL (1987) Early histopathologic and ultrastructural alterations in femorotibial joints of partial medial meniscectomised guinea pigs. Vet Pathol 24:436–443

24. Bendele AM (1987) Progressive chronic osteoarthritis in femorotibial joints of partial medial meniscectomised guinea pigs. Vet Pathol 24:444–448

25. Bendele AM, Hulman JF (1988) Spontaneous cartilage degeneration in guinea pigs. Arthritis Rheum 31:561–565

26. Bendele AM, White SL, Hulman JF (1989) Osteoarthritis in guinea pigs: histopathologic and scanning electron microscopic features. Lab Anim Sci 39:115–121

27. Silverstein E, Sokoloff K (1958) Natural history of degenerative joint disease in small laboratory animals. V. Osteoarthritis in guinea pigs. Arthritis Rheum I:82–86

28. Meacock SCR, Bodmer JL, Billingham MEJ (1990) Experimental osteoarthritis in guinea-pigs. J Exp Pathol 71:279–293

29. Bendele AM, Hulman JF (1991) Effects of body weight restriction on the development and progression of spontaneous osteoarthritis in guinea pigs. Arthritis Rheum 34:1180–1184

30. De Bri E, Rheinholt FP, Svensson O (1995) Primary osteoarthritis in guinea pigs: a stereological study. J Orthop Res 13:769–776

31. Greenwald RA, Chowdhury MH, Moak SA, et al (1994) Long term doxycycline treatment inhibits histologic and immunologic features of spontaneous osteoarthritis in guinea pigs. Trans Orthop Res Soc 19:473

32. Olszewski J, McDonnell J, Stevens K, et al (1996) A matrix-metalloprotease-generated aggrecan neopeptide as a marker of skeletal maturation and aging in cartilage. Arthritis Rheum 39:1234–1237
33. MacPherson LJ, Bayburt EK, Capparelli MP, et al (1997) Discovery of CGS 27023A, a non-peptidic, potent, and orally active stromelysin inhibitor that blocks cartilage degradation in rabbits. J Med Chem 40:2525–2532
34. O'Byrne EM, Parker DT, Roberts ED, et al (1995) Oral administration of a matrix metalloprotease inhibitor, CGS 27023A, protects the cartilage proteoglycan matrix in a partial meniscectomy model of osteoarthritis in rabbits. Inflamm Res 44S:S117–S118
35. O'Byrne E, Blancuzzi V, Singh HN, et al (1995) A matrix metalloprotease (MMP) inhibitor, CGS 27023A, in animal models of osteoarthritis. World Congress on Inflammation (abstract). Inflamm Res 44S3:W10/08.
36. Harrison R, Teahan J, Stein R (1989) A semicontinuous, high-performance liquid chromatography-based assay for stromelysin. Anal Biochem 180:110–113
37. Knight CG, Willenbrock F, Murphy G (1992) A novel coumarin-labelled peptide for sensitive continuous assays of the matrix metalloproteinases. FEBS 296:263–266
38. Goldberg RL, Parker D, MacPherson L, et al (1995) Intra-articular injection of stromelysin into rabbit knees as a model to evaluate matrix metalloprotease inhibitors. Inflamm Res 44S:2:S115–S116
39. O'Byrne EM, Blancuzzi V, Wilson DE, et al (1990) Elevated substance P and accelerated cartilage degradation in rabbit knees injected with interleukin-1 and tumor necrosis factor. Arthritis Rheum 33:1023–1028
40. Goldberg RL, Kolibas LM (1990) An improved method for the determination of proteoglycans synthesized by chondrocytes in culture. Connect Tissue Res 24:265–275
41. Farnesdale RW, Sayers CA, Barrett AJ (1982) A direct spectrophotometric microassay for sulfated glycosaminoglycans in cartilage cultures. Connect Tissue Res 9:247–248
42. Thonar EJ-M, Lenz ME, Klinsworth GK, et al (1985) Quantification of keratan sulfate in blood as a marker of cartilage metabolism. Arthritis Rheum 48:1367–1376

Protein Kinase C-Activator Inhibits Progression of Osteoarthritis by Inhibiting c-Fos Protein Expression in Articular Chondrocytes

Chiaki Hamanishi, Hiroshi Miyazaki, Hiroshi Satsuma, and Seisuke Tanaka

Summary. Expression of the c-Fos protein was examined by immunohistochemistry in rat knee joints with surgically induced osteoarthritis. Cells stained for the c-Fos protein were not observed in the control knees. However, in early osteoarthritic joints, chondrocytes that expressed c-Fos protein were observed in all the articular cartilage layers on day 3 and in the residual superficial layers 2 weeks after surgery. Safranin-O staining of the matrix decreased in the superficial layers in which c-Fos-positive chondrocytes were identified. In those knee joints in which potent protein kinase C (PKC) agonist 12-o-tetradecanoylphorbol-13-acetate (TPA) was injected intraarticularly, significantly fewer histological osteoarthritic changes developed 2 and 4 weeks after surgery, and the numbers of chondrocytes that expressed c-Fos protein generally decreased and were observed mainly in the superficial layers even on day 3 and were not observed in any of the articular cartilage layers 2 and 4 weeks after surgery. Safranin-O staining was normally observed even 2 weeks after surgery. These chondroprotective effects of exogenous TPA appeared to be related to the inhibition of c-Fos protein synthesis in chondrocytes.

Key Words. Experimental Osteoarthritis, Chondrocyte, c-Fos, Protein kinase C

Introduction

The c-*fos* gene is rapidly expressed in response to various external stimuli and acts as a tertiary messenger stimulating DNA synthesis for several proteins and cytokines [1–6]. Altered mechanical forces on articular cartilage should cause increased chondrocytic c-*fos* expression in response to changes involving various receptors and second messengers. The mitogenic effects of transforming growth factor-β (TGF-β) were mediated by c-*fos* in chondrocytes [4,5] and

Department of Orthopaedic Surgery, Kinki University School of Medicine, 377-2 Ohno-Higashi, Osaka-Sayama, Osaka 589-8511, Japan osteoblasts [6]. The induction of c-*fos* was also reported to mediate the stimulative effect of basic fibroblast growth factor (bFGF) on cell proliferation by preventing the terminal differentiation of chondrocytes [7]. Although the ultimate response of chondrocytes that express c-*fos* is not clear, the in vitro evidence suggests that c-*fos* expression in chondrocytes may lead to a chondrodestructive course by degrading matrix proteoglycans and by inducing the proliferation of immature chondrocytes. Induction or suppression of c-*fos* transcription is triggered by several distinct secondary messengers. TGF-β uses protein kinase C (PKC) as a secondary messenger in cultured fibroblasts [8] and chondrocytes [5] to induce c-*fos* gene expression. Epidermal growth factor stimulation of matrix metallo proteinase (MMP-3) mRNA in rat fibroblasts requires the induction of c-*fos* and the activation of PKC [9]. The c-*fos* serum response element responds to PKC-dependent signals [8].

We recently reported that intraarticularly injected 12-*o*-tetradecanoyl-phorbol-13-acetate (TPA) markedly inhibited the progression of osteoarthritis surgically induced in rabbit knee joints [10]. PKC-dependent phosphorylation has been reported to inhibit MMP-3 [11]. PKC, therefore, is one of the secondary messengers affecting c-*fos* expression in chondrocytes also. No reports, however, have found on in vivo interaction between PKC and c-*fos* concerning the initiation and progression of osteoarthritis. In this study, osteoarthritis was induced surgically in TPA-administered and nonadministered rat knee joints, and subsequent immunohistochemical expression of the c-Fos protein in articular chondrocytes was observed periodically.

Methods

Preparation of Materials

One milligram of TPA (Sigma Chemical, St. Louis, MO, USA) was dissolved in 1.6 ml dimethyl sulfoxide (DMSO; Wako-Junyaku, Osaka, Japan) and used to make a 1-mM TPA stock solution. Aliquots of $0.8\,\mu$l of this solution containing $0.5\,\mu$g of TPA were diluted with $500\,\mu$l of physiological saline and used for intraarticular injection.

Surgically Induced Osteoarthritis

The right knees of 40 male Sprague-Dawley rats weighing 160–200 g were opened after the induction of anesthesia by the intraperitoneal injection of pentobarbital (4 mg/100 g). Using a surgical microscope, the anterior cruciate, posterior cruciate, and medial collateral ligaments were dissected. Skin incisions and capsulotomies were performed on the left knees as sham-operated controls. The rats were fed and housed under standard conditions. Four groups composed of 5 rats respectively were injected with TPA intraarticularly 3 days preoperatively and killed 3 days after surgery, or injected 3 days postoperatively and killed after 1 week, or injected on both days 3 and 10 and killed after 2 weeks, or injected on days 3, 10, 17, and 24 and killed after 4 weeks.

Preparation of Tissue Sections

Either 3 days, 1 week, 2 weeks, or 4 weeks after surgery, the rats were anesthetized and perfused through the left ventricle with 30 ml of 0.9% NaCl, followed by 200 ml of fixative containing 4% paraformaldehyde and 0.2% picric acid in 0.1 M phosphate buffer at a flow rate of 120 ml/min. Both knee joints were excised, and articular cartilage blocks were trimmed to contain a thin layer of subchondral bone. Tissue was immersed in a fixative containing 4% paraformaldehyde and 0.2% picric acid for 3 days and washed with 30% sucrose in a 0.1 M phosphate buffer for 1 day. Next, blocks were decalcified with a 5% EDTA solution for 1 week and stored in 30% sucrose in 0.1 M phosphate buffer. The tissue blocks then were frozen and serially sectioned using a cryostat in the frontal plane at a thickness of 10–15 μm.

Histological and Histochemical Grading of Articular Cartilage Lesions

The sections were stained with safranin-O, and specimens showing the most advanced cartilaginous lesions were chosen and scored by the rating system shown in Table 1, which is a modification of that described by Yoshimi et al. [12] to evaluate the experimentally induced osteoarthritis in these animals.

TABLE 1. Histological and histochemical grading of articular cartilage lesions

Structure	
Normal	0
Surface irregularities	1
Irregular and pannus formation	2
Cleft formation	3
Disorganization	4
Cell	
Normal	0
Hypercellularity	1
Cloning	2
Hyopocellularity	3
Safranin Ostaining	
Normal	0
Slight reduction	1
Moderate reduction	2
Severe reduction	3
No dye noted	4
Tidemark	
Intact	0
Crossed by blood vessels	1

Immunohistochemical Staining

The sections were preincubated in 0.3% H_2O_2 and 5% normal rabbit serum in phosphate-buffered saline (PBS) containing 0.03% Triton X-100 (PBS-T) for 30 min to block endogenous peroxidase activity and nonspecific antibody binding, respectively. The sections were subsequently incubated with a primary monoclonal antibody to c-Fos (Ab-1, $1\mu g/ml$; Oncogene Science, Cambridge, MA, USA) for 1 h. After washing with PBS-T, the sections were incubated with biotinylated rabbit antimouse IgG (Vector Laboratories, Burlingame, CA, USA) for 1 h, and then with the avidin-biotin-complex kit (Vectastain Elite, Vector) for 1 h. After three rinses, the reaction was visualized with 0.02% 3,3'-diaminobenzidine (Sigma), 0.2% nickel ammonium sulfate, and 0.005% H_2O_2 in 50 mM Tris-HCL buffer (pH 7.4).

Results

Macroscopic Observation

Sham-Operated Joints

Joint effusion, joint swelling, or rough changes on the femoral and tibial surfaces of the cartilage were not observed at 3 days, 1 week, 2 weeks, and 4 weeks after surgery.

Osteoarthritic Joints

Three days after surgery, the articular surface had normal shine and color. One week after surgery, shine of the cartilage was partially lost. Two weeks after surgery, the synovial membrane was injected and edematous, and loss of shine of the articular surface and hyperplasia of the fibrous tissue at the marginal area of the tibial plateau were observed. Four weeks after surgery, granulomatous tissue and osteophytes were observed at the marginal area of the tibial plateau. The cartilage surface was rough, especially at the center of the medial condyle.

Histological Observation

Sham-Operated Joints

The articular cartilage surfaces were smooth with normal tangential, transitional, and radial chondrocyte layers at 3 days and 2 weeks after surgery. Safranin-O staining was evenly observed in the pericellular and extracellular matrix in all layers above the tidemark.

Osteoarthritic Joints

Three days after the procedure, the articular cartilage surfaces were smooth and contained normal tangential, transitional, and radial layers of

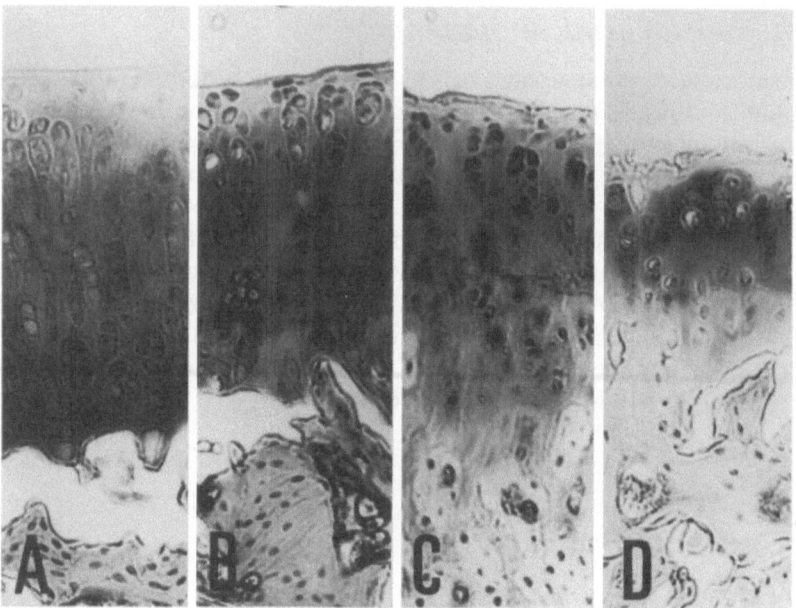

FIG. 1A–D. Safranin-O staining (×100). **A** Three days after the procedure, the articular cartilage surfaces were smooth and contained normal tangential, transitional, and radial layers of chondrocytes. The matrix generally stained less prominently with safranin-O, and normal staining was observed only in the deepest layers. **B** Osteoarthritic joints, 1 week after surgery. The articular surface showed some irregularity, and safranin-O stainability was less prominent in the superficial and middle layers. **C** Osteoarthritic joints, 2 weeks after surgery. Tangential layers were worn out, and hypocellularity and clonal proliferations of the chondrocytes in the residual transitional layers were observed. The tidemark was irregular and crossed by blood vessels. The cartilage matrix generally stained less prominently with safranin-O. **D** Osteoarthritic joints, 4 weeks after surgery. Superficial layers and half the middle layers were worn out. The tidemark was irregular, and subchondral bony trabeculae were thickened. Safranin-O stainability was observed in the residual radial layers

chondrocytes. The matrix generally stained less prominently with safranin-O, and normal staining was observed only in the deepest layers (Fig. 1A). One week after surgery, the articular surface showed some irregularity, and safranin-O stainability was less prominent in the superficial layers (Fig. 1B).

Two weeks after surgery, tangential layers were worn out, and hypocellularity and clonal proliferations of the chondrocytes in the residual transitional layers were observed. The tidemark was irregular and crossed by blood vessels. The cartilage matrix generally stained less prominently with safranin-O (Fig. 1C). Four weeks after surgery, the superficial layers and half of the middle layers were worn out. The tidemark was irregular and the subchondral bony trabeculae had thickened. Safranin-O stainability was observed in the residual radial layers (Fig. 1D).

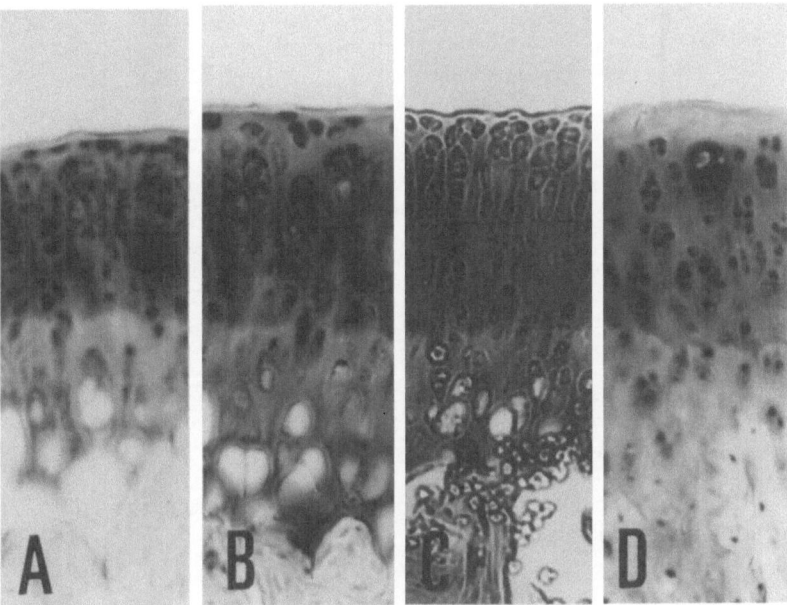

FIG. 2A–D. Safranin-O staining (×100). Osteoarthritic joints injected with TPA (12-*o*-tetradecanoylphorbol-13-acetate). **A** Three days after surgery, the cartilage matrix showed normal safranin-O staining. **B** One week after surgery, cartilage matrix showed normal safranin-O staining. **C** Two weeks after surgery, slight hypercellularity was observed. The gross histological and histochemical findings and safratin-O stainability were almost the same as those seen 1 week after surgery. **D** Four weeks after surgery, the thickness of the cartilage was still preserved. The articular surface was irregular and tangential layers were lost. Hypocellularity and clonal proliferations of the chondrocytes were observed. Matrix was less prominently stained, and the tidemark was intact

TPA-Injected Osteoarthritic Joints

At 3 days and 1 week after surgery, the cartilage matrix showed normal safranin-O staining (Fig. 2A,B). Two weeks after surgery, although slight hypercellularity was observed, the gross histological and histochemical findings and safranin-O stainability were almost the same as those 1 week after surgery (Fig. 2C). Four weeks after surgery, the thickness of the cartilage was still preserved although loss of the tangential layer, surface irregularity, hypocellularity, and clonal proliferations of the chondrocytes were observed in the less prominently stained matrix (Fig. 2D). The tidemark seemed to be intact.

Histological and Histochemical Grading of Articular Cartilage

The scores of the osteoarthritic groups were 1.2 ± 0.4 on day 3, 3.6 ± 0.5 after 1 week, 5.2 ± 0.4 after 2 weeks, and 5.6 ± 0.5 at 4 weeks after surgery, and

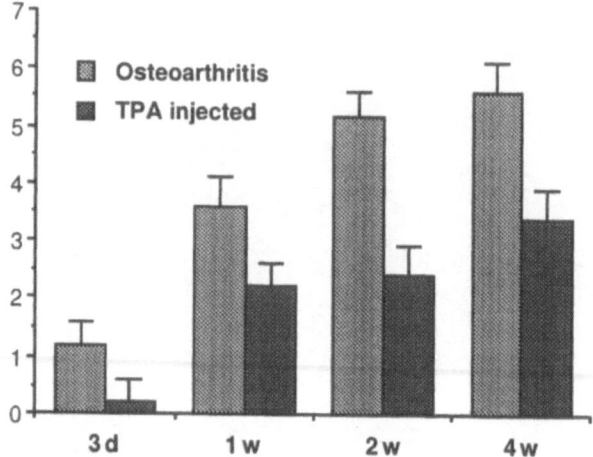

F IG. 3. Grading of articular cartilage lesions in non-TPA-injected and TPA-injected osteoarthritic rat knee joints

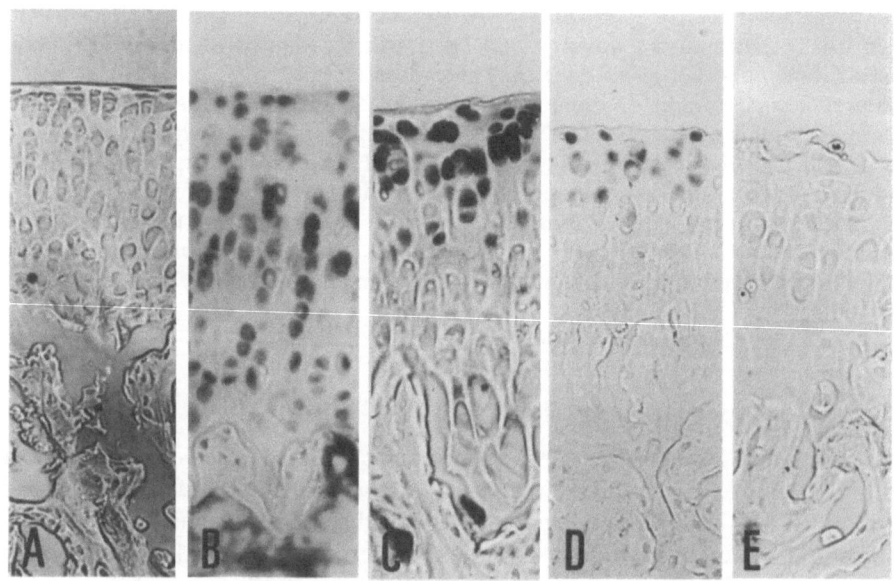

F IG. 4A–E. Immunohistochemistry for c-Fos in osteoarthritic joints (×100). **A** Two weeks after the sham operation, the chondrocytes were not stained in any cartilage layers. **B** Osteoarthritic joints, 3 days after surgery. The cytoplasm of the chondrocytes in all layers of articular cartilage including the calcified layer expressed the c-Fos protein. **C** Osteoarthritic joints, 1 week after surgery. Chondrocytes in the superficial and part of the radial layers expressed the c-Fos protein. **D** Osteoarthritic joints, 2 weeks after surgery. Only chondrocytes in the residual superficial layers showed cytoplasmic immunoreactivity. **E** Four weeks after surgery, no residual chondrocytes were immunoreactive those of TPA-injected groups were 0.2 on day 3, 2.2 ± 0.4 after 1 week, 2.4 ± 0.5 after 2 weeks, and 3.4 ± 0.5 at 4 weeks after surgery (Fig. 3). These differences were statistically significant at every time period (P values: 0.0077 on day 3, 0.0022 at 1 week after, 0.0001 at 2 weeks after, and 0.0002 at 4 weeks after surgery).

Immunohistochemistry for c-Fos

Sham-Operated Joints

The chondrocytes in all layers were not stained with anti-c-Fos antibodies 3 days or 2 weeks (Fig. 4A) after surgery.

Osteoarthritic Joints

Three days after the procedure, the nuclei and cytoplasm of the chondrocytes expressed c-Fos protein in all layers of the articular cartilage including the

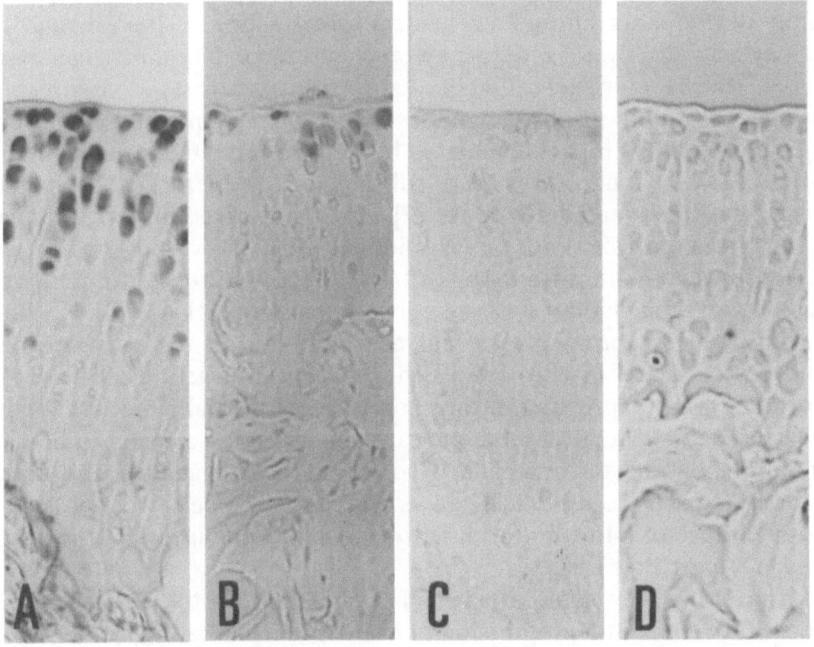

FIG. 5A–D. Immunohistochemistry for c-Fos in TPA-injected osteoarthritic joints (×100). **A** Six days after the injection of TPA and 3 days after surgery, chondrocytes in the superficial and part of the radial layers expressed the c-Fos protein. **B** One week after surgery and 4 days after the injection of TPA, the chondrocytes expressing the c-Fos protein were only observed in the most superficial layers. **C** Two weeks after surgery and 4 days and 10 days after the injections of TPA, the chondrocytes expressing the c-Fos protein were seen in hardly any of the articular cartilage layers. **D** Four weeks after surgery and 4, 10, 17, and 24 days after the injections of TPA, no chondrocytes in any layers showed c-Fos protein calcified cartilage layer (Fig. 4B). One week after surgery, chondrocytes in the superficial and part of the radial layers expressed the c-Fos protein (Fig. 4C). Two weeks after the operation, only chondrocytes in the residual superficial layers showed cytoplasmic immunoreactivity (Fig. 4D). No residual chondrocytes were immunoreactive 4 weeks after surgery (Fig. 4E).

TPA-Injected Osteoarthritic Joints

Three days after surgery, chondrocytes in the superficial and part of the radial layers expressed the c-Fos protein (Fig. 5A). One week after surgery, chondrocytes expressing the c-Fos protein were only observed in the most superficial layers (Fig. 5B). At 2 and 4 weeks after surgery, chondrocytes in all layers were not stained with anti-c-Fos antibodies (Fig. 5C,D).

Discussion

After the multiple ligament dissection, which compromises the mechanical stability of the joints, altered mechanical forces acting on the articular cartilage may activate several receptor systems and secondary messenger systems including those that trigger c-*fos* gene expression at early stages. Expression of c-*fos* and its protein product regulates cell proliferation when chondrocytes [4,5] and osteoblasts [6] are stimulated by TGF-β. Inhibited terminal differentiation of the chondrocytes and subsequent proliferation of immature chondrocytes are mediated by c-*fos* [7]. c-*fos* is involved in both stimulation and inhibition of MMP-3 gene expression [13]. The c-*fos* transfectants significantly increased their transcription of MMP-3 and suppressed transcription of aggrecan and tissue inhibitor of metalloproteinase (TIMP-1) [14]. [^{35}S]Sulfate incorporation into proteoglycan was also inhibited in the c-*fos*-transfected chondrocytes. These in vitro results suggest that destruction of the cartilage may follow c-Fos expression in the chondrocytes, partially because of stimulated degradation of matrix proteoglycans and induction of proliferation of the immature chondrocytes. In this in vivo study, the degradation and decay of the cartilage from the superficial layers after 1 and 2 weeks were preceded by the appearance of c-Fos in the chondrocytes in all the layers of the articular cartilage 3 days after surgery.

We have reported that intraarticular injections of the nonspecific PKC agonist, TPA, inhibited progression of osteoarthritis in rabbits [10]. The same chondroprotective effect of exogenous TPA was also observed in rat osteoarthritis in this study. In the TPA-injected group, the chondrocytes expressing c-Fos protein were markedly decreased in numbers and only observed in the superficial layer 3 days and 1 week after surgery, and then they were abolished from entire layers of normal-looking articular cartilage 2 weeks after surgery. The safranin-O stainability tended to decrease in the layers where c-Fos-positive chondrocytes appeared, whereas the stainability remained normal in all the layers of TPA-treated cartilage.

Using the same experimental rat osteoarthritis model, we have reported that a subspecies of calcium-independent PKC, ε-PKC, is evident in chondrocytes of the deep layers of articular cartilage, and that calcium-dependent α-PKC is newly synthesized in the superficial layers 2 weeks after surgery [15]. Exogenous TPA might activate these subspecies of PKC and stimulate production of matrix prostaglandins (PGs) through the inhibition of c-Fos expression.

Acknowledgments. This study was supported by a grant from the Ministry of Education, Science and Culture (grant-in-aid for scientific research-C, no. 07671630).

References

1. Greenberg ME, Ziff EB (1984) Stimulation of 3T3 cells induces transcription of the c-*fos* proto-oncogene. Nature (Lond) 311:433–438
2. Kruijer W, Cooper JA, Hunter T, Verma IM (1984) Platelet-derived growth factor induces rapid but transient expression of the c-*fos* gene and protein. Nature (Lond) 312:711–716
3. Raab-Cullen DM, Thiede MA, Petersen DN, Kimmel DB, Recker RR (1994) Mechanical loading stimulates rapid changes in periosteal gene expression. Calcif Tissue Int 55:473–478
4. Boumediene K, Vivien D, Macro M, Bogdanowicz P, Lebrun E, Pujol J-P (1995) Modulation of rabbit articular chondrocyte (RAC) proliferation by TGF-β isoforms. Cell Prolif 28:221–224
5. Osaki M, Tsukazaki T, Okano K, Yamasita T, Iwasaki K (1995) c-*fos* gene regulation by TGF-β in rat articular chondrocytes. Nippon Seikeigeka Gakkai Zasshi (J Jpn Orthop Assoc) 69:S1738
6. Machwate M, Jullienne A, Moukhtar M, Lomri A, Marie P (1995) c-*fos* protooncogene is involved in the mitogenic effect of transforming growth factor-β in osteoblastic cells. Mol Endocrinol 9:187–198
7. Wroblewski J, Edwall-Arvidsson C (1995) Inhibitory effects of basic fibroblast growth factor on chondrocyte differentiation. J Bone Miner Res 10:735–742
8. Gilman MZ (1988) The c-*fos* serum response element responds to protein kinase C-dependent and -independent signals but not to cyclic AMP. Genes Dev 2:394–402
9. McDonnell SE, Kerr LD, Matrisian LM (1990) Epidermal growth factor stimulation of stromelysin mRNA in rat fibroblasts requires induction of proto-oncogenes c-*fos* and c-*jun* and activation of protein kinase C. Mol Cell Bio 10:4284–4293
10. Hamanishi C, Hashima M, Satsuma H, Tanaka S (1996) Protein kinase C-activator inhibits progression of osteoarthritis induced in rabbit knee joints. J Clin Lab Med 127:540–544
11. Schmitz JP, Schwartz Z, Sylvia VL, Dean DD, Calderon F, Boyan BD (1996) Vitamin D$_3$ regulation of stromelysin-1 (MMP-3) in chondrocyte cultures is mediated by protein kinase C. J Cell Physiol 168:570–579

184 C. Hamanishi et al.

12. Yoshimi T, Kikuchi T, Obara T, et al (1994) Effects of high-molecular-weight sodium hyaluronate on experimental osteoarthrosis induced by the resection of rabbit anterior cruciate ligament. Clin Orthop Relat Res 298:296–304
13. Kerr LD, Magun BE, Matrisian LM (1992) The role of C-Fos in growth factor regulation of stromelysin/transin gene expression. Matrix 1(suppl):176–183
14. Tsuji M, Funahashi S, Takigawa M, Seiki M, Fujii K, Yoshida T (1996) Expression of c-*fos* gene inhibits proteoglycan synthesis in transfected chondrocyte. FEBS Lett 381:222–226
15. Satsuma H, Saitou N, Hamanishi C, Hashima M, Tanaka S (1996) Alpha and epsilon isozymes of protein kinase C in the chondrocytes in normal and early osteoarthritic articular cartilage. Calcif Tissue Int 58:192–194

E. Promising Treatments 2: Cartilage Repair

Articular Cartilage Repair

Ernst B. Hunziker

Summary. Partial-thickness articular cartilage defects, analogous to the clefts and fissures that characterize the early stages of human osteoarthritis, do not heal. It was the aim of our study to identify the innate limitations of this biological system, which are operative in impeding regeneration, and to establish a treatment protocol by means of which the intrinsic tissue repair potential may be triggered to induce a healing response. Superficial defects of defined dimensions, created in adult rabbits and Goettingen miniature pigs, were investigated histologically and immunohistochemically at various time intervals after surgical intervention. The absence of cartilage repair was found to be attributable to a number of factors, including poor adhesion of repair cells to the lesion surface, limited migration and proliferative capacity of repair cells, poor spatial awareness of the aforesaid repair cells, and the incapacity of these to undergo differentiation into chondrocytes. All these limitations can be overcome by instigating a single-step treatment protocol based on the following principles: enzymatic degradation of superficial proteoglycans to expose the underlying collagenous network and thereby to improve the adhesion of repair cells to native tissue; deposition of a space-filling matrix to define the defect void and hence to facilitate its population by repair cells; inclusion of a mitogenic or chemotactic factor to attract a sufficient number of repair cells into the defect void and to induce their proliferation therein; and introduction of an encapsulated tissue-transformation factor to be released as a chondrogenic switch at an appropriate juncture during the healing process. To optimize such a treatment protocol for use in the clinical setting, many technical difficulties remain to be solved: the control of cell recruitment and numerical density, an adequate matrix scaffold, bonding of the repair to parent tissue, and triggering of a homogeneously distributed chondrogenic switch. The problems, however, are not insurmountable.

Key Words. Cartilage, Superficial defects, Repair, Growth factor, Glue

---

M.E. Müller Institute for Biomechanics, University of Bern, Murtenstrasse 35, P.O. Box 30, 3010 Bern, Switzerland

187

Introduction

Synovial joints of the human skeleton fulfill several functions, which include load transmission, assurance of friction-free movement between paired skeletal elements, the distribution of forces over a broad area of cartilaginous tissue by virtue of the extensive surface contact between, and the closely contiguous contours of, the opposing skeletal components, and the minimization of peak focal stress phenomena. This latter property is attributable to the viscoelastic properties of articular cartilage tissue, operative in all functional and anatomical positions of the joint. The functions of articular cartilage tissue itself are thus primarily biomechanical in nature. However, this tissue represents but one of several components comprising the synovial joint complex; the others are the synovial membrane, the subchondral bone plate and marrow space, and the mantling ligamentous/muscular/capsular apparatus. Optimal functioning of the joint naturally depends on the concerted action of each of these structural members. Hence, endeavors to understand physiological as well as pathological processes must take into account the active interplay of these tissue components. Under the latter conditions, repair usually involves the activity of several of these.

The articular cartilage layer is nonetheless a key component, the well-regulated activity of which is vital for optimal functioning of the joint. A cursory inspection of its structural organization in adult organisms reveals a deceptively simple architecture, being composed of a mere scantling of cells (chondrocytes) embedded within an abundant extracellular matrix (Fig. 1) [1,2]. The aforesaid matrix constitutes an astounding 98% of the total tissue volume while the chondrocytes themselves represent the remaining 2%. From this circumstance, it is evident that each cell must exert metabolic control over a very large domain. This in turn immediately raises the question as to how these chondrocytes communicate with one another under physiological conditions and whether signaling over such a protracted pathway is impaired during injury and disease.

It is the extracellular matrix that is answerable for the mechanical properties of articular cartilage [3,4], albeit that its principal component is water, which accounts for approximately 70% of the tissue volume; of its organic constituents, fibrillar collagens (types II, IX, and XI) [5,6] represent the main ingredients. Nonfibrillar collagens (types IX, VI, and X) and proteoglycans [7] are also present. The latter belong principally to the chondroitin sulfate and keratan sulfate classes of these macromolecules, but a lesser proportion of the smaller ones (dermatan sulfate types) [8,9] also exists. The matrix additionally contains small quantities of diverse proteins [10,11], among which are numbered oligometric matrix protein [12], fibronectin [13], fibromodulin [14], and chondroadherin [15]; but the precise function of these latter remains largely unknown.

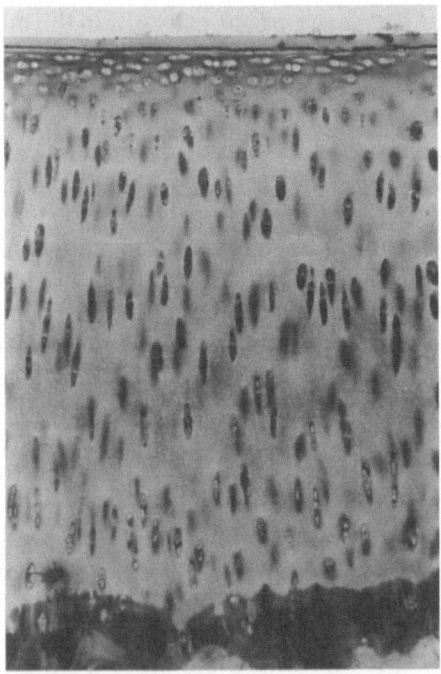

FIG. 1. Light photomicrograph of normal adult articular cartilage (Goettingen miniature pig) illustrating its highly ordered structure. In the horizontal direction, chondrocytes are organized into distinct strata (superficial layer, transitional layer, upper and lower radial zones); in the vertical one, they form radial stacks in the upper and lower radial zones. In this species, cells occupy a mere 8% of the tissue volume, the bulk of which consists of intercellular matrix (approximately 92%). Thick (150-μm) section stained with McNeil's tetrachrome, toluidine blue O, and acid fuchsin

When an appropriately stained longitudinal section through articular cartilage tissue is examined with the light microscope, one is immediately struck by the highly anisotropic organization of both its cells and matrix (Fig. 1). There exists a distinct horizontal stratification, which reflects the grouping of chondrocytes of like morphology into successive layers, known as the superficial, transitional, radial, and calcified cartilage zones; the latter interdigitates with the subchondral bone plate [1,16]. Chondrocytes within each layer are characterized by a distinctive size, profile, and orientation in space. There exists a gradient of increasing cell size from the superficial to the radial zone [2]. Chondrocytes in the former are flat and elliptical in shape, with their long axis orientated parallel to the cartilage surface, whereas those in the latter assume the form of oblate spheroids, their long axis being orientated perpendicular to the articular cartilage surface; cells within the interposed transitional zone have a roundish profile.

Electron microscopic analysis of articular cartilage tissue corroborates and extends these anisotropic structural principles at the macromolecular level. Collagen fibrils of the articular cartilage matrix follow a highly characteristic course: in the superficial zone they form a network running in a predominantly parallel direction relative to the tissue surface [17]; those in the underlying transitional zone are arranged in an arcade-like manner, and in the remaining ones (down to the level of the subchondral bone) they are disposed perpendicular to the articular cartilage surface [18,19]. These fibrils manifest a gradient of increasing caliber from the superficial to the deep radial zone, the difference in girth spanned from the finest to the coarsest being of the order of approximately tenfold [20]. This zone-specific fibril architecture [21] is confined to the matrix compartment furthest removed from individual chondrocytes, namely, the interterritorium, which constitutes approximately 95% of the entire cartilage matrix volume [1].

In the region immediately surrounding single cells (pericellular matrix) and groups of chondrocytes (territorium) (which together represent 2%–3% of the matrix volume), fibrils form a basket-like arrangement [22,23]. Cryotechnical tissue processing has recently revealed a network of filamentous structures, probably collagenous in nature, which are present within all matrix compartments [24–26]. The interstices of the entire fibrillar meshwork are filled with proteoglycans at an exceedingly high concentration (approximately 100 mg/ml) [27] and in an underhydrated state; in association with these macromolecules a very high density of fixed negative charges is present in the cartilage matrix. During deformation or loading of articular cartilage, the interplay among tissue components—water flow, free ions, and fixed charges (streaming potentials)—, as well as osmotic phenomena, play key roles in determining its mechanical properties [3,4,28]. The matrix of adult articular cartilage contains neither blood vessels, lymphatics, nor neural components, which circumstance has an important bearing on this tissue's very limited capacity to undergo repair [29,30].

The highly anisotropic organization of adult articular cartilage is, of course, not merely fortuitous; it is indeed of considerable importance in optimizing the mechanical properties of this tissue, both the confined (aggregate modulus) and unconfined (Young's modulus) stiffness of mature anisotropic tissue being much greater than those of the immature isotropic one [31,32]. Hence, any attempts to induce cartilage repair should aim at reestablishing optimal structural organization at both cellular and molecular levels. Unless this is achieved, the mechanical competence of the repair tissue will always fall short of that of native articular cartilage. There will be, moreover, an abrupt change in this property at the interface between the former and the latter.

The intrinsic capacity of articular cartilage to repair structural lesions appearing within its substance is extremely limited; unfortunately, such defects are all too common. They frequently occur in active young individuals as a result of trauma following professional injuries or sports accidents and in older persons during the course of diseases such as osteoarthritis; this latter is a severely debilitating condition which affects aged individuals in all populations [33–35]. The development of a suitable treatment strategy, truly effective in restoring the structural and functional integrity of articular cartilage following trauma or in disease states, would thus have far-reaching consequences.

It was the aim of our own studies to determine the "critical size" of an articular cartilage lesion, that is, the dimensional limits beyond which a defect fails to heal spontaneously; to ascertain the nature of the intrinsic limitations that undermine this tissue's capacity to undergo spontaneous repair, and by so doing, to delineate a treatment protocol whereby these limitations may be overcome.

Materials and Methods

Critical-Size Defects

Our aim was to define the range of critical-size defects in the mature articular cartilage of adult Goettingen miniature pigs. Nonpenetrating lesions were created in the patellar groove of the stifle joint in 5 groups of animals, the width of the defect being increased in 25-μm increments between the second (width, 25μm) and the fifth (width, 100μm) group; in the first, mere scalpel splits were produced. All lesions were then rinsed briefly to remove tissue remnants from their void. They were left untreated, and analyzed either 1 or 3 months after surgery by histological, stereological, and electron micro-scopical means (unpublished data).

Biological Limitations of Repair

To ascertain the nature of the intrinsic limitations undermining spontaneous repair, we set up a small, superficial defect model in mature rabbits or mature miniature pigs. A custom-built planing instrument was developed to create lesions of specific dimensions in each animal model: 1 mm (width) $\times$ 0.2 mm (depth) in rabbits and 0.5 mm (width) $\times$ 0.5 mm (depth) in miniature pigs. Defect length was controlled by the surgeon to lie within the range 8–10 mm [29,36].

Our initial premise in undertaking this investigation was that cells recruited to the defect site fail to gain a foothold and establish themselves therein owing to the anti-cell-adhesive properties of the cartilage tissue forming the lesion walls [29,30]. The series of experiments thereby set in train revealed this to be but one of the impediments to repair. Indeed, it became abundantly clear that multifarious and interconnected factors were involved, and that a systematic, stepwise analysis of these was absolutely essential before we could hope to invoke an enduring healing response within articular cartilage defects. We embarked upon this course of study about 10 years ago, and it is only recently that we have been in a position to forward our findings with confidence [29,30,37; Hunziker, manuscript submitted for publication]. A summary of the intrinsic biological factors elucidated and of the measures taken to overcome these follows.

Poor Adhesion of Potential Repair Cells

The defect surface was treated with chondroitinase avidin-biotin-peroxidase complex (ABC) or trypsin to remove the superficial layer of proteoglycans, which are known to have anti-cell-adhesive properties. By so doing, the underlying collagenous network would be exposed and the adhesion of potential repair cells thereby facilitated [36,38].

Poor Recruitment and Proliferation of Potential Repair Cells

Mitogenic or chemotactic growth factors, such as insulin-like growth factor (IGF-1), epidermal growth factor (EGF), basic fibroblast growth factor (bFGF), and transforming growth factor-β (TGF-β), were administered topically at low levels of activity in an endeavor to improve cell coverage of the defect surfaces and to promote filling of the lesion void [29].

Poor Spatial Awareness of the Repair Cell Population

A space-filling biodegradable matrix (such as fibrin, gelatin, or collagen) was introduced into the defect void to furnish a scaffolding for its invasion by repair cells [29].

Chemotactic Attraction of Potential Repair Cells to, and Mitogenic Stimulation of Resident Cells within, the Space-Filling Matrix

A chemotactic or mitogenic growth factor was incorporated into the biodegradable matrix to enhance the population density of repair cells therein.

Poor Capacity of Repair Cells to Differentiate into Chondrocytes

A liposome-encapsulated differentiation factor (such as TGF-β), at a high activity level, was introduced into the space-filling matrix which the invading mesenchymal type of repair cells started to remodel, thereby causing its release and promoting cell transformation into chondrocytes [30; Hunziker, manuscript submitted for publication].

Improvement of Integration between Repair and Native Tissue

The usefulness of a biological glue (tissue transglutaminase) [37] to act in this capacity was tested.

Results and Discussion

It has been often reported in the literature that only full-thickness defects, that is, those which penetrate the subchondral bone plate, undergo spontaneous repair. In these cases, the lesion makes an inroad into the marrow space; bleeding into its void ensues, and first a hematoma and then a blood clot forms within. The latter becomes invaded by blood vessels and mesenchymal cells, and the primitive type of repair tissue initially laid down subsequently transforms into fibrous cartilage and bone [39–42]. Such spontaneous repair responses have been well characterized in rabbits, dogs, and other animal models. The mechanical properties of the fibrous cartilage formed have never been found to attain physiological competence [43,44]. With respect to its biochemical composition, type I collagen fibrils, in particular, persist throughout the entire course of the observation period. The stiffness of this repair tissue is also unsatisfactory, and its permeability compared to that of normal articular cartilage significantly increased. It is, moreover, unstable; in the rabbit model, proteoglycan loss and degeneration have been observed to occur after 6 months in virtually all cases [40,42]. Experimental findings pertaining to this spontaneous repair model are thus by no means encouraging; even so, it still forms the rationale behind a number of empirical surgical approaches (e.g., abrasive chondroplasty, Bridie drillhole formation, and the microfracturing protocol) adopted to treat osteoarthritic conditions [45].

The poor outcome of the spontaneous repair response [29,46,47] may have been one of the reasons why such a large number of empirical approaches have been developed for the induction of healing since the end of the last century. These are largely based on transplantation concepts, utilizing cartilage-bone cylinders [48–52], cartilage tissue itself, and periosteal or perichondrial flaps, to name but a few [53–56]. The idea of introducing chondrocytes or mesenchymal stem cells (Fig. 2) embedded within a space-filling matrix into the defect void—in an endeavor to promote the formation of a more stable cartilage-like tissue with enduring functional properties—has attracted considerable attention in recent years, and the progress thus far made is quite encouraging [57].

Defects that are confined to the substance of articular cartilage itself (i.e., partial-thickness or superficial lesions) fail to undergo anything more than an abortive spontaneous repair response, at best. Our own experiments were restricted to the investigation of such defects, and our data consistently confirmed this previous observation. This finding prompted us to ascertain whether there exists for cartilage tissue something like the critical-size defect that has been well characterized in the field of bone repair. To this end, we created exceedingly narrow partial-thickness lesions, down to a width of a mere 25 μm. Even though such tiny defects lay within the size range of a single chondrocyte, these gaps were not bridged by cells from the adjacent native tissue or by matrix material, and no substantial repair response was set in train.

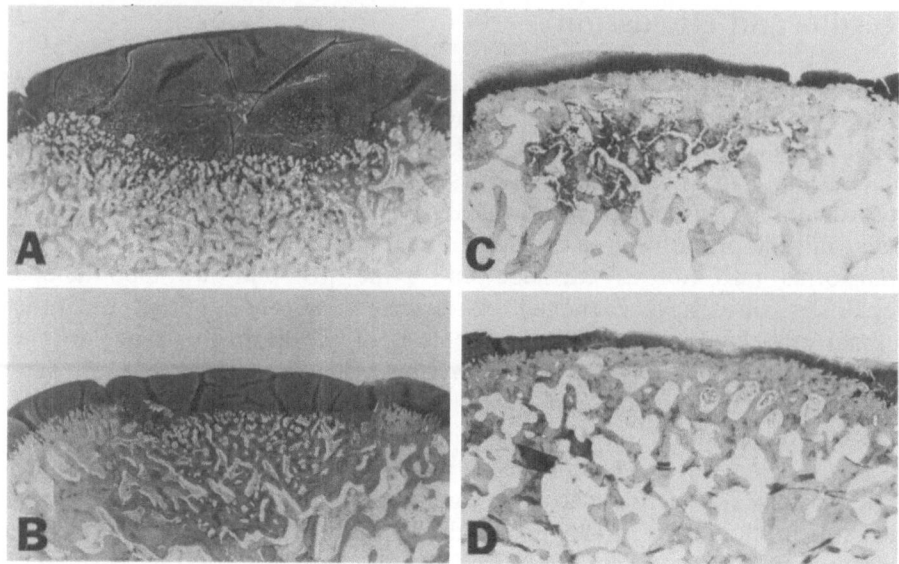

Fig. 2A–D. Light photomicrographs illustrating the characteristics of repair tissue filling full-thickness defects 2 weeks (**A**), 4 weeks (**B**), 12 weeks (**C**), and 24 weeks (**D**) after implantation of bone-marrow-derived mesenchymal stem cells in a collagen gel. (From [57], with permission)

75% of the lesion volume remained completely devoid of repair cells or tissue of any description and contained only remnants of cartilage chipped off during surgery; the remaining 25% of the defect volume became filled with a mesenchymal type of repair tissue, probably of synovial origin (unpublished data). These disappointing results prompted us to examine the consequences of producing mere slits in the articular cartilage tissue, effected with a fine diamond scalpel, but even in these instances healing did not occur.

We then undertook a systematic investigation to elucidate the reasons for this absence of spontaneous repair in superficial defects [29]. Detailed histological analysis revealed that native tissue in the immediate vicinity of such lesions was not completely devoid of cell activity. In these regions, a limited degree of chondrocyte proliferation was evidenced by the presence of cell clusters, which may have been indicative of an abortive repair response. However, even in the smallest defects, this process, if extant, never led to healing. Indeed, these focal proliferations occurred only sporadically; in no instance were they observed around the entire defect periphery. Careful inspection of the corners of such superficial defects, or of the microgrooves inadvertently created in the walls of these during surgery, revealed the presence of small groups of mesenchymal-like cells which had become established therein and laid down a fibrous type of connective tissue. The presence even of such small numbers of nonchondrocytic repair cells indicated that these lesions are accessible to an extrinsic source of these, which were probably transported within the synovial fluid and thus most likely originated from the synovial membrane or subsynovial spaces.

One of the reasons why so few cells became lodged within the superficial defects may be that their adherence therein was inhibited by the intrinsic properties of the cartilage matrix itself [36,38]. The aforesaid matrix is very rich in proteoglycans and aggrecans which are well known to have anti-cell-adhesive properties. We therefore hypothesized that superficial removal of such molecules from the defect surface (down to a depth of approximately 1μm) by brief enzymatic degradation would, by exposing the underlying network of collagen fibrils, promote the adhesion of repair cells (Fig. 3). Such was found to be the case: coverage of the defect surface could be increased by up to 54% 1 month after surgery [36]. However, this effect was only transient; by the third month, the degree of coverage had reverted to that manifested in nonenzymatically treated controls. Although not useful as a means of establishing a successful repair response, such a measure may prove to be beneficial in promoting adhesion of an extrinsic matrix deposited within the defect space. Indeed, recent experiments conducted in vitro using the biological glue, tissue transglutaminase, have shown that such an enzymatic step may be useful in this capacity [37]. Hence, although a long-term potentiation of tissue adhesiveness is clearly not achievable, probably owing to the reestablishment of the original proteoglycan population by underlying cell activity, enzymatic degradation of a superficial layer of these macromolecules may be a useful initial step in treatment protocols involving the deposition of a matrix.

Although coverage of the defect surface by repair cells could be enhanced temporarily by enzymatic degradation of matrix proteoglycans, even at the 1-month stage the lining was incomplete, and cells failed to spread into the lesion void. Their spontaneous proliferative activity is thus very low. We therefore investigated the effects of introducing a mitogenic growth factor into the defect space. A number of such substances that have been shown in vitro to have mitogenic or chemotactic activities were tested, that is, TGF-β (4ng/ml), IGF-1 (40ng/ml), bFGF (10ng/ml), and EGF (20ng/ml). Each of these substances significantly improved the coverage of defect surfaces by repair cells (Fig. 3), and in most instances, the lining was complete. Indeed, not only mono- but also bi- and sometimes even multilayers of mesenchymal-like repair cells were built up. Unfortunately, however, inward growth proceeded no further than this. And although these cells laid down a narrow sheet of connective tissue along the lesion wall, this did not transform into cartilage (Fig. 3). This result points to another intrinsic limitation undermining spontaneous repair; namely, that repair cells recruited into the defect area have a very limited spatial awareness. This is, perhaps, not surprising given their mesodermal origin. In epithelia or epithelial-like tissue (such as skin or liver), which contain cells of ectodermal origin, the situation is quite different; in these, lesions may become more or less completely obliterated by repair tissue.

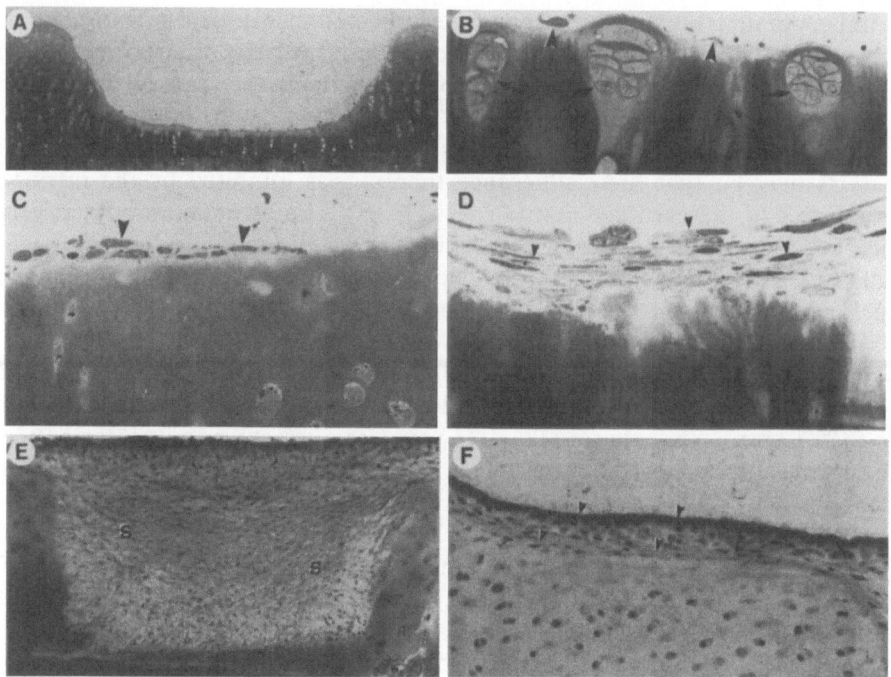

Fig. 3A–F. Light photomicrographs of superficial articular cartilage defects, 4 weeks after creation in mature rabbits (**A–D**) and miniature pigs (**E,F**). When left untreated, such lesions do not heal (**A,B**). A few mesenchymal cells may occur sporadically along the defect surface (*arrowheads* in **B**), and within the native tissue, some proliferating chondrocyte clusters may be observed (*arrows* in **B**). After controlled removal of cartilage matrix proteoglycan molecules by enzymatic digestion with chondroitinase ABC, adhesion of repair cells to the lesion surface is improved (*arrowheads* in **C**), but filling of the defect void is not achieved. Addition of the mitogenic factor, insulin-like growth factor (IGF-I) (**D**), to chondroitinase ABC-treated defects elicits the formation of mesenchymal cell multilayers (*arrowheads* in **D**), which lay down a fibrous connective tissue, but the defect space is still not completely filled. Deposition of a space-filling biodegradable matrix (**E**), such as fibrin, and concomitant application of a chemotactic/mitogenic growth factor, such as TGF-β, leads to complete filling of the lesion volume with a primitive type of scar tissue (*S* in **E**). Mesenchymal cells appear to be chemotactically attracted from the synovial and subsynovial tissue compartment, as evidenced by the migrating cell tracks (*arrowheads* in **F**) located along the normal articular cartilage surface [29]. **A–D**, semithin sections, stained with toluidine blue O; **E,F**, thick, surface-polished saw cuts, stained with McNeil's tetrachrome, toluidine blue O, and acid fuchsin

It thus became clear that the entire defect void needed to be defined by an appropriate space-filling matrix. This matrix must fulfill certain requirements: it should be porous, so that cells can migrate freely into and within it, its internal supporting framework should be of such a nature as to facilitate cell adhesion, and it should preferably be biodegradable. We chose fibrin. This matrix, when deposited within superficial defects, became populated with repair cells throughout its volume, albeit at low numerical density. The cells spontaneously remodeled the fibrin and laid down a loose, avascular connective tissue which occupied the entire void. The numerical density of cells could be increased by introducing a mitogenic factor (TGF-β or IGF-1), at low concentration, together with the fibrin matrix.

Fibrin is not, however, the ideal choice for use in cartilage repair, because clot retraction occurs during the polymerization of fibrinogen, and matrices thus shrank to approximately 58% of their original extent. Hence, defect-filling to the extent of 58% in our experimental model would represent a success rate of 100% [Hunziker, manuscript submitted for publication]. This does not, of course, mitigate the retraction problem itself, which is a serious one, as it sets up conditions of instability and hence lessens the chances of achieving a good integration between repair and native tissue from the outset. Even when tissue adhesiveness was enhanced by enzymatic degradation of superficial proteoglycans, loss of fibrin matrices occurred in 12% of cases [Hunziker, manuscript submitted for publication].

The loose connective tissue laid down within the fibrin-filled defects persisted up to the end of the observation period, 1 year, but in no instance did it transform into cartilage. The mesenchymal-like repair cells thus lack the capacity to differentiate spontaneously into chondrocytes. Although it became clear that we needed to introduce a chondrogenic factor into the matrix, it is not so easy to achieve the desired result. Such factors, for example, TGF-β, which act in this capacity at high concentration, are none other than those which, at low concentration, act mitogenically or chemotactically. Hence, they must become available only after the peak phase of cell proliferation has passed.

In our initial attempt, we simply injected TGF-β at high concentration (500 ng/ml) into the joint cavity at the time when we deemed that it would be required. However, intra-articular application of such a potent growth factor immediately precipitated adverse effects, such as joint effusion, synovial inflammation, and osteophyte formation, and we had to terminate our experiments. Obviously, then, TGF-β needed to be incorporated into the deposited matrix, so as to assure only a very local action, but it nevertheless had to be introduced in such a form that it would become available at high activity only after the peak proliferative phase had passed. To this end, we encapsulated TGF-β at high concentration within liposomes, which were introduced together with the fibrin matrix. By so doing, the desired chondrogenic switch was triggered: a cartilage-like tissue was formed (Fig. 4) [Hunziker, manuscript submitted for publication].

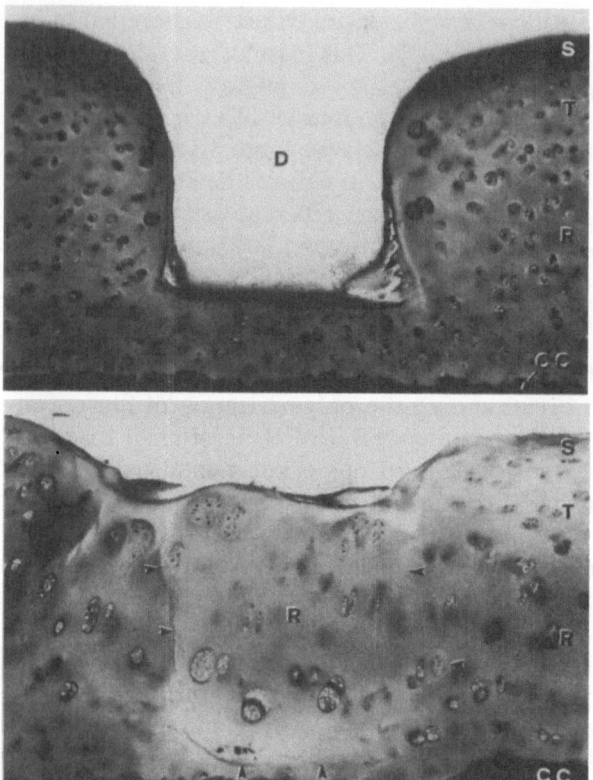

FIG. 4. Partial-thickness articular cartilage defect, 6 weeks after creation in miniature pig knee joints. *Top*: Control defect (*D*), no treatment; absence of a healing response. *Bottom*: Application of a space-filling, biodegradable matrix containing TGF-β at low concentration, to act as a chemotactic/mitogenic factor, and at high concentration, in a liposome-encapsulated form, to promote tissue differentiation by its timely release (Hunziker, manuscript submitted for publication), elicits the formation of a cartilage-like repair tissue. *Arrowheads*, original defect edges; *S*, superficial layer; *T*, transitional layer; *R*, radial zone; *CC*, calcified cartilage. Thick, polished saw cuts, surface-stained with McNeil's tetrachrome, toluidine blue O, and acid fuchsin

Our investigation has thus delineated the principles of a protocol that could be instigated for the induction of repair in partial-thickness defects. Most importantly, our findings reveal that a joint-intrinsic repair reaction can be set in train without having recourse to the transplantation of cells or tissue. Although the results look promising, it should nonetheless be borne in mind that our system needs to be optimized and placed on a firm, reproducible basis before it can be considered for clinical use.

One of several unresolved problems relates to the presence of microcracks between repair and native tissue. It was this circumstance that prompted us to further explore the possibility of improving adhesion of the fibrin matrix to the walls of the defect. The biological glue, tissue transglutaminase, is a potential candidate [37]. This enzyme is present physiologically in most tissues of the body, above all in the skin, but also in differentiated cartilage tissues. It induces the formation of stable isopeptide bonds between proteins, thereby leading to the formation of stable interproteinacious networks. We undertook a series of in vitro experiments to test the efficacy of this enzyme to act as a biological adhesive by using it to glue together two apposing cylinders of cartilage under well-defined conditions. When employed at 1 U/ml, tissue transglutaminase had a gluing effect similar to that achievable using a commercially available fibrin adhesive. Furthermore, the gluing effect, measured as a function of the maximal shear force required to displace one cartilage cylinder from the other, increased linearly with increasing concentrations of the enzyme.

In summary, defects restricted to the substance of articular cartilage tissue do not heal spontaneously. This circumstance is attributable to a number of factors, including poor adhesion of repair cells to the lesion surface, limited migration and proliferative capacity of repair cells, poor spatial awareness of the aforesaid repair cells, and the incapacity of these to undergo differentiation into chondrocytes. All these limitations can be overcome by instigating a single-step treatment protocol based on the following principles: enzymatic degradation of superficial proteoglycans to expose the underlying collagenous network and thereby to improve the adhesion of repair cells to native tissue; deposition of a space-filling matrix to define the defect void and hence to facilitate its population by repair cells; inclusion of a mitogenic or chemotactic factor to attract a sufficient number of repair cells into the defect void and to induce their proliferation therein; and introduction of an encapsulated tissue-transformation factor to be released as a chondrogenic switch at an appropriate juncture during the healing process.

To optimize such a treatment protocol for use in the clinical situation, many technical difficulties remain to be solved: the control of cell recruitment and numerical density, and the triggering of a homogeneously distributed chondrogenic switch. Perhaps the major unsolved problem relates to the choice of an appropriate matrix, which should adhere well to the defect surface, have an adequate porosity to permit cell infiltration, and furnish a surface to which cells may readily adhere; it should also be biologically degradable, deformable, and resistant to swelling/shrinking during the early stages of repair. We thus still have much to achieve. The problems, however, are not insurmountable, and I think we may be sanguine about the future of articular cartilage repair.

Acknowledgment. The author thanks Prof. Tanaka and Dr. Hamanishi for their kind invitation to participate in the International Symposium "Advance in Osteoarthritis" held on October 2, 1997, at Kobe, Japan. This article is based on the presentation given at the aforesaid meeting.

References

1. Hunziker EB (1992) Articular cartilage structure in humans and experimental animals. In: Kuettner KE, Schleyerbach R, Peyron JG, Hascall VC (eds) Articular cartilage and osteoarthritis. Raven, New York, pp 183–199
2. Eggli PS, Hunziker EB, Schenk RK (1988) Quantitation of structural features characterizing weight- and less-weight-bearing regions in articular cartilage: a stereological analysis of medial femoral condyles in young adult rabbits. Anat Rec 222(3):217–227
3. Grodzinsky AJ, Frank EH (1990) Electromechanical and physicochemical regulation of cartilage strength and metabolism. In: Hukins DWL (ed) Connective tissue matrix. Macmillan, London, pp 91–126
4. Grodzinsky AJ, Kim YJ, Buschmann MD, Garcia ML, Hunziker EB (1998) Response of the chondrocyte to mechanical stimuli. In: Lohmander, Brandt, Doherty (eds) Osteoarthritis. Oxford University Press, Oxford (in press)
5. Bruckner P, van der Rest M (1994) Structure and function of cartilage collagens. Microsc Res Technique 28(5):378–384
6. van der Rest M, Dublet B (1996) Type XII and type XIV collagens: interfibrillar constituents of dense connective tissues. Semin Cell Dev Biol 7(5):639–648
7. Hardingham TE, Fosang AJ (1995) The structure of aggrecan and its turnover in cartilage. J Rheumatol 22(suppl 43):86–90
8. Kresse H, Hausser H, Schonherr E (1993) Small proteoglycans. Experientia (Basel) 49(5):403–416
9. Stanescu V (1990) The small proteoglycans of cartilage matrix. Semin Arthritis Rheum 20(3 suppl 1):51–64
10. Heinegard D, Oldberg A (1989) Structure and biology of cartilage and bone matrix noncollagenous macromolecules. FASEB J 3(9):2042–2051
11. Roughley PJ, Lee ER (1994) Cartilage proteoglycans: structure and potential functions. Microsc Res Technique 28(5):385–397
12. Oldberg A, Antonsson P, Lindblom K, Heinegard D (1992) COMP (cartilage oligomeric matrix protein) is structurally related to the thrombospondins. J Biol Chem 267(31):22346–22350
13. Jasin HE (1995) Structure and function of the articular cartilage surface. Scand J Rheumatol Suppl 101:51–55
14. Hedlund H, Mengarelliwidholm S, Heinegard D, Reinholt FP, Svensson O (1994) Fibromodulin distribution and association with collagen. Matrix Biol 14(3):227–232
15. Neame PJ, Sommarin Y, Boynton RE, Heinegard D (1994) The structure of a 38-kDa leucine-rich protein (chondroadherin) isolated from bovine cartilage. J Biol Chem 269(34):21547–21554
16. Stockwell RA (ed) (1979) Biology of cartilage cells. Cambridge University Press, Cambridge
17. Jurvelin JS, Muller DJ, Wong M, Studer D, Engel A, Hunziker EB (1996) Surface and subsurface morphology of bovine humeral articular cartilage as assessed by atomic force and transmission electron microscopy. J Struct Biol 117(1):45–54
18. Benninghoff A (1922) Ueber den funktionellen Bau des Knorpels. Anat Anz Ergeb Heft 55:250–267
19. Benninghoff A (1925) Form und Bau der Gelenkknorpel in ihren Beziehungen zur Funktion. II. Der Aufbau des Gelenknorpels in seinen Beziehungen zur Funktion. Z Zellforsch Mikrosk Anat 2:783–862

20. Hedlund H, Mengarelli Widholm S, Reinholt FP, Svensson O (1993) Stereologic studies on collagen in bovine articular cartilage. APMIS 101(2):133–140

21. Clark JM (1985) The organization of collagen in cryofractured rabbit articular cartilage: a scanning electron microscopic study. J Orthop Res 3(1):17–29

22. Szirmai JA (1963) Quantitative approaches in the histochemistry of mucopoly-saccharides. J Histochem Cytochem 11(1):24–34

23. Szirmai JA (1969) Structure of cartilage. In: Engel A, Larsson T (eds) Thule international symposium on aging of connective and skeletal tissue. Nordiska Boekhandelns, Stockholm, pp 163–184

24. Hunziker EB, Wagner J, Studer D (1996) Vitrified articular cartilage reveals novel ultrastructural features respecting extracellular matrix architecture. Histochem Cell Biol 106(4):375–382

25. Studer D, Chiquet M, Hunziker EB (1996) Evidence for a distinct water-rich layer surrounding collagen fibrils in articular cartilage extracellular matrix. J Struct Biol 117(2):81–85

26. Hunziker EB, Michel M, Studer D (1997) Ultrastructure of adult human articular cartilage matrix after cryotechnical processing. Microsc Res Technique 37(4):271–284

27. Hascall VC (1977) Interactions of cartilage proteoglycans with hyaluronic acid. J Supramol Struct 7:101–120

28. Grodzinsky AJ (1983) Electromechanical and physicochemical properties of connective tissue. Crit Rev Biomed Eng 9(2):133–199

29. Hunziker EB, Rosenberg LC (1996) Repair of partial-thickness articular cartilage defects. Cell recruitment from the synovium. J Bone Joint Surg 78A(5):721–733

30. Hunziker EB, Rosenberg LC (1997) Articular cartilage repair. In: McCarty DJ, Koopman WJ (eds) Arthritis and allied conditions—a textbook of rheumatology. Lea & Febiger, Philadelphia, pp 2027–2038

31. Wong M, Wuethrich P, Eggli P, Hunziker E (1996) Zone-specific cell biosynthetic activity in mature bovine articular cartilage: a new method using confocal micro-scopic stereology and quantitative autoradiography. J Orthop Res 14(3):424–432

32. Wong M, Wuethrich P, Buschmann MD, Eggli P, Hunziker E (1997) Chondrocyte biosynthesis correlates with local tissue strain in statically compressed adult articu-lar cartilage. J Orthop Res 15(2):189–196

33. Howell DS (1986) Pathogenesis of osteoarthritis. Am J Med 80(4B):24–28

34. Hamerman D (1989) The biology of osteoarthritis. N Engl J Med 320(20):1322–1330

35. Kraus VB (1997) Pathogenesis and treatment of osteoarthritis. Med Clin North Am 81(1):85

36. Hunziker EB, Kapfinger E (1998) Removal of proteoglycans from the surfaces of articular cartilage defects promotes adhesion of repair cells. J Bone Joint Surg

37. Jürgensen K, Aeschlimann D, Cavin V, Genge M, Hunziker EB (1997) A new biological glue for cartilage-cartilage interfaces: tissue transglutaminase. J Bone Joint Surg 79A(2):185–193

38. Rosenberg L, Hunziker EB (1995) Cartilage repair in osteoarthritis. The role of the dermatan sulfate proteoglycans. In: Kuettner KE, Goldberg VM (eds) Osteoarthritic disorders. American Academy of Orthopaedic Surgeons, Monterey, CA, pp 341–356

39. Mankin HJ (1974) The reaction of articular cartilage to injury and osteoarthritis (first of two parts). N Engl J Med 291(24):1285–1292

40. Altman RD, Kates J, Chun LE, Dean DD, Eyre D (1992) Preliminary observations of chondral abrasion in a canine model. Ann Rheum Dis 51(9):1056–1062
41. Mitchell N, Shepard N (1976) The resurfacing of adult rabbit articular cartilage by multiple perforations through the subchondral bone. J Bone Joint Surg (Am Vol) 58(2):230–233
42. Shapiro F, Koide S, Glimcher MJ (1993) Cell origin and differentiation in the repair of full-thickness defects of articular cartilage. J Bone Joint Surg (Am Vol) 75(4):532–553
43. Furukawa T, Koide S, Eyre DR, Glimcher MJ (eds) (1979) The biochemical properties of repair articular cartilage induced surgically in the rabbit knee. In: Transactions of the 25th annual meeting of the Orthopaedic Research Society. Orthopaedic Research Society, pp 134–134
44. Furukawa T, Eyre DR, Koide S, Glimcher MJ (1980) Biochemical studies on repair cartilage resurfacing experimental defects in the rabbit knee. J Bone Joint Surg 62A(1):79–89
45. Hunziker EB (1998) Articular cartilage repair: are the intrinsic biological constraints undermining repair insuperable? Osteoarthritis and Cartilage (in press)
46. Mankin HJ (1962) Localization of tritiated thymidine in articular cartilage of rabbits. I. Growth in immature cartilage. J Bone Joint Surg 44A(4):682–688
47. Meachim G (1963) The effect of scarification on articular cartilage in the rabbit. J Bone Joint Surg 45B:150–161
48. Axhausen G (1909) Die histologischen und klinischen Gesetze der freien Osteoplastik auf Grund von Tierversuchen. Arch Klin Chir 99:13, 23–145, 286
49. Beresford WA (1981) Chondroid bone, secondary cartilage and metaplasia. Urban & Schwarzenburg, Baltimore-Münich, pp 1–88
50. Buckwalter JA, Rosenberg LC, Coutts RD, Hunziker EB, Reddi AH, Mow V (1987) Articular cartilage: injury and repair. In: Woo SLY, Buckwalter JA (eds) Injury and repair of the musculoskeletal soft tissues. American Academy of Orthopaedic Surgeons, Park Ridge, NJ, pp 465–482
51. Buckwalter JA, Mankin HJ (1997) Articular cartilage. 2: Degeneration and osteoarthritis, repair, regeneration, and transplantation. J Bone Joint Surg 79A(4):612–632
52. Brent B (1992) Auricular repair with autogenous rib cartilage grafts—two decades of experience with 600 cases. Plast Reconstr Surg 90(3):355–374
53. Engkvist O, Wilander E (1979) Formation of cartilage from rib perichondrium grafted to an articular defect in the femur condyle of the rabbit. Scand J Plast Reconstr Surg 13(3):371–376
54. Ohlsen L (1976) Cartilage formation from free perichondrial grafts: an experimental study in rabbits. Br J Plast Surg 29(3):262–267
55. Skoog T, Ohlsen L, Sohn SA (1972) Perichondral potential for cartilagenous regeneration. Scand J Plast Reconstr Surg 6:123–125
56. Skoog T, Ohlsen L, Sohn SA (1975) The chondrogenic potential of the perichondrium. Chir Plast (Berl) 3:91–103
57. Wakitani S, Goto T, Pineda SJ, Young RG, Mansour JM, Caplan AI, Goldberg VM (1994) Mesenchymal cell-based repair of large, full-thickness defects of articular cartilage. J Bone Joint Surg 76A(4):579–592

Knee Washout for Osteoarthritis

Richard H. Edelson

Summary. Twenty-nine knees in 23 patients with symptomatic osteoarthritis refractory to treatment with medication underwent washout with lactated Ringer's solution made hypertonic with mannitol. Two arthroscopic cannulas were placed under local anesthesia into the knee. Three liters of fluid were run through the knee, varying inflow and outflow to alternately inflate and deflate the knee. Following washout, patients were injected intraarticularly with hyaluronic acid or placebo; patients were blinded as to which injection they received. Patient were followed prospectively with Hospital for Special Surgery (HSS) knee scores, Knee Society (KS) pain and function ratings, visual analog pain scales, and physical examination obtained before and up to 2 years afterwashout. At 1 year, the mean HSS score increased from 72 to 87, KS pain rating from 64 to 89, and KS function from 62 to 82. Visual analog pain score showed significant improvement in rising from a chair and walking 10m, 100m, and 1km. At 1 year, 25 knees (86%) had a good or excellent result. When 21 of these were observed at 2 years, 17 (81%) had good or excellent results. Overall, 61% of knee washouts had a good or excellent result at 2 years postwashout. Injection with hyaluronic acid gave no additional clinical benefit following washout. This study confirms the value of a fluid washout in an arthritic knee for some patients. This result may explain some of the symptom relief seen with arthroscopic procedures in this condition.

Key Words. Knee lavage, Hyaluronic acid, Washout, Osteoarthritis, Hypertonic Saline

Introduction

The role of arthroscopic procedures for treatment of degenerative conditions of the knee remains unclear. Burman et al. [1] first reported good results with arthroscopic examination of arthritic knees in 1934. Their instruments were

---

[1] Oregon Sports Medicine Associates, 19250 SW 65th Avenue, #245, Tualatin, OR 97062, U.S.A.

primarily for diagnostic purposes only, and had not evolved technologically to allow for surgical debridement or bone abrasion. Because of this, one could presume the patient's relief was from the fluid washout alone. Thus, in a certain percentage of osteoarthritic knees, short-term pain relief provided by arthroscopy may result from mechanical fluid washout alone and not specific arthroscopic treatment. Other authors have also noted that arthroscopy alone, without debridement or other surgical intervention, can result in marked improvement of symptoms [2–4]. Particulate debris from autologous articular cartilage has been shown to promote symptomatic synovitis and osteophyte formation in dogs when injected intraarticularly [5]. Also, Dahl et al. [6] showed a significant increase in the total amount of polysaccharide in synovial fluid from patients with joint diseases. Removal of these particles could explain why mechanical washout alone provides relief.

Previous studies have shown that hyaluronic acid is altered and its concentration decreased in patients with degenerative joint disease [7–9]. One could hypothesize that the arthritic knee might be returned to a healthy, more pain-free state by the injection of physiologically adjusted hyaluronic acid. Our prospective study was performed with two aims [10]. The first goal was to evaluate prospectively the effectiveness of fluid washout alone in the treatment of degenerative or osteoarthritic knees. The hypothesis tested was that knee washout with an osmotically adjusted lactated Ringer's solution would provide short-term relief of pain in patients with osteoarthritis. The second goal was to determine if any additional benefit could be obtained by injecting the knee with hyaluronic acid after the washout treatment. This design tested the hypothesis that physiologically adjusted hyaluronic acid would improve the clinical outcome in patients undergoing knee lavage.

Materials and Methods

To be included in this study, patients had to have symptomatic osteoarthritis in the knee that was no longer adequately responding to nonsteroidal anti-inflammatory drug therapy. This was determined by the patient having enough pain, in spite of medication, that he or she wanted additional treatment of the knee. These patients also had no clinical signs or symptoms of meniscal tear or obvious mechanical abnormalities. The patients had grade I to grade III radiographic changes of osteoarthritis as described by Holden et al. [12].

Twenty-three patients (29 knees) with symptomatic degenerative joint disease underwent knee washout after giving informed consent and were observed prospectively. The average age of patients undergoing knee washout, 20 men and 3 women, was 58 years (range, 39–79), and their average weight was 194 pounds (88 kg). Thirteen right knees and 16 left knees underwent washout, and 6 patients had bilateral washouts performed. Sixteen knees were randomly selected to receive an injection of hyaluronic acid after the washout and 13 received an injection of placebo (lactated Ringer's solution). The patients were blinded as to which they received.

Knee surgeries before washout had been performed in several patients: eight open meniscectomies, one arthroscopic meniscectomy, one open reduction, internal fixation of a lateral tibial plateau fracture, and two arthroscopic debridements. Three patients had more than one procedure on their knee.

Patients were evaluated with the Hospital for Special Surgery (HSS) knee score [12], the Knee Society (KS) clinical rating system for pain and function [13], and a visual analog pain scale. The visual analog scale was a 10-cm line on which the patients registered their amount of pain at rest, rising from a chair, walking 10 m, walking 100 m, walking 1 km, and running or sports participation. Zero was equal to no pain, and 10 was unbearable pain. Medication use was also documented.

Physical examination of the knee included measurement of active range of motion, effusion, thigh circumference at the proximal pole of the patella and 10 cm above the proximal pole of the patella, alignment, ligamentous stability, and muscle strength. Effusion was graded by the examiner as 0, none; I, slight; II, moderate; or III, tense effusion. Patients were seen before the washout and at 2 weeks, 6 weeks, 3 months, 6 months, 9 months, 1 year, and 2 years of follow-up.

Radiographs were graded as follows: grade I, slight narrowing of the joint, minimum osteophyte formation, slight sclerosis; grade II, moderate joint narrowing, spur formation, and sclerosis; grade III, some bone-on-bone changes and sclerosis, but no loss of bone stock; and grade IV, complete obliteration of joint, loss of bone stock, and severe sclerosis [11]. Radiographic evaluation was performed in a blinded fashion by two orthopedic surgeons. There were 11 knees with grade I, 13 with grade II, and 5 with grade III osteoarthritic changes. Patients with grade IV changes were excluded from the study.

The knee lavage solution consisted of 3 l of lactated Ringer's solution made hypertonic by adding 75 g of mannitol to raise the osmolality to 375 mmol/kg, which was done so that the fluid was as close as possible to the normal osmolality level of synovial fluid in healthy, young volunteers [14]. Osmolality was measured with a freezing point depression osmometer. To determine if mannitol was absorbed into the circulation, serum osmolality was measured before and after washout from synovial samples taken immediately following placement of the arthroscopic needles into the joint.

Washout was performed in all patients with 3 l of sterile hypertonic lactated Ringer's solution in the following manner. The patient was placed supine on the examination table. The knee to be lavaged was scrubbed with a standard Betadine prep and paint solution. The knee was draped in a sterile fashion with disposable paper drapes. The area superolateral to the patella was infiltrated with 1% Lidocaine. A 2.3-mm cannulated arthroscopic needle was inserted and joint fluid obtained for synovial analysis. The needle was then connected to a 3-l bag of hypertonic lactated Ringer's solution, and the knee was inflated with gravity flow. Using a similar technique, a superomedial needle was placed and the outflow connected to an empty, sterile 3-l bag. The knee was sequentially inflated and drained until the 3 l of solution had been used. Any tissue fragments were collected for histological examination.

A randomized table was used to determine which patients received a 3-ml injection of hyaluronic acid with a molecular mass range of 500 000–1 000 000 daltons (Lifecore Biomedical, Minneapolis, MN, and Biomet, Warsaw, IN, USA) or placebo (hypertonic lactated Ringer's solution). The hyaluronic acid or placebo was injected directly through the inflow needle immediately following knee lavage. Patients were blinded as to which injection they received. All patients undergoing bilateral washout received hyaluronic acid in one knee and placebo in the other (randomized based on severity of symptoms).

Following washout, patients were instructed to apply ice to the knee and avoid activity overnight to reduce the risk of hemarthrosis. Weight-bearing as tolerated was allowed immediately. Patients were instructed to stop all antiinflammatory medication use for the duration of the study.

Statistical analysis was performed using the Wilcoxon signed rank test for paired nonparametric data and the Mann–Whitney test for paired nonparametric data. A P value less than .05 was considered significant.

Results

Knee washouts were performed on 33 knees in 26 patients. One patient was lost to follow-up immediately after washout. One patient reinjured his knee 3 months following washout, required surgical intervention, and was dropped from the study. This patient had an excellent result until his injury. A third patient required bilateral knee arthroscopies, which prevented him from completing the study. Therefore, 29 knees in 23 patients were included in the study. Patients tolerated the washout well. There were no immediate adverse effects. No patient required ambulation supports. There were no complications at the needle insertion sites.

The results of HSS and KS knee scores are shown in Fig. 1. The mean prewashout HSS score for all knees was 72, and at 1 year was 87. The patients with good or excellent results at 1 year were examined again at 2 years, and the mean score remained 87. The average KS pain score improved from 64 to 89 at 1 year. The average KS function score similarly was improved from 62 to 82 at 1 year. For those patients having good or excellent results at 1 year, the 2-year results were 88 for pain and 86 for function.

The analog pain scale results are shown in Fig. 2. Again, the 2-year results are only for those patients with good or excellent results at 1 year. No significant differences were noted between 1 and 2 years. Pain rising from a chair and at walking 10 m, 100 m, and 1 km were all significantly different from baseline.

There was no statistically significant difference in outcome at 1 or 2 years after washout between those knees that received hyaluronic acid injection after washout versus those that received placebo. In those two groups, there were no statistical differences between age, weight, radiographic classification, or prewashout scores. Additionally, of those patients undergoing bilateral knee washouts (each patient had placebo injection in one knee and hyaluronic

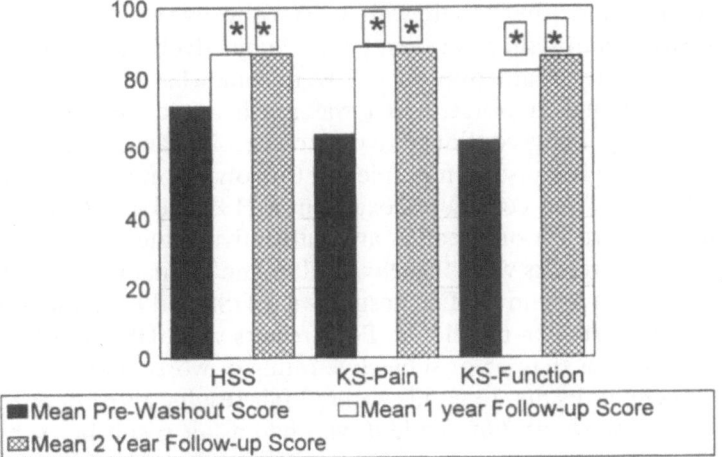

FIG. 1. Results of the Hospital for Special Surgery (HSS) and Knee Society (KS) scores. Note that the 2-year scores are for patients with good and excellent results at 1 year.
*, $P < .001$

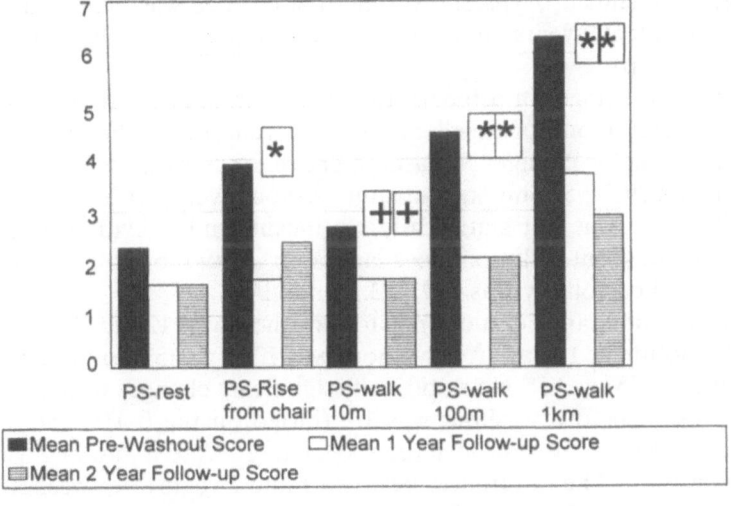

FIG 2. Results of the analog pain scales for different activities. Note that the 2-year scores are for patients with good and excellent results at 1 year.
*, $P < .001$; +, $P < .005$

acid injection in the other), there were no statistically significant differences in pre- or postwashout scores between knees. Subjectively, at 1 year after washout, 15 knees were greatly improved, 7 were somewhat improved, 5 were the same, 1 was somewhat worse, and 1 was much worse when compared with baseline. Seven patients continued to use nonsteroidal antiinflammatory medications, primarily because of multiple joint involvement with osteoarthritis.

Overall results were considered excellent if HSS and KS pain and function rating scores were 90 or greater, and subjectively the patient felt greatly improved. Good results were those with HSS and KS pain and function score averages between 80 and 89. Fair results were HSS and KS pain and function score averages between 65 and 79. Poor results were HSS and KS pain and function scores less than 65 or subjective rating of worse than baseline. There were 12 excellent results, 13 good results, 2 fair results, and 2 poor results at 1 year following washout. One patient who had a fair result has subsequently gone on to total knee arthroplasty. Twenty-five of the 29 knees (86%) treated with washout had a good or excellent result at 1 year.

Of the 25 knees with good or excellent results at 1 year after washout, 21 knees in 18 patients were seen at 2-year follow-up after washout. There were 9 excellent, 8 good, 2 fair, and 2 poor results. Three knees (2 patients) were lost to follow-up. One patient with an excellent result at 1 year was killed in a motor vehicle accident before her 2-year followup; at her 18-month followup, she was considered a good result. Seventeen of the 21 knees (81%) had good or excellent results at 2 years. Overall, 61% of knee washouts had a good or excellent result at 2 years after washout (assuming fair or poor results in those lost to followup).

Radiographic stages of osteoarthritis had no statistically significant correlation with result. Good or excellent results were not more likely in those with fewer radiographic changes. Measurement of serum osmolality before washout averaged 293 ± 5 mmol/kg and after washout averaged 294 ± 1.5 mmol/kg. This difference was not statistically significant, and is evidence that use of hypertonic washout solution does not alter serum osmolality. The mean synovial fluid osmolality was 299 ± 3.1 mmol/kg.

The mean total range of motion before washout was $123° \pm 2.3°$. Mean total range of motion at 1 year after washout was $126° \pm 2.5°$, and at 2 years after washout was $125° \pm 3.5°$. No statistically significant changes were present. The mean effusion before washout was 1.1 (based on the 0–III scale described previously). Mean effusion at 1 year was 0.6 ($P < .05$), and at 2 years after washout was 0.7. The differences between 1 and 2 years after washout, as well as baseline versus 2 years after washout, were not statistically significant. There was no statistically significant difference in age among patients who had a fair or poor result and those who had a good or excellent result at either 1 or 2 years after washout.

There was one complication. A 63-year-old man underwent washout and placebo injection in his left knee, and 3 months later he underwent washout and hyaluronic injection in his right knee. Approximately 24h after the right knee washout the patient developed a painful, sterile effusion in his right knee. He had no fevers, chills, or elevated white blood cell count. Cultures of the right knee and blood were negative. Cell count in the synovial fluid was 85000, with 95% polymorphonuclear neutrophil leukocytes (PMNs). He underwent arthroscopic debridement, and his symptoms resolved. However, he developed a sterile effusion of the left knee 12h later (3 months after left knee washout) with similar laboratory findings and negative cultures. The left knee was also treated with arthroscopic debridement, and the symptoms resolved; the patient was removed from the study. Because one knee flared 3 months after washout and appeared identical to the opposite knee, the exact cause was not determined.

Discussion

Arthroscopic treatment of osteoarthritis of the knee is usually performed in the hope of avoiding or delaying more extensive surgery, such as total knee arthroplasty or osteotomy. Surgery ranges from diagnostic in nature to aggressive debridement of osseous or soft tissues. Most reports on arthroscopic debridement have reported fair to good results for pain relief in 50%–80% of patients [2,15–29]. However, many authors have noted surprisingly good results from arthroscopic lavage alone [1,2,4,21]. Eriksson and Haggmark [21] reported ten avid runners with significant knee osteoarthritis who improved with arthroscopy and were then able to continue jogging with repeated needle lavage of the knee every 4–12 months.

It remains unclear how much of the relief seen after an arthroscopic procedure is the result of to mechanical washout. In this study, 86% of patients had good or excellent results, with significant pain relief and functional improvement by objective measures at 1 year after washout, and 81% of those (61% of all patients) had good or excellent results at 2 years. This proved the first hypothesis: in a select patient population with knee osteoarthritis, that is, without evidence of other internal derangements, mechanical washout can provide significant palliation. Additionally, this procedure was very well tolerated, with minimal recovery, and most patients returned to full activities within 1–2 days.

Moseley et al. [22] reported on results of a pilot study that included a placebo arthroscopy group for treatment of osteoarthritis. Although the small numbers of patients precluded a valid statistical analysis, the issue of placebo effect was raised. By the nature of the washout procedure, it would be impossible to have blinded controls with a placebo washout. It is, therefore, possible that some placebo effect may have contributed to perceived benefits of knee washout. However, most patients who did well had a dramatic benefit that lasted 1–2 years.

Decreased use or complete cessation of antiinflammatory medications is an additional benefit to the use of knee lavage. Most patients in this study completely discontinued use of antiinflammatory medications for the duration of the study (seven were unable to do so, primarily because of multiple joint involvement). Gastrointestinal and renal complications from long-term use of nonsteroidal antiinflammatory drugs are well known. Significant costs are also associated with long-term use of antiinflammatory medications.

Radiographic stage of osteoarthritis did not reliably predict who would have a beneficial effect from knee washout. However, radiographic stage also did not correlate with severity of symptoms before washout. The underlying mechanism for symptomatic relief from washout is unknown. Evidence exists that removal of water-soluble mediators of inflammation, as well as fragments of articular cartilage, could explain the therapeutic effect [4–6,23,24] Histological analysis of fluid collected from washouts showed fragments of articular cartilage in various stages of degradation in several patients.

Baumgarten et al. [14], measuring osmolality (a measure of the concentration of ions and particles in solution), demonstrated that synovial fluid from knees in young, healthy individuals at rest was hypertonic (mean, 404 mmol/kg) when compared with their serum (mean, 305 mmol/kg). Shanfield et al. [24] subsequently showed that patients with degenerative arthritis have decreased synovial fluid osmolality (mean, 297 mmol/kg) when compared with normal controls. The mean synovial fluid osmolality in our patients was 298 mmol/kg, which supports the findings of Shanfield et al. Bloebaum and Wilson [25] found that variation of osmotic concentration of solutions results in scanning electron microscopic changes in the surface of articular cartilage. Both normal saline and lactated Ringer's solution have been shown to cause at least transient changes in articular cartilage [26,27]. Use of hypertonic lactated Ringer's solution results in morphologically normal chondrocytes [28]. For these reasons, it was chosen to irrigate knees with a hypertonic solution that was as close to normal synovial fluid as possible. Comparison of pre- and postwashout serum osmolality showed no significant difference.

There are numerous reports of beneficial effects from injection of Hyaluronic acid in osteoarthritic knees, but none of these studies are definitive [3,8,9]. The decrease in osmolality of osteoarthritic synovial fluid has been shown, at least in part, to be secondary to the alteration and decreased concentrations of hyaluronic acid [6]. In this washout study, there were no significant differences in results between patients who received an injection of hyaluronic acid and those who did not. Furthermore, patients undergoing bilateral washouts and blinded as to which knee received hyaluronic acid stated there was no difference between the knees. This disproved our hypothesis that hyaluronic acid would give additional clinical benefit to the patient. This study did not evaluate the role of treatment with hyaluronic acid alone for knee osteoarthritis, nor did it evaluate a range of doses for the hyaluronic acid.

Controls for the study essentially consisted of the failure of antiinflammatory medications in the patients, as well as literature controls of arthroscopic procedures [29]. Prior prospective short-term studies have shown a statistically significant improvement in pain relief and function with tidal irrigation compared with conservative medical management [30].

The results at 1 and 2 years from nonoperative washouts of osteoarthritic knees have given results comparable to those reported for arthroscopic treatment.

Knee washout can be considered another palliative treatment option for osteoarthritis. Minimal procedural discomfort and the possibility of obviating the need for, or eliminating the use of, nonsteroidal antiinflammatory medications are potential benefits. This study confirms the value of a fluid washout in an arthritic knee for some patients. The relatively short-term relief from discomfort provided by arthroscopy in a certain percentage of osteoarthritic knees may be the result of mechanical fluid washout alone and not specific arthroscopic treatment. This same benefit can potentially be achieved without the expense, risk, and postoperative recovery by simple lavage under local anesthetic in a clinic setting.

References

1. Burman M, Finkelstein H, Mayer L (1934) Arthroscopy of the knee joint. J Bone Joint Surg 16:255
2. Jackson R (1974) The role of arthroscopy in the management of the arthritic knee. Clin Orthop 101:28–35
3. Jackson RW, Abe I (1972) The role of arthroscopy in the management of disorders of the knee. J Bone Joint Surg 54B:310–322
4. O'Connor RL (1973) The arthroscope in the management of crystal-induced synovitis of the knee. J Bone Joint Surg 55A:1443–1449
5. Chrisman O, Fessell J, Southwick W (1965) Experimental production of synovitis and marginal articular exostosis in the knee joint of dogs. Yale J Biol Med 37:409–412
6. Dahl LB, Dahl IMS, Engstrom-Laurent A, et al (1985) Concentration and molecular weight of sodium hyaluronate in synovial fluid from patients with rheumatoid arthritis and other arthropathies. Ann Rheum Dis 44:817–822
7. Namiki O, Toyoshima H, Morisaki N (1982) Therapeutic effect of intraarticular injection of high molecular weight hyaluronic acid on osteoarthritis of the knee. Int J Clin Pharmacol 20:501–507
8. Peyron JG, Balazs EA (1974) Preliminary clinical assessment of Na-hyaluronate Injection into human arthritic joints. Pathol Biol 8:731–736
9. Weiss C, Balazs EA, St Onge R, et al (1985) Clinical studies of the intraarticular injection of healon (sodium hyaluronate) in the treatment of osteoarthritis of human knees. Osteoarthritis Sympos 143–144
10. Edelson RH, Burks RT, Bloebaum RD (1995) Short-term effects of knee washout for osteoarthritis. Am J Sports Med 23(3):345–349
11. Holden DL, James S, Larson RL, et al (1988) Proximal tibial ostotomy in patients who are fifty years old or less. J Bone Joint Surg 70A:977–982
12. Insall JN, Ranawat CS, Aglietti P, et al (1976) A comparison of four models of total knee replacement prostheses. J Bone Joint Surg 58A:754–756
13. Insall J, Dorr L, Scott R, et al (1989) Rationale of the Knee Society clinical rating system. Clin Orthop 248:13–14
14. Baumgarten M, Bloebaum RD, Ross SDK, et al (1985) Normal human synovial fluid: osmolality and exercise-induced changes. J Bone Joint Surg 67A:1336–1339

15. Bert J, Maschka K (1986) The arthroscopic treatment of unicompartmental gonarthrosis: a five-year followup study of abrasion arthroplasty plus arthroscopic debridement and arthroscopic debridement alone. Arthroscopy 2:54–69
16. Friedman MJ, Berasi CC, Fox JM, et al (1984) Preliminary results with abrasion arthroplasty in the osteoarthritic knee. Clin Orthop 182:200–205
17. Oglivie-Harris DJ, Fitsialos DP (1991) Arthroscopic management of the degenerative knee. J Arthrosc 7:151–157
18. Salisbury R, Nottage W, Gardner V (1985) The effect of alignment on results in arthroscopic debridement of the degenerative knee. Clin Orthop 198:268–272
19. Sprague NF III (1981) Arthroscopic debridement for degenerative knee joint disease (1981) Clin Orthop 160:118–123
20. Timoney JM, Kneisl JS, Barrack RL, et al (1990) Arthroscopy in the osteoarthritic knee. Orthop Rev 29:371–379
21. Eriksson E, Haggmark T (1980) Knee pain in the middle-aged runner. In: AAOS symposium on the foot and leg in running sports. American Academy of Orthopedic Surgeons, Atlanta, pp 106–108
22. Moseley JB, Wray NP, Kuykendall D, et al (1996) Arthroscopic treatment of osteoarthritis of the knee: a prospective, randomized, placebo-controlled trial. Am J Sports Med 24(1):28–34
23. Forrester JV, Balazs EA (1980) Inhibition of phagocytosis by high molecular weight hyaluronate. Immunology 40:435–446
24. Shanfield S, Campbell P, Baumgarten M, et al (1988) Synovial fluid osmolality in osteoarthritis and rheumatoid arthritis. Clin Orthop 235:1–7
25. Bloebaum RD, Wilson AS (1980) The morphology of the surface of the articular cartilage in adult rats. J Anat 131:333–346
26. Reagan BF, McInerny VK, Treadwell BV, et al (1983) Irrigating solutions for arthroscopy. J Bone Joint Surg 65A:629–631
27. Straehley D, Heller A, Solomons C, et al (1985) The effect of arthroscopic irrigating solutions on cartilage and synovium. In: 31st annual meeting, Orthopedic Research Society, February, 1985, Las Vegas, NV, p 260
28. Bloebaum RD, Rubman M, Merrell M, et al (1992) Hyaluronate solution as a cartilage antidesiccant. J Biomed Mat Res 26:303–317
29. Burks RT (1990) Arthroscopy and degenerative arthritis of the knee: a review of the literature. J Arthrosc 6:43–47
30. Ike R, Arnold W, Rothschild E, et al (1992) Tidal irrigation vs conservative medical management in patients with osteoarthritis of the knee: a prospective randomized study. J Rheumatol 19:772–779

Viscosupplementation for the Treatment of Osteoarthritis of the Knee with Hyaluronan and Hylans: Rationale and State of the Art

JACQUES G. PEYRON

Summary. Hyaluronan is essential in maintaining the homeostasis of joint tissues and synovial fluid through its elastoviscosity, lubricating properties, protection of cells and nerves, molecular sieving effect, and metabolic influence on synovial cells. These properties are molecular weight- and concentration dependent. In osteoarthritis (OA), synovial fluid hyaluronan becomes less effective because of dilution and a decrease in molecular weight. Through viscosupplementation, a therapeutic procedure of serial intra-articular injections of high molecular weight hyaluronan or its derivatives, hylans, the normal elastoviscous properties of synovial fluid may be restored. The reported tolerance of viscosupplementation is very good, with similar results for the three available products. Local adverse effects occur after approximately 2% of the injections in 2%–4% of the patients; these are typically short lived and have no sequelae. This efficacious and safe treatment is the only therapy for osteoarthritis that addresses the mechanorheological homeostasis of joint tissues.

Key Words. Hyaluronan, Hylans, Osteoarthritis, Knee

Introduction

Viscosupplementation with hyaluronan was introduced in medicine in the late 1960s. The first hyaluronan preparation used for viscosupplementation was the highly purified fraction of sodium hyaluronan (NIF-NaHA, the noninflammatory fraction of sodium hyaluronan, Healon) developed during the 1960s and tested clinically in the early 1970s. This preparation of hyaluronan was never marketed for viscosupplementation. Two hyaluronan preparations (average molecular weight [M_w], 500 000–750 000) have been

Centre de Rhumathologie, Hôpital de la Pitié. 3 Rue des Dames Augustines, 92200 Neuilly sur Seine, 75013 Paris, France marketed for viscosupplementation since 1987. Published short-term studies (3 months) show that about twice as many osteoarthritis (OA) patients respond positively to hyaluronan as to saline injections; 20%–40% of the results are termed "very good," and in some patients longlasting effects may result.

The second-generation hyaluronan preparations are derivatives of hyaluronan called hylans. Hylans are cross-linked hyaluronan that display a very high elastoviscosity and a prolonged residence time in the joint tissues, allowing greater therapeutic benefit after fewer injections. Controlled trials with hylans showed that three injections have a significant pain-reducing effect compared to control injections for as long as 6 months; 60% of patients report a very good result. A retrospective study of 336 patients over 2.5 years in a clinical practice setting showed 76% responders, with 35% reporting very good results. Duration of effect was greater than 6 months in most patients. The mean time lag before a second treatment was required was 8.2 months, with a range of 3–18 months.

Hyaluronan and Hyaluronan Solutions

Physicochemistry

Hyaluronan (hyaluronic acid) is a ubiquitous and essential component of all intercellular matrices of connective tissues [1,2]. It is a glycosaminoglycan composed of linear, unbranched chains of disaccharide units. Each disaccharide unit contains one molecule of N-acetylglucosamine and one of β-1,4-glucuronic acid. In solution, the large hyaluronan molecules adopt a highly hydrated random coil conformation, occupying a large spherical domain. At a concentration of 0.2 mg/ml, there is no room for the individual hyaluronan molecules to exist separately, so they overlap to form an entangled polymer network.

Recent nuclear magnetic resonance (NMR) and electron microscopic studies suggest that the hyaluronan molecules in physiological solution, internally bound by hydrogen bonds, can interact with one another to form tubular or sheetlike structures [3]. The fact that hyaluronan molecules occupy the space between collagen fibers and proteoglycan molecules in the intercellular matrix confers to hyaluronan a controlling effect on the traffic of small and large molecules. The hyaluronan polymer network can exclude other very large molecules such as globulins from the intercellular fluid and slow down the transit of mid-size molecules such as albumin [4–7]. Small solutes circulate freely, and the migration of some of them can even be paradoxically facilitated [8]. Hyaluronan solutions have a buffering effect against osmotic variations. They tend to inhibit the nucleation and growth of hydroxyapatite crystals in vitro [9], although in synovial fluid other factors may influence this effect [10].

Hyaluronan solutions exhibit both elastic and viscous behavior. The transi-

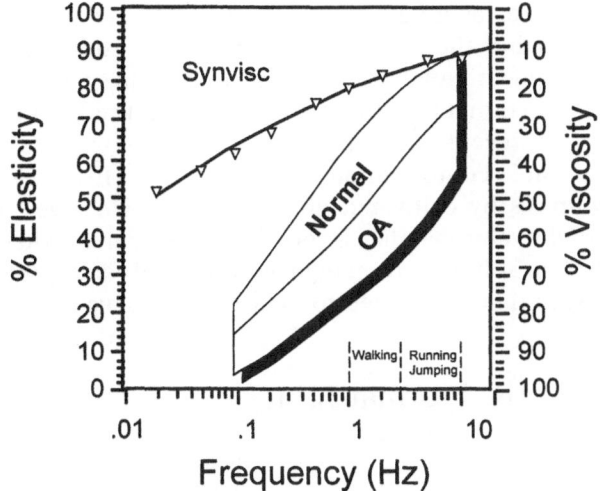

FIG. 1. Energy dissipation in human synovial fluids at different frequencies of movement. The fraction of the applied energy converted to elastic storage vs. viscous flow is
illustrated on the *left* and *right* axes, respectively. The high percent elasticity of Synvisc
allows it to raise the elasticity of osteoarthritis (OA) synovial fluid into a normal range

tion from viscous to elastic behavior occurs rapidly, a feature unique to
hyaluronan solutions among other polymers [5,11]. For example, hyaluronan
in synovial fluid is predominantly viscous under low deformation frequencies
(i.e., walking) because of the entanglement of molecules. In the case of high
deformation frequency (running, jumping), the synovial fluid hyaluronan
is mostly elastic and behaves as a shock absorber, transiently storing energy
(Fig. 1) [5]. The ability of such hyaluronan solutions to adapt from elastic to
viscous behavior provides the cells and tissues with a protection that allows
them to function normally under a large variety of mechanical stresses.

Biological Properties

High-viscosity hyaluronan solutions in vitro inhibit lymphocyte–lymphoblast
transformation [12], phagocytic activity of macrophages and leukocytes, and
release of prostaglandin [13–15]. In vitro they protect chondrocytes or cartilage explants in culture against degradation by enzymes, interleukin-I (Il-l),
and oxygen-derived free radicals, and they stimulate the production of tissue
inhibitor of metallo proteases (TIMP). These protective activities, which
include protection against physical damage, are concentration- and molecular
weight dependent [13–20].

Hyaluronan solutions can stimulate the synthesis of hyaluronan in synovial
cell cultures [21]. This effect reaches a maximum 48 h after hyaluronan is

added to the culture medium and is concentration- and molecular weight dependent. The higher the molecular weight of the added hyaluronan, the more pronounced this stimulatory effect on hyaluronan synthesis. A proposed possible explanation is that this stimulatory effect is caused by the activation of several cell-surface receptors at the same time, thus requiring a particular molecular size and conformation. Interleukin-1 (Il-1) also stimulates hyaluronan synthesis by cultivated fibroblasts [22]. However, much of this newly synthesized hyaluronan has a very low molecular weight [23].

Thus, hyaluronan solutions display many regulatory and protective effects on cells and tissues that are related to their elastoviscous properties.

Hyaluronan in the Normal Joint

Metabolism

Hyaluronan is continuously distributed within the joint spaces and tissues, from the cartilage surface through the joint fluid to the intercellular matrix of the synovial tissue and the capsule. There are no barriers between these compartments [24]. It is secreted by the synovial cells lining the synovial tissue and moves into the joint fluid and back through the synovial tissue [25]. The degradation of hyaluronan does not occur until the hyaluronan molecules move into the lymph and reach the lymph nodes where some degradation occurs. The lymph carries the hyaluronan to the blood and ultimately to the liver where hyaluronan is fully degraded [26,27]. The intravenous half-life is only a few minutes.

The original metabolic studies of therapeutic hyaluronan preparations in the joint (NIF-NaHA, Healon) found a half-life of 24h [28]. Subsequent studies using different preparations and methods yielded generally similar results in terms of half-life in the joint and the speed of systemic elimination. Studies using a radiotracer in the rabbit knee joint found the half-life to be 13.2h for a preparation of M_w = 3 million and 10.2h for a preparation of M_w = 900000, M_w a significant difference [29]. Another publication reported a half-life of 10.8h in the sheep hock joint [30]. Use of radiolabeled hyaluronan confirmed the dependence of hyaluronan elimination on molecular weight in the rabbit knee, finding that the half-life of a preparation of M_w = 900000 is approximately 20h in the joint cavity and 40h in the synovial tissues, as compared to approximately 40h (cavity) and 60h (tissues) for a preparation of M_w = 1.8 million [31].

Articular Cartilage

Hyaluronan is an important constituent of cartilage, contributing to this tissue's unique mechanical properties. At the cartilage surface, hyaluronan is concentrated in the superficial layer of cartilage (*lamina splendens*) [32]. Exogenous hyaluronan (Healon) injected in the joint also accumulates in the lamina splendens where it remains for an extended period of time [28]. The Injection of fluoresceinated hyaluronan in the rabbit shoulder shows that it condenses as a highly fluorescent thin layer on the surfaces of the synovial tissue and of the articular cartilage, where it can still be seen 7 days later. This residual hyaluronan can be washed off by buffer [33]. The hyaluronan of the middle and deep layers of the cartilage is secreted by the chondrocytes and immobilized in complexes with specific proteoglycans (e.g., aggrecan). It is unlikely that the hyaluronan in synovial fluid freely exchanges with hyaluronan in the deeper layers of cartilage when the cartilage is intact.

Synovial Fluid

The remarkable viscoelastic properties of the synovial fluid are entirely the result of its high hyaluronan content. Elasticity and viscosity are directly related to hyaluronan concentration and molecular weight [34,35].

In normal human synovial fluid, the concentration of hyaluronan varies from 3.8 mg/ml in the young adult to 2.5 g/ml later on, with a rather sharp drop after the age of 30 years [34]. Thus a normal knee containing 1–2 ml of fluid would contain 2.5–8 mg of hyaluronan. Its molecular weight is very polydisperse, with a mean in the range of M_w = 4–5 million and with no detectable change between age groups [34]. High molecular weight hyaluronan in the joint tissues is responsible for the exclusion of large proteins, lipoproteins, and fibrinogen, as well as granulocytes from normal synovial fluid [36].

Synovial Tissue

Within the synovial tissue, the major deposits of hyaluronan are seen at the surface and surrounding the synovial cells lining the cavity [28,32]. There are lighter deposits in the area around the blood vessels and in areolar areas [37,38]. Hyaluronan concentration in the synovium has been found to be 1.07 mg/ml, with about 60% of it "free" (buffer extractable), possibly a lower molecular weight fraction [37,39]. Studies of synovial flow suggest that hyaluronan at and near the synovial surface is in a state of entanglement and aggregation [40] and that it could act as a "filtercake" [41].

In the synovial tissue, pain arises from the free nerve endings of thin unmyelinated nerve fibers [42]. In the normal joint these nociceptive terminals discharge signals only when the joint movement is beyond the normal range of motion. During articular inflammation, these nociceptive fibers may discharge during normal movement and even when the joint is at rest [43]. Hyaluronan exerts a protective buffering role on these nociceptors [43]. In the rat knee, hyaluronan solutions injected simultaneously with bradykinin exert a protection against gait disturbances resulting from the painful joint. This effect is concentration- and molecular weight dependent, requiring a minimal M_w of 400 000, and increasing at 860 000 and 2.1 million. If injected before bradykinin, high concentrations of hyaluronan (M_w = 860000 and 2.3 million) display a protective effect lasting up to 3 days [44]. In dogs, the duration of the protective effect against a subsequent bradykinin injection was found to be 2 days with a hyaluronan solution of M_w = 2 million but negligible with a solution of M_w = 1 million [45]. In the anesthetized cat, measuring the electrical potentials of the sensory nerves of the overextended joint, it was found that the protection against this mechanical nerve stimulation was also molecular weight dependent [43]. If joint pain is induced by local injection of urate crystals in a dog's knee, a hyaluronan solution of M_w = 2 million injected before the crystals prevents the appearance of pain symptoms, but not if it was injected after them, suggesting an effect on the first steps of the crystal-induced reaction [45].

Lubrication

The synovial fluid and the hyaluronan films on the tissue surfaces are important components of the joint's remarkable lubrication system. It can be noticed that nearly all the usual weight-bearing movements of the knee occur at a deformation frequency of at least 1 Hz and higher, which illustrates the importance of the elastic behavior of the synovial fluid (see Fig. 1).

Elastohydrodynamic lubrication, implying a "liquid wedge" and "squeeze film" separating the opposing surfaces [46], applies mostly during rapid movements and particularly in the sliding synovial tissues [47]. It is dependent on the elastoviscosity, concentration, and molecular weight of the hyaluronan. Boundary lubrication has been suggested to result from the reciprocal repulsion of glycoproteins adsorbed to the opposing cartilage surfaces [48,49]. In this mechanism, hyaluronan has the important role of maintenance of this thin molecular layer by interacting with the active glycoproteins [50].

In experiments on isolated hip joints, the lubricating effectiveness of diverse hyaluronan solutions is clearly related to the molecular weight of the hyaluronan. Only solutions of hyaluronan of M_w = 3.3 million and greater approach the lubricating power of natural synovial fluid [51].

Hyaluronan in the Osteoarthritic Joint

Synovial Fluid

The changes of hyaluronan in the synovial fluid of osteoarthritis patients are well known [14,24,34,52,53]. Although hyaluronan varies considerably from one patient to another, there is a consistent tendency toward decreased concentration or molecular weight of hyaluronan in osteoarthritic synovial fluids. Whether this lower molecular weight is caused by faulty synthesis by synovial cells or rather by the action of degradative factors, especially oxygen-derived free radicals [54], or both is unclear. This decrease in concentration and molecular weight significantly affects the elastoviscous properties of the fluid, thus jeopardizing its lubricating and protective effects (Fig. 1) [34]. The decreased rheological properties could be all the more deleterious because the osteoarthritic cartilage surface displays, even in intact areas, an increased roughness [55]. The decreased protective and molecular exclusion capacities might be especially damaging in view of the numerous proinflammatory and degradative substances found in osteoarthritic synovial fluid and tissue. Degradative enzymes and cytokines [56–58], prostaglandins apparently coming from the synovial tissue [59,60], calcium crystals [61,62], and cartilage proteoglycan fragments [63–65] have been repeatedly described in osteoarthritic synovial fluid. In osteoarthritic cartilage, synovial fluid carrying fluorescein-labeled hyaluronan was described as reaching within the damaged cartilage throughout the fibrillated superficial layer and still deeper through clefts and fissures [66].

Synovial Tissue

In the thickened hyperproliferative synovium, hyaluronan deposition was found to be increased throughout the tissue, particularly around proliferating synovial cells and blood vessels. The hyaluronan concentration in the inflamed joint tissue is decreased by dilution, despite increased hyaluronic acid (HA) synthesis [39]. Cultured fibroblasts from osteoarthritic synovial tissue showed a decreased level of hyaluronan synthesis, but proved highly sensitive to the stimulatory effect of exogenous hyaluronan solution added to the culture medium. This effect was marginal with preparations of hyaluronan of $M_w = 620\,000$ and $900\,000$ but was clearly significant with preparations of 3.8 and 4.7 million [21].

In explants of synovial tissue infiltrated with granulocytes, hyaluronan synthesis is increased but the hyaluronan is low in molecular weight [67]. Inhibition of the oxygen free radicals prevents hyaluronan degradation [68]. The bradykinin-induced release of the prostaglandin precursor arachidonic acid from osteoarthritic fibroblasts in culture is decreased by hyaluronan in a molecular weight-dependent manner: hyaluronan of $M_w = 2$ million is significantly more inhibitory than a preparation of $980\,000$ [69]. In a culture of osteoarthritic synovial cells, hyaluronan inhibited the production of mterleukm-1- (IL-1-) induced prostaglandin E2 in a dose- and molecular weight dependent manner: hyaluronan of $M_w = 2$ million proved significantly more active than that of $M_w = 1.6$ million [19].

Thus, in the osteoarthritic joint and tissues, hyaluronan has lost many of its normal biological properties related to its high molecular weight and the resulting elastoviscous character.

Experimental Osteoarthritis

In experimental arthritis produced by surgically induced instability of the joint or intraarticular papain injection, hyaluronan injections, usually begun early after arthritis inception, have shown a retarding effect [28]. Hyaluronan injections have shown a retarding effect on the development of degenerative cartilage lesions compared to the nontreated joint [70–73]. This effect was recently confirmed in a rabbit cruciate ligament transection model in which hyaluronan injections protected the articular cartilage from the loss of proteoglycans and collagen and decreased synovial hyperplasia [28,74]. In a rabbit meniscetomy model, a preparation of M_w = 1.9 million was found more protective than a preparation of M_w = 800 000 [75]. After transection of the anterior cruciate ligament in the rabbit knee, the protective effect of hyaluronan of M_w = 2 million was found superior to that of a compound of M_w = 950 000 [76].

In a study using synovectomy to induce cartilage degeneration, hyaluronan injections maintained the presence of the amorphous substance layered at the surface of the cartilage [77]. In rabbit knees injected with papain, loss of sulfated proteoglycans from the cartilage is significantly diminished by injecting hyaluronan of M_w = 2 million into the joint, but not that of M_w = 900 000 [78]. In two models of degenerative arthritis induced by immobilization of the rabbit's knee, hyaluronan injections significantly helped to maintain or to restore joint mobility and decreased the loss of sulfated glycosaminoglycans from the articular cartilage [28,79]. In both cases, a hyaluronan preparation of M_w = 2 million proved more effective than a preparation of M_w = 1 million [75,79].

Cartilage degradation induced by fibronectin fragments (which is likely to be proteinase mediated) is prevented by hyaluronan both in vitro and in vivo, possibly by the protective coating of hyaluronan on the cartilage surface [80]. In the synovial membrane of dogs with experimental osteoarthritis, hyaluronan injections to the joint decreased vacuolar degeneration of synovial cells and increased their expression of heat-shock protein (Hsp) 72, a cell—protective protein [81].

Thus, there is ample evidence showing that hyaluronan plays a major role in maintaining the homeostasis of joint tissues and functions by protecting them against aggressive factors. Moreover, whenever the effect of molecular weight was analyzed, the data demonstrated that the measured benefits increased significantly with increasing average molecular weight of hyaluronan and thus depend on the increasing elastoviscosity of the hyaluronan solutions used.

Hylan A, with considerably higher average molecular weight (~6 million), forms solutions with significantly greater elastoviscous properties than hyaluronan solutions [82]. Hylan A solutions are significantly more effective in protecting cartilage explants against the degradation effect of mononuclear cell-conditioned medium and in protecting against the damaging effect of oxygen-derived free radicals [83]. Moreover, hylan A has proved three times more stable than hyaluronan to degradation by oxygen radicals [84]. Moreover, there is evidence that increased molecular weight prolongs the residence time of hyaluronan in joint fluid and tissues [28,29] as well as the duration of its preventive effect against joint pain [43]. The higher molecular weight of hylan therefore improves many characteristics related to its clinical benefits.

Veterinary investigations on traumatic arthritis in racehorses confirm the importance of elastoviscosity to the therapeutic benefit [85]. In a study that compared the duration of clinical benefit after one injection of different hyaluronan preparations, results showed that the mean duration of symptomatic relief was less than 2 months for three hyaluronan preparations of $M_w < 2$ million, but increased to more that 4 months (137 days) for a $M_w = 2.1$ million preparation and to 5 months (160 days) following the use of a preparation of $M_w = 3.3$ million [86].

Taken together, the data we have reviewed show that the therapeutic application of hyaluronan and its derivatives (hylans) is based on using preparations with sufficiently high molecular weight to provide solutions with high elastoviscosity. Cell- and joint-protective properties, as well as lubricating capacities, have all been observed to require solutions with high molecular weight and high elastoviscosity to produce a therapeutic effect [53,87].

Clinical Use of Hyaluronan and Hylans

The clinical use of hyaluronan was made possible by the development of a non-inflammatory preparation with sufficient purity, molecular weight, and elastoviscous properties to be medically useful. This preparation, developed in the 1960s by E.A. Balazs, was called by its acronym NIF-NaHA or noninflammatory sodium hyaluronan [88]. The use of intraarticular injections of high elastoviscous solutions of hyaluronan or hylans to treat arthritis is called viscosupplementation [87].

The first clinical evaluations of intraarticularly injected hyaluronan were carried out in the early 1970s using a 1% solution of hyaluronan of average molecular weight of 2-3 million (NIF-NaHA, manufactured by Biotrics, Arlington, MA, USA), which is slightly less than the molecular weight of hyaluronan in normal synovial fluid [89–91]. The patients noticed decreased pain and improved joint function during several weeks after one or two injections. No noticeable side effects were observed. This hyaluronan product was not marketed for human intraarticular use, but it has been marketed worldwide for ophthalmic viscosurgery in human eyes under the trade name of Healon (Pharmacia & Upjohn, Uppsala, Sweden). The same hyaluronan preparation was also marketed worldwide for the treatment of equine arthritis under the tradename Hylartin (Pharmacia & Upjohn).

Artz

The first hyaluronan preparation marketed in 1987 for the treatment of human osteoarthritis is tradenamed Artz (Seikagaku, Japan). It is a 1% solution of hyaluronan extracted from rooster combs with an average molecular weight of 600000–800000. Clinical trials show efficacy for a treatment series of 5–16 injections, depending on the patient population and the investigators. The recommended treatment is a series of five weekly injections of 25mg (2.5ml) each. Clinical trials are summarized in Table 1. Early short-term trials [92–95] in 135 patients showed that 50%–84% of the patients improved and 20.4%–38% were graded "much better." In one controlled trial in which 60% of the patients responded to hyaluronan, 34% were also improved by placebo injections. One study using multiple injections over 6 months [96] showed 80% responders (43.5% "excellent") with an average of 13.7 injections per patient, suggesting that repeat injections may increase the effectiveness and the duration of the treatment's effect.

However, the clinical data are mixed. A recent 14-week controlled trial [97] showed a significant benefit of hyaluronan, while a 1-year trial in patients selected by arthroscopic criteria failed to show a positive result [98]. Lohmander et al. [99], in a 20-week trial, found significant benefit for hyaluronan only in the subgroup of patients more than 60 years of age with a Lequesne index greater than 10, while the intent-to-treat analysis showed no difference between hyaluronan and control.

Hyalgan

Hyalgan (Fidia, Italy) is a 1% solution of hyaluronan of $M_w = 500000–730000$. The recommended treatment consists of five weekly injections of 20mg (2ml) [100–106] (Table 2). Six placebo-controlled studies have been published (Table 2) as well as two studies comparing Hyalgan to corticosteroid injections [107,108]. Short-term controlled studies [100–102] totaling 130 patients show that 74%–88% of the patients respond to test injections as opposed to 30%–50% placebo responders. It also appears that 40-mg injections were not significantly more successful than those of 20mg, and that a series of five injections had a better result over 2 months than a series of three injections [102]. Outside Italy, a 5-month study of a five injection regimen [103] failed to show a significant advantage of hyaluronan over placebo except with respect to the consumption of escape antiinflammatory drugs. A 48-week trial [104] found the benefit of Hyalgan compared to placebo very effective on rest pain and mildly effective on pain on movement. A study of 38 patients [106] (19 on Hyalga, nine injections over 6 months) entailed an arthroscopic evaluation of the joint before the treatment and 1 year later. At that time, the progression of the arthroscopically evaluated joint lesions was less in the Hyalgan-treated patients than in the control group, thus raising the possibility of a retarding effect on joint degradation [106]. However, no placebo

TABLE 1. Clinical trials with Artz

Reference(s)	Trial duration	Number of patients	Number of injections	Results	Remarks
[92–95]	4–8 weeks	435	1–16	50%–84% Responders 20.4%–38% Excellent	Summary of four early short-term studies of which only one was placebo controlled. In the latter, 60% responders to Artz vs. 34% responders to placebo
[96]	26 weeks	33	7–20	88% Responders 45.5 Excellent	Study of multiple injections; average, 13.7 injections per patient
[97]	14 weeks	95	5	Lequesne index improved by 4.4 in Artz group, 2.8 in placebo group	$P < .005$
[98]	52 weeks	28	5	Improvement from baseline not statistically different from placebo	Patients all had prior arthroscopy
[99]	20 weeks	96	5	Improvement from baseline not statistically different from placebo	Artz was only significantly better than placebo in the patient subgroup age 60 and over, having a Lequesne index of 10 or greater

TABLE 2. Clinical trials with Hyalgan

References	Trial duration	Number of patients	Number of injections	Results	Remarks
[100–102]	8 weeks	189	3–5	75%–88% Hyalgan responders vs. 30%–50% placebo responders	Single injection of 40mg no better than 20mg Five injections better than three
[103]	20 weeks	91	5	No statistical difference between Hyalgan and placebo except for use of escape NSAID	Numerous dropouts Numerous side effects
[104]	48 weeks	63	4	Hyalgan statistically better than placebo	Patients improved more for pain at rest than for pain on movement or activity.
[106]	52 weeks	36	9	Hyalgan statistically better than placebo	Chondroscopy used to assess disease progression

injections were administered in the later trial, making it difficult to interpret the results. Comparisons with methylprednisolone injections showed that pain decrease induced by hyaluronan was slower to appear but ultimately as effective as with corticosteroids and lasted considerably longer [107,108].

Taken together, the studies with Artz and with Hyalgan, two preparations of similar molecular weight, show that the useful unit dose is 20–25 mg, and that a series of five consecutive weekly injections is necessary to produce a significant effect over several weeks or months. Used in this way, hyaluronan injections are generally more effective than placebo injections. The effect is of longer duration than that of corticosteroids. Details within the studies tend to show that pain symptoms are better influenced than examination signs, and that the best results are obtained in patients with mild to moderate radiologic changes (Kellgran Lawrence grades II and III) and with no or only small effusions.

Finally, tolerance of hyaluronan has proved to be very good. Thus, this type of treatment has gained wide acceptance in countries where it is available. However, long-term studies evaluating repeat treatments and possible influence of this therapy on the natural history of knee osteoarthritis are still to be made.

Synvisc

Recently, more elastoviscous derivatives of hyaluronan have been introduced to clinical medicine. Hylans are polymers of hyaluronan cross-linked through their hydroxyl groups [82,87]. They are very highly hydrated [109] and are very powerful scavengers of hydroxyl radicals [84].

Synvisc (Biomatrix, Ridgefield, NJ, USA), a mixture of two hylan polymers (hylan A fluid, hylan B gel), was developed specifically for the treatment of human OA by viscosupplementation. Synvisc contains hylan A, an elastoviscous fluid with an average molecular weight of 6 million. Hylan A makes up 90% (per weight) of Synvisc. Hylan B is a viscoelastic gel also derived from hyaluronan. Because it is a gel, it has an infinite molecular weight, and it is extremely hydrated (~99.5% solvent content) but is not water soluble. Hylan B gel constitutes 10% (per weight) of Synvisc. The elastic modulus of Synvisc is greater than that of normal synovial fluid (see Fig. 1), and its residence time in the joint fluid space and tissues is longer than that of hyaluronan. Hylan B contributes to the elastoviscosity of Synvisc and increases the residence time of hylan A in the joint. The unit dose of Synvisc is 2 ml (16 mg of hylans), and the recommended therapeutic regimen is 3 weekly injections during a 2-week period.

Several clinical studies with Synvisc have been reported (Table 3) [110–113]. Two dose-ranging, placebo-controlled, double-blind trials showed that two injections of Synvisc are significantly better than placebo on most criteria, but that three injections were significantly better than two at 8 and 12 weeks. Some

TABLE 3. Clinical trials with Synvisc

References	Trial duration	Number of patients	Number of Injections	Results	Remarks
[110]	12 weeks	80	2 or 3	Both the 2-injection and 3-injection treatments are statistically superior to placebo	3-injection treatment regimen statistically superior to 2-injection regimen
[111]	26 weeks	118	3	Synvisc is statistically superior to placebo for all outcome measures	At 6 months, 53% of the Synvisc patients still have "excellent" improvement vs. 22% with placebo
[112]	26 weeks	93	3	Synvisc is as good or better than continuous NSAID therapy	Synvisc is statistically superior to NSAID when using a repeat measures analysis corrected for covariates
[113]	2.5 years (retrospective)	336 (122 treated bilaterally)	3	77% of patients rated "much better" or "better"	Mean time to retreatment was 8.2 months. Improvement lasted more than 6 months in the majority of patients

statistical differences from placebo were evident after the first Synvisc injection. A telephone survey at 26 weeks confirmed the duration of these effects. It was concluded that three injections was the optimum treatment schedule.

A double-blind, placebo-controlled, multicenter efficacy study of 118 patients [111] confirmed that most outcome measures were significantly improved after the first injection, and this effect continued to week 26. At 3 months, 71% of the Synvisc-injected patients had an excellent result (Visual Analog Scale pain scores decrease: 20 mm) versus 29% of control patients (at 6 months; 53% and 22%, respectively).

A comparison of Synvisc to continuous nonsteroidal antimflammatory drug (NSAID) therapy was performed in 93 patients [112]. One group continued their usual NSAID therapy and received three weekly arthrocenteses as an intraarticular control. A second group continued their usual NSAID therapy, but additionally received three Synvisc injections; the third group discontinued their usual NSAIDs and instead received three Synvisc injections. In a repeated measures analysis corrected for covariates, the Synvisc group was significantly better than the NSAID group [114]. At 26 weeks, telephone-evaluated outcome measures were significantly better in the two Synvisc-injected groups than in the NSAID-alone group. It was concluded that three Synvisc injections were as good or better than continued NSAID therapy and could be used to replace continuous NSAID therapy, providing pain relief for more than 6 months. No interference between the two treatments was observed.

Finally, a retrospective study collected all cases treated by five Canadian rheumatologists during a period of 2.5 years [113]. The files of 336 patients (458 knees) were reviewed. Fifty-six knees required a second treatment. Responders to the treatment were 76% after a first series and 84% after the second. About half of the patients were graded "much better." Clinical benefits after a first treatment lasted more than 3 months in 65% of the patients and more than 6 months in more than half the patients. The mean lag time before a second treatment was required was 8.2 months.

Safety of Hyaluronan and Hylan Injections

Safety is obviously a major concern for a therapy aimed at a chronic non-life-threatening condition that may require many repeat administrations. A comprehensive review of available data shows that local injections of hyaluronan or hylans largely meet this safety requirement (Table 4).

The only adverse effects (AEs) of significance are transient local reactions in the injected joint, which are typically benign, short lived, without sequelae, and similar to those observed with any intraarticular treatment. The mean prevalence of local AEs in controlled clinical trials is generally between 2% and 4% of the injections. In controlled clinical studies, the frequency of AEs after control injections (usually saline) falls within the same range.

TABLE 4. Rates of local adverse effects (AEs) reported for the available hyaluronan and hylan products

Product	Rate (%) of local AE per injection (range)		Percent of patients who discontinued clinical trials
	Clinical trials	Postmarked surveys	
Artz	2.6 (2–4.4)	0.5	1.4
Hyalgan	4.2 (1.6–15)	0.4[a]	3.4
Synvisc	2.3 (0–3.5)	0.16	1.5

[a] Calculated from the rate per patient, assuming 5 injections per course of treatment. Data courtesy of Laboratories Fournier, Dijon, France.

Intraarticular injections of corticosteroids are known to cause painful reactions with approximately 3% frequency per injection [115,116].

These local AEs are very much the same with all intraarticular injection products. The AEs include joint pain occurring a few hours or within 2 days after the injection. The joint may be swollen, and is rarely warm. An effusion may be present and, in a few instances, has been reported to be abundant and rich in mononuclear cells. These symptoms, in most cases, resolve spontaneously in a few days, often before the next weekly injection. Rest, cold packs, analgesics, sometimes NSAIDs, and occasionally corticosteroid injections or arthrocentesis to remove the effusion have been found helpful as treatments. No lasting sequelae have been described. This local reaction does not necessarily recur with subsequent injections, so discontinuation of the treatment is generally unnecessary and clinical benefits can often be significant after the local reaction subsides.

The mechanism of these local AEs is poorly understood. The absence of recurrence after further injections seem to preclude allergic mechanisms. It has been suggested that these local reactions may resuit from misplacement of the needle in the soft periarticular tissues [113], causing tissue swelling and possible decrease of synovial fluid outflow. In a few cases, large and highly cellular effusions have been reported and the possibility of crystal arthritis has been raised. Presently, these mechanisms remain conjectural.

No alteration of blood or urine tests related to the hyaluronan and hylan products has been observed. No interaction with drugs taken by the patients for coincident conditions are known, nor are they expected because intraarticular hyaluronan has no systemic pharmacological activity. Infection remains a threat, as for all intraarticular procedures. Manufacturers insist on the strictness of aseptic conditions while performing the injections. Reports of septic arthritis after hyaluronan or hylan injections are very rare.

Finally, it is notable that in several million patients who received hyaluronan or hylan preparations intraarticularly in Japan, Italy, Canada, Sweden, and Germany in the past 10 years, as well as in an estimated 40 million people treated with hyaluronan preparations in ophthalmic surgical procedures worldwide during the past 25 years, no case of viral infection has been reported.

Conclusions

Intraarticular therapy with elastoviscous solutions of hyaluronan or hylans (viscosupplementation) is among the safest and most effective treatments for osteoarthritis of the knee. It reduces pain and improves joint function for several months after a series of three to five injections and can significantly decrease the patient's dependence on NSAIDs and corticosteroid injections and the hazards associated with them. It is increasingly evident, from preclinical and clinical studies, that the greater the elastoviscosity (molecular weight) of the viscosupplementation product, the greater the effectiveness of the treatment. By reestablishing elastoviscous homeostatic conditions in the joint, viscosupplementation has the potential to influence the natural course of osteoarthritis.

Acknowledgments. The help of Agnes Pilliard, Jean Bonomo, Raquel Newton, and Jennifer Bagley is gratefully acknowledged.

References

1. Laurent TC (1987) Biochemistry of hyaluronan. Acta Otolaryngol Suppl 442:7–24
2. Laurent TC, Fraser RE (1992) Hyaluronan. FASEB J 6:2397–2404
3. Mikelsaar R, Scott JE (1994) Molecular modeling of secondary and tertiary structures of hyaluronan, compared with electron microscopy and NMR data. Possible sheet and tabular structures in aqueous solution. Glycoconj J 11:65–71
4. Ghosh P (1994) The role of hyaluronic acid (hyaluronan) in health and disease: interactions with cells, cartilage, and components of synovial fluid. Clin Exp Rheumatol 12:75–82
5. Balazs EA, Gibbs DA (1970) The rheological properties and biological function of hyaluronic acid. In: Balazs EA (ed) Chemistry and molecular biology of the intercellular matrix. Academic, London, pp 1241–1254
6. Levick JR, McDonald JN (1990) Influence of intra-articular hyaluronan on flow across the synovial lining of knees in anesthetized rabbits. J Physiol (Camb) 422:23
7. Levick JR (1992) Synovial fluid. Determinants of volume turnover and material concentration. In: Kuettner K, Schleilrbach R, Peyron J, Hascall V (eds) Articular cartilage and osteoarthritis. Raven, New York, pp 529–541
8. Hadler NM, Napier MA (1977) Structure of hyaluronic acid in synovial fluid and its influence on the movement of solutes. Semin Arthritis Rheum 7:141–152

9. Paschalakis P, Vynios DH, Tsiganos CP, et al (1993) Effects of proteoglycans on hydroxyapatite growth in vitro: the role of hyaluronan. Biochim Biophys Acta 1158:129–136

10. Campion GV, Shellis RP, Dieppe PA (1990) The effect of synovial fluid and serum on the growth of calcium hydroxyapatite crystals. J Rheumatol 17:515–520

11. Ogston AG, Stanier JE (1953) The physiological function of hyaluronic acid in synovial fluid: viscous, elastic, and lubricant properties. J Physiol (Camb) 115:244–252

12. Darzynkiewicz Z, Balazs EA (1971) Effect of connective tissue intercellular matrix on lymphocyte stimulation. I. Suppression of lymphocyte stimulation by hyaluronic acid. Exp Cell Res 66:113–123

13. Balazs EA, Darzynkiewicz Z (1973) The effect of hyaluronic acid on fibroblast, mononuclear phagocytes, and lymphocytes. In: Kuionen E, Pikkarainen J (eds) Biology of the fibroblast. Academic, London, pp 237–252

14. Forrester JV, Balazs EA (1980) Inhibition of phagocytosis by high molecular weight hyaluronate. Immunology 40:435–446

15. Forrester JV, Wilkinson PC (1981) Inhibition of leukocyte locomotion by hyaluronic acid. J Cell Sci 48:315–331

16. Brandt K (1970) Modification of chemotaction by synovial fluid hyaluronate. Arthritis Rheum 13:308

17. Piako EJ, Turner RA, Soderstrom LP, et al (1983) Inhibition of neutrophil phagocytosis and enzyme release by hyaluronic acid. Clin Exp Rheumatol 1:41–44

18. Larsen NE, Lombard KM, Parent EG, et al (1992) Effect of hylan on cartilage and chondrocyte culture. J Orthop Res 10:23–32

19. Yasui Y, Akatsuka M, Tobetto K, et al (1992) Effects of hyaluronan on the production of stromelysin and tissue inhibitor of metalloproteinase 1 (TIMP 1) in bovine articular chondrocytes. Agents Actions 37:155–156

20. Kikuchi T, Denda S, Yamaguchi T (1993) Effect of sodium hyaluronate (SL 1010) on glycosaminoglycan synthesis and release in rabbit articular cartilage (in Japanese, summary in English). Jpn Pharmacol Ther 21(suppl 1):157–163

21. Smith MM, Ghosh P (1987) The synthesis of hyaluronic acid by human synovial fibroblasts is influenced by the nature of the hyaluronate in the extra cellular environment. Rheumatol Int 7:114–122

22. Hammerman D, Wood DD (1984) Interleukins enhance synovial cell hyaluronate synthesis. Proc Soc Exp Biol Med 177:205–210

23. Konttinen YT, Saari H, Nordstrom DC (1991) Effect of interleukin 1 on hyaluronate synthesis by synovial fibroblastic cells. Clin Rheumatol 10:151–154

24. Balazs EA (1974) The physical properties of the synovial fluid and the special role of hyaluronic acid. In: Helfet A (ed) Disorders of the knee. Lippincott, Philadelphia, pp 63–75

25. Hiori K, Kikawa M, Takaichi K, et al (1993) Autoradiography of the knee joint after intra-articular administration of ^{14}C sodium hyaluronate (^{14}C-SL-1010) in rabbits (in Japanese, summary in English). Jpn Pharmacol Ther 21:201–206

26. Antonas KM, Fraser JRE, Muirden KD (1973) Distribution of biologically labeled hyaluronic acid injected into joints. Ann Rheum Dis 32:102–111

27. Laurent UBG, Fraser RE, Engstrom-Laurent A, et al (1992) Catabolism of hyaluronan in the knee joint of the rabbit. Matrix 12:130–136

28. Denlinger JL (1982) Metabolism of sodium hyaluronate in articular and ocular tissues. Ph.D. thesis, Université des Sciences et Techniques de Lille, Lille, France

29. Brown TJ, Laurent UBG, Fraser JRE (1991) Turnover of hyaluronan in synovial joints: elimination of labeled hyaluronan from the knee joint of the rabbit. Exp Physiol 76:125–134

30. Fraser JRE, Kimpton WG, Pierscionek BK, et al (1993) The kinetics of hyaluronan in normal and acutely inflamed synovial joints. Observations with experimental arthritis in sheep. Semin Arthritis Rheum 22(suppl 1):9–17

31. Sato I, Matsuo K, Akima K (1992) Studies on metabolic fate of sodium hyaluronate (SL 1010) after intra-articular administration. Jpn Pharmacol Ther 21 (suppl 2):185–193

32. Balazs EA, Bloom GD, Swann DA (1966) Fine structure and glycosamino-glycan content of the surface layer of articular cartilage. Fed Proc 25:1813–1816

33. Akima K, Matsuo K, Watari N, et al (1993) Studies on the metabolic fate of sodium hyaluronate after intra-articular administration (in Japanese, summary in English). Jpn Pharmacol Ther 21:173–183

34. Balazs EA, Watson D, Duff IF, et al (1967) Hyaluronic acid in synovial fluid, molecular parameters of hyaluronic acid in normal and arthritic human fluids. Arthritis Rheum 10:357–376

35. Saari H, Kontinen YT (1989) Determination of the concentration and polymer-ization of synovial fluid hyaluronate using high performance liquid chromatogra-phy. Ann Rheum Dis 48:565–570

36. Balazs EA, Briller S, Denlinger JL (1981) Na-hyaluronate molecular size variations in equine and arthritic synovial fluid and effect on phagocytic cells. Semin Arthritis Rheum 11:141–143

37. Worall JG, Bayliss MT, Edwards JC (1990) Morphological localization of hyaluronan in normal and diseased synovium. J Rheum 18:1466–1472

38. Wells AF, Klareskog L, Lindblad S, et al (1992) Correlation between increased hyaluronan localized in arthritic synovium and the presence of proliferating cells. Arthritis Rheum 35:391–396

39. Pitsillides AA, Worall JG, Wilkinson LS, et al (1994) Hyaluronan concentration in non-inflamed and rheumatoid synovium. Br J Rheumatol 33:5–10

40. McDonald JN, Levick JR (1994) Hyaluronan reduces fluid escape from rabbit knee joints disparately from its effect on fluidity. Exp Physiol 79:103–106

41. Levick JR (1996) Synovial fluid hydraulics. Sci Med 11:52–61

42. Mapp PI (1995) Innervations of the synovium. Ann Rheum Dis 54:398–403

43. Pozo A, Balazs EA, Belmonte C (1997) Reduction of sensory responses to passive movements of inflamed knee joints by hylan, a hyaluronan derivative. Exp Brain Res 116:3–9

44. Gotoh S, Onaya J, Abe M, et al (1993) Effects of the molecular weight of hyaluronic acid and its action mechanisms on experimental joint pain in rats. Ann Rheum Dis 52:817–822

45. Shimizu N, Matsui Y, Masaki F, et al (1993) Analgesic effect of high molecular weight sodium hyaluronate (SL 1010) on bradykinin-induced knee pain in beagles (in Japanese, summary in English). Jpn Pharmacol Ther 21:133–141

46. Maroudas A (1969) Studies on the formation of hyaluronic acid films. In: Wright V (ed) Lubrication and wear in joints. Sector, London, pp 124–133
47. Cooke AF, Dowson D, Wright V (1976) Lubrication of synovial membrane. Ann Rheum Dis 35:56–59
48. Radin EL, Paul JL (1972) A consolidated concept of joint lubrication. J Bone Joint Surg 54A:607–616
49. Swann DA, Radin EL, Nazimiec M, et al (1974) Role of hyaluronic acid in joint lubrication. Ann Rheum Dis 33:318–326
50. Jay GD, Lane BP, Sokoloff L (1992) Characterization of a bovine synovial fluid lubricating factor. III. The interaction with hyaluronic acid. Connect Tissue Res 28:245–255
51. Altman S, Zeidler H, Langer HE (1985) The frictional behavior of articular cartilage in relation to the lubricant (abstract). In: Transactions of the 15th symposium of the European Society of Osteoarthrology. University of Kuopio, Finland, p 525
52. Davies DY, Palfrey AJ (1968) Some of the physical properties of normal and pathological synovial fluid. J Biomech 1:79–88
53. Balazs EA, Denlinger JL (1984) The role of hyaluronic acid in arthritis and its therapeutic use in osteoarthritis. In: Peyron JG (ed) Current clinical and fundamental problems. Geigy, Paris, pp 165–174
54. Greenwald RA, Moy WW (1980) Effect of oxygen derived free radicals on hyaluronic acid. J Clin Invest 66:298–305
55. Wright V, Dowson D, Unsworth A (1971) The role of lubrication in osteoarthrosis. In: Abstracts, VII European congress on rheumatology, Brighton. Arthritis and Rheumatism Council, London, 36:17
56. Martel-Pelletier J, Cloutier JM, Pelletier JP (1986) Neutral proteases in human osteoarthritic synovium. Arthritis Rheum 29:1112–1123
57. Westacott CI, Whicher JT, Barnes TC, et al (1990) Synovial fluid concentration of five different cytokines in rheumatic diseases. Ann Rheum Dis 49:676–681
58. Vignon E, Mathieu P, Conrozier T, et al (1990) Cytokines, phospholipase A2, prostaglandin E_2 et metalloproteases du ciquide synovial dans la gonarthrose (abstract). Rev Rhum Mal Osteo Artic 57:682
59. Egg D (1984) Concentration of prostaglandin D2, E2, F(2), 6-keto-F (1), and thromboxane B2 in synovial fluid from patients with inflammatory disorders and osteoarthritis. J Rheumatol 43:89–96
60. Wittenberg RH, Willburger RE, Kleemeyerk S (1993) In vitro release of prostaglandins and leukotrienes from synovial tissue, cartilage, and bone in degenerative joint diseases. Arthritis Rheum 36:1444–1450
61. Gibilisco PA, Schumacher HR, Hollander JK, et al (1985) Synovial fluid crystals in osteoarthritis. Arthritis Rheum 28:511–515
62. Dieppe PA, Aiwan W (1987) Synovial fluid in osteoarthritis (abstract). Arthritis Rheum 30:S130
63. Heinegard D, Inerot S, Wieslander O (1985) A method for the quantification of cartilage proteoglycan structures liberated to the synovial fluid during developing degenerative joint disease. Scand J Clin Invest 45:421–427
64. Witter J, Roughley PJ, Webber C, et al (1987) The immunologic detection and characterization of cartilage proteoglycan degradation in synovial fluid of patients with arthritis. Arthritis Rheum 30:519–529

65. Shinmei M, Miyauchi S, Machida A, et al (1992) Quantitation of chondroitin 4-sulfate and chondroitin 6-sulfate in pathologic joint fluid. Arthritis Rheum 34:1304–1308
66. Obara T, Yamaguchi T, Moriya Y, et al (1993) Tissue distribution of fluorescein labeled sodium hyaluronate in experimentally induced osteoarthritis (in Japanese, summary in English). Jpn Pharmacol Ther 21:193–201
67. Greenwald RA (1991) Oxygen radicals, inflammation and arthritis: pathophysiological considerations and implication for treatment. Semin Arthritis Rheum 20:219–240
68. Schenck P, Schneider S, Miehlke R, et al (1995) Synthesis and degradation of hyaluronate by synovia from patients with rheumatoid arthritis. J Rheumatol 22:400–405
69. Tobetto K, Yasui T, Ando T, et al (1992) Inhibitory effects of hyaluronan on ^{14}C arachidonic acid release from labeled human synovial fibroblasts. Jpn J Pharmacol 60:79–84
70. Wigren A, Wik O, Falk J (1976) Intra-articular injection of high molecular weight hyaluronic acid. An experimental study on normal adult rabbit knee joints. Acta Orthop Scand 47:480–485
71. Abatangelo G, Botti P, Delbue M, et al (1989) Intra-articular sodium hyaluronate injections in the Pond-Nuki experimental model of osteoarthritis in dogs. Clin Orthop 241:278–285
72. Schiavinato A, Lini E, Guidolin D, et al (1989) Intra-articular sodium hyaluronate injections in the Pond-Nuki experimental model of osteoarthritis in dogs. Clin Orthop 241:286–299
73. Armstrong S, Read R, Ghosh P (1994) The effects of intra-articular hyaluronan on cartilage and subchondral bone changes in an ovine model of early osteoarthritis. J Rheumatol 21:680–688
74. Yoshioka M, Shimizue C, Hardwood FL, et al (1997) The effect of hyaluronan during the development of osteoarthritis. Osteoarthritis Cartil 5:251–260
75. Kikushi T, Yamagushi T, Sakakibard Y, et al (1993) Therapeutic effect of high molecular weight sodium hyaluronate (SL 1010) on the experimental osteoarthritis induced by rabbit knee immobilization (in Japanese, summary in English). Jpn Pharmacol Ther 21:123–131
76. Yoshimi T, Kikuchi T, Obaka T, et al (1994) Effects of high molecular weight sodium hyaluronate on experimental osteoarthrosis induced by the resolution of rabbit anterior cruciate ligament. Clin Orthop 298:296–304
77. Toyoshima H (1978) The influence of synovectomy on articular cartilage of rabbit knee and preventive effects of hyaluronic acid on degenerative changes of the cartilage. J Tokyo Womens Med Coll 48:890
78. Kitoh Y, Katsurmaki T, Tanaka H, et al (1992) Effect of SL 1010 (sodium hyaluronate with high molecular weight) on experimental osteoarthritis induced by intra-articularly applied papain in rabbits (in Japanese, summary in English). Folia Pharmacol Jpn 100:67–76
79. Kido H, Maeyama K, Tagawa T, et al (1993) Effect of high molecular weight sodium hyaluronate (SL 1010) on experimental osteoarthritis induced by immobilization of rabbit knee joint (in Japanese, summary in English). Jpn Pharmacol Ther 24:115–121
80. Williams JM, Plaza V, Hui F, et al (1997) Hyaluronan suppresses fibronectin fragment mediated cartilage chondrolysis II in vivo. Osteoarthritis Cartil 5:235–240

81. Asari A, Miyauchi S, Matsuzaka S, et al (1996) Hyaluronate on heat shock protein and synovial cells in a canine model of osteoarthritis. Osteoarthritis Cartil 4:213–215

82. Balazs EA, Leshchiner EA (1989) Hyaluronan, its crosslinked derivative Hylan, and their medical applications. In: Inagaki H, Phillips GO (eds) Cellulosics utilization: research and rewards in cellulosics. Elsevier, New York, pp 233–241

83. Larsen NE, Lombard KM, Parent EG, Balazs EA (1992) Effect of hylan on cartilage and chondrocyte cultures. J Orthop Res 10:23–32

84. Al-Assaf S, Phillips GO, Deeble DJ, et al (1995) The enhanced stability of the cross-links hylan structure to hydroxyl (OH) radicals compared with the uncross-linked hyaluronan. Radiat Phys Chem 46:207–217

85. Balazs EA, Denlinger JL (1985) Sodium hyaluronate and joint function. J Equine Vet Sci 5:217–228

86. Philips MW (1989) Clinical trial comparison of intra-articular sodium hyaluronate products in the horse. J Equine Vet Sci 9:39–40

87. Balazs EA, Denlinger JL (1993) Viscosupplementation. A new concept in the treatment of osteoarthritis. J Rheumatol 20(suppl 39):3–9

88. Balazs EA (ed) (1971) Hyaluronic acid and matrix implantation. Biotrics, Arlington, MA

89. Helfet J (1974) Management of osteoarthritis of the knee joint. In: Helfet J (ed) Disorders of the knee. Lippincott, Philadelphia, p 179

90. Peyron JG, Balazs EA (1974) Preliminary assessment of Na-hyaluronate injection into human arthritic joints. Pathol Biol 22:731–736

91. Weiss C, Balazs EA, St. Onge R, et al (1981) Clinical studies of the intra-articular injection of Healon (sodium hyaluronate) in the treatment of osteoarthritis of human knees. Semin Arthritis Rheum 11:143–144

92. Namiki O, Toyoshima H, Morisaki N (1982) Therapeutic effect of intra-articular injection of high molecular weight hyaluronic acid on osteoarthritis of the knee. Int Clin Pharmacol Ther Toxicol 20:501–507

93. Oshima Y (1983) Intra-articular injection therapy of high molecular sodium hyaluronate on osteoarthritis of the knee joint. Phase II clinical study. Jpn Pharmacol Ther II:2253–2257

94. Shichikawa AK and the drug evaluation committee of the Japanese Rheumatic Association (1983) Evaluation of the effect of sodium hyaluronate on osteoarthritis of the knee. Ryumachi 23:280–290

95. Honma T (1989) Clinical effect of high molecular weight sodium hyaluronate (Artz) injected into osteoarthritic knee joints. Jpn Pharmacol Ther 17:5057–5072

96. Igarashi M (1983) Multicenter clinical studies of high molecular weight sodium hyaluronate in the long-term treatment of osteoarthritis of the knee. Jpn Pharmacol Ther II:4871–4888

97. Puhl W, Bernau A, Greiling H, et al (1993) Intra-articular sodium hyaluronate in osteoarthritis of the knee: a multicenter double-blind study. Osteoarthritis Cartil I:219–232

98. Dahlberg L, Lodhander LS, Ryd L (1994) Intra-articular injections of hyaluronan in patients with cartilage abnormalities and knee pain. A one-year double-blind, placebo-controlled study. Arthritis Rheum 37:521–528

99. Lohmander LS, Dalen N, Englund G, et al (1996) Intra-articular hyaluronan injections in the treatment of osteoarthritis of the knee. A randomized

double-blind, placebo-controlled multicentre trial. Ann Rheum Dis 55:424–431

100. Bragantini A, Gassini M, Debastiani G, et al (1982) Controlled single blind trial of intra-articularly injected hyaluronic acid (Hyalgan) in osteoarthritis of the knee. Clin Trials J 24:333–340

101. Grecomoro G, Martorana J, Dimarco C (1987) Intra-articular treatment with sodium hyaluronate in gonarthrosis: a controlled clinical trial versus placebo. Pharmatherapeutica 5:137–141

102. Carabba M, Paresce E, Angelin M, et al (1992) Efficacy and safety of different dose-schedules of intra-articular injections of hyaluronic acid in painful and hydarthrodial osteoarthritis of the knee. Results of a prospective randomized, placebo and arthrocentesis controlled study (abstract). In: Transactions of the VIIth Eular scientific symposium, London, pp 22–24

103. Henderson EB, Smith EC, Pegley F, et al (1994) Intra-articular injections of 750 KD hyaluronan in the treatment of osteoarthritis: a randomized single center double-blind, placebo-controlled trial of 91 patients demonstrating lack of efficacy. Ann Rheum Dis 53:529–534

104. St. John Dixon A, Jacoby RK, Berry H, et al (1988) Clinical trials of intra-articular injections of sodium hyaluronate in patients with osteoarthritis of the knee. Curr Med Res Opin II:205–213

105. Dougados M, Nguyen M, Listrat V, et al (1993) High molecular weight sodium hyaluronate (Hyalectin) in osteoarthritis of the knee. A one-year placebo-controlled trial. Osteoarthritis Cartil 1:97–104

106. Listrat V, Ayral X, Patarnello F, et al (1997) Arthroscopic evaluation of potential structure modifying activity of hyaluronan (Hyalgan) in osteoarthritis of the knee. Osteoarthritis Cartil 5:153–160

107. Pietrogrande V, Leonardi M, Ulivi M, et al (1989) Confronto clinico della efficacia e tolerabilita del acido ialuronico e 6 metilprednisolone sommistrato per via intra-articolare nel trattamento della gonartrosi. Ortop Traum Oggi 9:275–280

108. Leardini G, Matara L, Franceschini M, et al (1991) Intra-articular treatment of knee osteoarthritis. A comparative study between hyaluronic acid and 6-methyl prednisolone acetate. Clin Exp Rheumatol 9:375–381

109. Takigami S, Takigami M, Phillips GO (1993) Hydration characteristics of the cross-linked hyaluronan derivative hylan. Carbohydr Polym 22:153–160

110. Scale D, Wobig M, Wolpert W (1994) Viscosupplementation of osteoarthritic knees with hylan-A treatment schedule study. Curr Ther Res 55:220–232

111. Adams ME (1993) An analysis of clinical studies of the use of cross-linked hyaluronan, hylan, in the treatment of OA. J Rheum 20(suppl 39):16–18.

112. Adams ME, Atkinson MH, Lussier A, et al (1995) The role of viscosupplementation with hylan G-F 20 (Synvisc) in the treatment of osteoarthritis of the knee. A Canadian multicenter trial comparing hylan G-F 20 alone, hylan G-F 20 with non-steroidal anti-inflammatory drugs (NSAIDs) and NSAIDs alone. Osteoarthritis Cartil 3:213–226

113. Lussier A, Cividino AA, McFarlane CA, et al (1996) Viscosupplementation with hylan for the treatment of osteoarthritis: findings from clinical practice in Canada. J Rheumatol 23:1579–1585

114. Adams ME (1997) Viscosupplementation with hylan vs. NSAID therapy: clinical trial experience. Osteoarthritis Cartil 5(suppl A):71

115. Hollander JL, Jessar RA, Brown EM (1961) Intra-synovial corticosteroid therapy: a decade of use. Bull Rheum Dis II:239–240
116. Gray RG, Gottlieb NL (1983) Intra-articular corticosteroids. Clin Orthop 177:235–263

Effects of Sodium Hyaluronic Acid on Fibrinolytic Factors in Humans with Arthropathies

HIRAKU KIKUCHI, TOHGO NONAKA, WATARU SHIMADA, ICHIRO MIYAGI,
HIROAKI ITAGANE, TERUMASA IKEDA, CHIAKI HAMANISHI,
and SEISUKE TANAKA

Summary. High molecular weight (90- to 100-kDa) plasminogen activator
(PA) urokinase-type/inhibitor-1 ([u-PA/PAI-1] complex) and 55-kDa u-PA
were identified in synovial fluid collected from 12 osteoarthritis (OA) patients
given hyaluronic acid (HA) into the knee joint. HA administration led
to an increase in levels of u-PA and PAI-1 antigen as well as increases
in the u-PA:PAI-1 ratio. In inhibition of their symptoms, the fibrinolytic
activity was progressively suppressed. The u-PA content was higher
at the weight-bearing site in OA and rheumatoid arthritis (RA) patients
compared to cartilage tissue from controls. The PAI-1 content was higher
in osteophyte-forming sites and in RA, compared to controls. Weight-
bearing sites in OA patients expressed a high u-PA mRNA level but a low
PAI-1 mRNA level. Osteophyte-forming sites in OA patients expressed a
low u-PA mRNA level but a high PAI-1 mRNA level. The levels of u-PA
and PAI-1 antigen increased in cartilage tissues exposed to mechanical
stress. In contrast, the release of u-PA and PAI-1 antigens from specimens
was suppressed with HA. At the weight-bearing site, the levels of
matrix metalloproteinase (MMP) were high and levels of TIMP (tissue
inhibitor of metalloproteinase) mRNA expression were low. In osteophyte-
formed sites, the levels of TIMP were high and the levels of MMP
mRNA expression low. These findings suggest that regulation of fibrinolysis may play a important role in the matrix of articular cartilage with
arthropathy.

Key Words. Arthropathy, Hyaluronic acid, Urokinase-type plasminogen
activator, PA inhibitor-1, Metalloproteinase, Tissue inhibitor of
metalloproteinase

Department of Orthopaedic Surgery, Kinki University School of Medicine, 377-2
Ohno-Higashi, Osaka-Sayama, Osaka 589-8511, Japan

Introduction

Destruction of articular cartilage is induced by such factors as stress, aging, permeability, angiogenesis, gas and chemical mediators, cytokines, proteinases, and adhesion [1]. Organic proteinases can be classified into four types, depending on their activity: metallo-, serine, cysteine, and aspartate proteinases. Of these, metalloproteinases [2–4] and serine proteinases [5] play leading roles in the decomposition of cartilage matrix. These proteinases have an optimum pH in the neutral range [3].

In the three kinds of matrix metalloproteinase (MMP), MMP-1 decomposes collagens types I, II, and III and MMP-3 decomposes proteoglycans and activates latent MMP-1. Typical inhibitors of these MMPs are tissue inhibitors of MMP-1 (TIMP-1) and MMP-2 (TIMP-2), which are produced in the synovium and cartilage and released into the joint spaces to inhibit decomposition of the matrix [3]. Plasmin and plasminogen activator (PA) are involved in decomposition in serine proteinases [5]. PA activates plasminogen to produce plasmin, which decomposes proteoglycans (PG) and also activates latent MMP-1 and MMP-3 [2,3].

There are two types of physiological PAs, which are immunologically and biologically distinct: tissue-type plasminogen activator (t-PA) and urokinase-type plasminogen activator (u-PA). The former has a higher affinity for fibrin and enhances enzymatic activity in the presence of fibrin or fibrin degradation products. On the other hand, u-PA is predominantly involved in extravascular fibrinolysis, which occurs in cell migration, in tissue remodeling, and in cell invasion and metastasis of cancer cells. U-PA secreted with a single strand but having no activity is linked to a u-PA receptor [6,7] (U-PAR) on the surface of chondrocytes or synovium, and these are activated with proteinases, as plasmin is activated to produce double strands. Double-strand u-PA has no affinity for fibrin. The PA-plasmin system has been implicated in turnover under physiological and pathological conditions. The system has been detected in mineralized tissues and appears to be involved in degradation of connective tissue. Such PA activity is inactivated by its specific fast-acting inhibitors, PA inhibitor-1 (PAI-1) and PAI-2, which bind to and limit the activity of t-PA and u-PA. The extracellular fibrinolytic system is regulated by the balance of PA and PAI. Both t-PA and u-PA, and u-PAR, PAI-1, and PAI-2, are produced in the synovium and cartilage and released into the joint space.

The main structural components of articular cartilage are fibrillar collagen and soluble PG. The collagen network provides mechanical stress [1], and PG is responsible for the transmission and dissipation of compressive loads during movement and weight-bearing [8]. PGs are present primarily in the form of aggregates in which monomers are noncovalently bound to HA, as a linear high molecular weight glycosaminoglycan. In osteoarthritis (OA), the pathophysiological changes within the cartilage matrix are progressive breakdown of collagen and degradation of PG macromolecules [9]. Destruction of the collagen network occurs initially around the pericellular zone of the chondrocytes, and with progression of the disease, the collagen network is completely disrupted.

Intraarticular administration of hyaluronic acid (HA) is widely prescribed for the treatment of OA [10,11]. When injected HA is introduced into the extracellular matrix (ECM), it acts to protect the injured ECM and to reduce friction. Although HA has clinical efficacy and is used in the treatment of subjects with arthropathy, there are few data on the effects of HA on fibrinolytic factors in the knee joint with OA.

In this study, we investigated the influence of HA on PA, PAI, MMP, and TIMP levels in the synovial fluid and cartilage tissue of humans with osteoarthritis.

Materials and Methods

Reagents

The following materials were purchased from the sources indicated: bovine thrombin (Mochida Pharmaceuticals, Tokyo, Japan), plasminogen-containing bovine fibrinogen (Organon Technika, Boxtel, The Nethelands), molecular weight 800 000 HA (80 HA, Artze^R; Kaken Seiyaku, Tokyo, Japan), molecular weight 1 800 000 HA (180 HA, NRD101; Denkikagaku Kogyo, Tokyo, Japan). The purified high molecular weight two-chain u-PA was a gift from Dr. N. Nobuhara (Mochida) and u-PAR was provided by Dr. O. Matsuo (Physiology, Kinki University, Osaka, Japan). Antibodies against u-PA (Mochida), t-PA (Sumitomo Pharmaceuticals, Tokyo, Japan). PAI-1 (Technoclone, Vienna, Austria), and PAI-2 (Technoclone) were purchased. [α-^{32}P]dCTP deoxycytidine triphosphate was purchased from Amersham (Buckinghamshire, UK) and the u-PA probe from the JCRB Gene Bank (Tokyo, Japan). The cDNA probes from MMP-1, MMP-3, TIMP-1, TIMP-2, and glyceraldehyde 3-phosphate dehydrogenase (GAPDH) were purchased from ATCC (Rockville, MD, USA). All other reagents and chemicals were of the highest grade available.

Patients and Collection of Synovial Fluid

Three men and nine women, all Japanese and with OA of the knee accompanied by effusion, agreed to participate in this study. Ages ranged from 55 to 83 years (average, 74.3 years). The methods used in this study were as follows: 3 ml of synovial fluid was collected before the introduction of 80 HA. Subsequently, a 25 mg dose of 80 HA was given and total synovial fluid was collected 3 h later. This procedure was repeated over a 4 week period. The collected synovial fluid was centrifuged for 5 min at 3000 $\times$ g and the cellular components were discarded. These fluid samples were then preserved at $-80°C$ until analyzed.

Collection of Cartilage Tissue from Patients

Cartilage tissues were obtained from OA and RA patients for whom total knee arthroplasty (TKA) had been carried out or who had undergone above-knee amputation (AK) as a result of peripheral circulatory disorders. In patients with OA (18 women; mean age, 68 years), samples (10 × 10mm) were taken from the weight-bearing site (WS) and the osteophyte-formed site (OS), without subchondral bone. In those with RA (10 women; mean age, 65 years) where no osteophytes had formed, samples were taken only from the WS. Control cartilage specimens were obtained from patients who had to undergo AK because of peripheral circulatory disorders (2 men and 4 women; mean age, 67 years). All specimens were stained with haematoxylin-eosin stain.

Cartilage tissue samples were immersed in 4ml of 50mmol/l Tris buffer solution (pH 7.4) per 100g of tissue and homogenized for 10min, followed by ultrasonication. The samples were then centrifuged at 2000 × g for 30min at 4°C, and the supernatant was dialyzed in 50mmol/l. The supernatant was then immersed in Tris buffer solution (pH 7.4) containing 10mmol/l (CaCl$_2$, 0.2mol/l NaCl, and 0.05% Tween 80 for 2 × 12h to obtain the extract. Absorbance was determined at 280nm with spectrometry, and this was converted to a protein concentration, in terms of albumin. The extracts were frozen at −80°C until use.

Measurement of PA and PAI activities in Synovial Fluid

PA activity and molecular weights were analyzed by electrophoretic enzymography [5,6] and those for PAI by reversed electrophoretic enzymography [2]. For preparation of the separation gel, 2ml of acrylamide (30g/100ml) and bisacrylamide (1g/100ml), 240μl of bovine plasminogen-rich fibrinogen (1.5mg/ml), and 1.5ml of 1.5M Tris-HCl buffer (pH 8.8) were mixed. Then, 24μl of thrombin (10MIH U/ml), 60μl of 10% sodium dodecyl sulfate (SDS), 10μl of N,N,N,N'-tetramethylethylenediamine (THEMED), and 60μl of 10% ammonium peroxydisulfate were further mixed. For preparation of the stacking gel, the usual method was used [5,6]. After electrophoresis, the gel was soaked in 2.5% Triton X-100 for 2h and incubated in 0.1M glycine buffer (pH 8.3) at 37°C. After soaking in 50% trichloroacetic acid (TCA) solution for 1h and in 7% ethanol for 1h, the gel was stained with Coomassie brilliant blue solution. After destaining with 7% acetic acid, the gels so produced developed a lysis zone when plasminogen activator (PA) was present in the sample solution.

Measurement of Antigens

The amount of t-PA, u-PA, PAI-1, and PAI-2 antigen in the synovial fluid from patients given HA treatment was determined using a t-PA ELISA kit (Technoclone), a u-PA ELISA kit (Monozyme, Virum, Denmark), and a PAI-

1 and PAI-2 ELISA kit (Technoclone), respectively. The amount of t-PA, u-PA, PAI-1, and TIMP-1 antigen in the cartilage from patients given TKA treatment was determined by a t-PA, u-PA, and PAI-1 ELISA kit and a TIMP-1 ELISA kit (Fujiyakuhin Kogyo, Tokyo, Japan).

Northern Blot Analysis

cDNA probes of u-PA, PAI-1, MMP-1, MMP-3, TIMP-1, TIMP-2, and GAPDH were labeled and the total RNA of each cartilage tissue sample was extracted with guanidium thiocyanate-phenolchloroform. The preparation was subjected to electrophoresis in a formaldehyde-modified agarose gel, followed by blotting on a BA 80 nitrocellulose membrane (Schleir & Schuell, Dassel, Germany). Hybridization was undertaken using each labeled probe, and a BA 80 nitrocellulose membrane was then washed three times for 30 min with 2× solution of sodium citrate containing 0.1% SDS before autoradiography. The concentrations of each autograph band were analyzed with a densitometer CS-900 (Shimadzu, Kyoto, Japan).

Mechanical Stress

Mechanical stress of $5 kg/0.25 cm^2$ was applied for 10 min to the cartilage samples using compression, and the quantity of u-PA and PAI-1 released was measured with 80 HA and 180 HA treatment overnight at 37°C.

Clinical Parameters

Pain, ballotment of the patella, range of motion, and activities of daily living were assessed before and after each weekly interarticular injection of HA and following the final administration of HA. Clinical parameters that showed improvement were labeled "positive" and those which showed either no improvement or worsening were labeled "negative."

Statistical Analysis

Data are presented as the mean ± SD, and Student's t-test was used to determine the statistical significance.

Results

Clinical Results

Nine of 12 patients showed improvement while receiving 80 HA. The joint effusion totally subsided in 1 of 12 patients by the third week and in another patient by the fourth week. Therefore, synovial fluid could not be obtained from these patients.

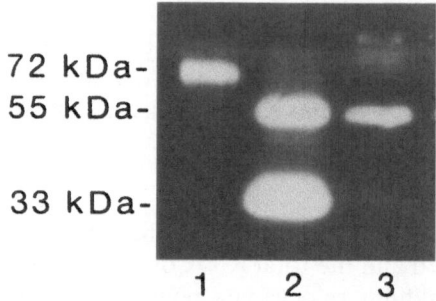

FIG. 1. Activity of plasminogen activator (PA) in synovial fluid. Electrophoretic enzymography of synovial fluid collected from knee joint of patients with osteoarthritis. The gel was incubated with 0.1 M glicine buffer, pH 8.3, at 37°C for 48 h. *Lane 1*, tissue-type PA (t-PA); *lane 2*, urokinase-type PA (u-PA); *lane 3*, synovial fluid

Analysis of PA Activity in Synovial Fluid and After Administration of 80 HA

Figure 1 shows electrophoretic enzymography of the synovial fluid. A major lysis band at 55 kDa and a trace lysis band at 90–100 kDa were observed (lane 3). In the presence of anti-u-PA IgG, all lysis bands disappeared; however, anti-t-PA IgG did not affect the lysis bands. The lysis band at 90–100 kDa was regarded as the u-PA/PAI-1 complex. The calculated MW was regarded as being the same as u-PA and PAI. PAI-1 antigen was present in this complex. Thus, u-PA and a small amount of u-PA and a complex formed with PAI-1 were secreted into the synovial fluid; t-PA was not detected.

Setting the value of u-PA activity before the 80 HA administration at 100%, u-PA activity increased to 147% ± 26% at 3 h after the administration of 80 HA. This phenomenon was observed for all 12 patients. However, the activity of u-PA gradually decreased from the first to fourth administration of 80 HA in 9 of 12 patients in whom the clinical parameters improved. On the other hand, in the 3 patients showing no improvement, u-PA activity was not affected by 80 HA at any time. The enzymograph of a typical case of improvement (Fig. 2) shows that u-PA activity was enhanced 3 h after the administration of 80 HA (lanes 3, 4) and that the u-PA and u-PA/PAI-1 complex activity gradually decreased from the second to the third week (lanes 5, 6). In the fourth week, the u-PA/PAI-1 complex disappeared and u-PA activity was observed as only a minor trace band (lane 7).

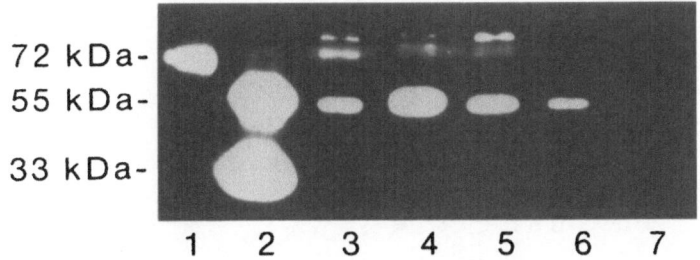

FIG. 2. Level of u-PA activity of the administration with hyaluronic acid (HA) (a typical case of improvement). Synovial fluid, 3 ml, was collected before administration of HA and total synovial fluid was collected after 3 h. This procedure was repeated over a 4-week period. The collected synovial fluid was centrifuged for 5 min at 3000 × g and the cellular components were discarded. *Lane 1*, t-PA; *lane 2*, u-PA; *lane 3*, synovial fluid, first week before administration of HA; *lane 4*, synovial fluid, first week after administration of HA; *lane 5*, synovial fluid, second week after introduction of HA; *lane 6*, synovial fluid, third week after administration of HA; *lane 7*, synovial fluid, fourth week after administration of HA

TABLE 1. Antigens of urokinase-type plasminogen activator (u-PA) and plasminogen activator inhibitor (PAI-1) in synovial fluid after administration of hyaluronic acid (HA) to patients

Protocol	Cases improved		Cases not improved	
	Before[a]	After[a]	Before[a]	After[a]
u-PA (ng/ml)	0.80 ± 0.27	1.29 ± 0.41	0.76 ± 0.24	0.79 ± 0.28
PAI-1 (ng/ml)	4.02 ± 2.06	9.84 ± 4.29*	4.88 ± 2.94	6.45 ± 3.62

Synovial fluid, 3 ml, was collected before the intraarticular administration of HA. Total synovial fluid collected after 3 h was centrifuged for 5 min at 3000 × g, and cellular components were discarded. These fluid samples were then preserved at −80°C until analyzed.
Nine patients showed improvement and three did not.
[a] Before and after refer to administration of HA.
* $P < .05$. Data are expressed as mean ± SD.

Changes in u-PA and PAI-1 Antigens after Administration of HA

The antigen of u-PA showed an increasing tendency 3 h after the administration of HA, and PAI-1 antigen was significantly increased in patients showing improvement. On the other hand, in cases of no improvement, u-PA and PAI-1 antigens showed only a slightly increased tendency (Table 1).

Changes in PAI-2 Antigen After Administration of 80 HA

The PAI-2 antigen was detected in 6 of 12 patients. In 5 of these 6, there was a gradual decrease in PAI-2 level, with improvement in symptoms. In only 1

244   H. Kikuchi et al.

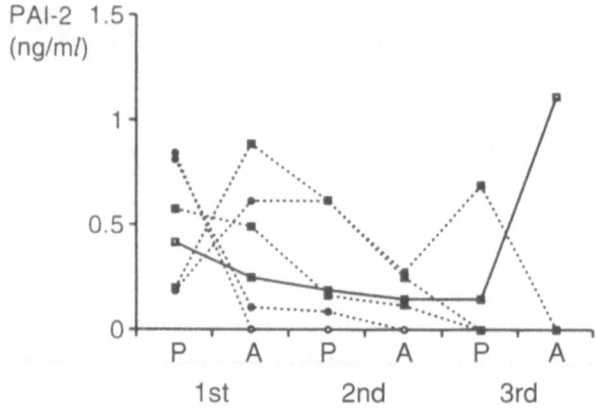

FIG. 3. Level of plasminogen activator inhibitor (PAI-2) antigen after administration of 80 HA. The amount of PAI-2 antigen in the synovial fluid from patients receiving 80 HA treatment was determined using ELISA kits. In five of six patients, the level of PAI-2 antigen decreased with improvement in symptoms. *P*, pretreatment with 80 HA; *A*, after treatment with 80 HA. *Dotted lines*, improved; *solid lines*, unchanged

patient there was an increase in PAI-2 with no improvement in the symptoms (Fig. 3).

Measurement of PA and PAI Antigens and Activities in Cartilage Tissue

Tissue extracts were prepared from cartilage tissues obtained from 11 patients with OA (70 ± 6 years of age), 5 with RA (68 ± 6 years of age), and 3 normal subjects with above knee amputation (60 ± 12 years of age). The antigens of t-PA, u-PA, PAI-1, and TIMP-1 were measured, and correction was made on the basis of the concentration of total protein.

The amount of u-PA antigen in the normal articular cartilage was 1.18 ± 0.24 ng/mg protein. Cartilage affected with OA contained 3.09 ± 0.62 ng/mg protein of u-PA in the WS and 1.26 ± 0.28 ng/mg protein in the OS, while that of RA contained 3.31 ± 0.48 ng/mg protein. The amount of u-PA antigen rose significantly in the WS group in whom the articular cartilage was affected with RA ($P < .001$) and the WS ($P < .01$), compared to the control cartilage. t-PA was not detected.

In the control group, the amount of PAI-1 antigen was 95.1 ± 10.3 ng/mg protein. In the OA group, the value was 33.0 ± 14.6 ng/mg protein for the WS and 145.1 ± 24.9 ng/mg protein for the OS, while in the RA group the value was 367.0 ± 91.4 ng/mg protein. Extracts from cartilage with RA ($P < .001$) and from the WS ($P < .01$) showed a significant increase in the amount of PAI-1 antigen, compared with the control. In the contrast, the articular carti-

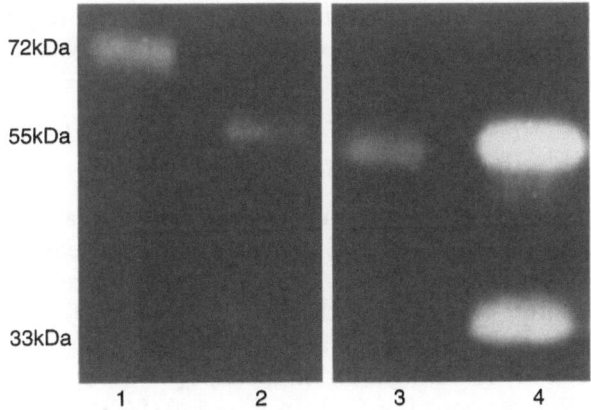

FIG. 4. Activity of u-PA in articular cartilage from patients with osteoarthritis and rheumatoid arthritis of the knee were measured by electrophoretic enzymography. *Lane 1*, t-PA; *lane 2*, u-PA; *lane 3*, osteoarthritis, *lane 4*; rheumatoid arthritis

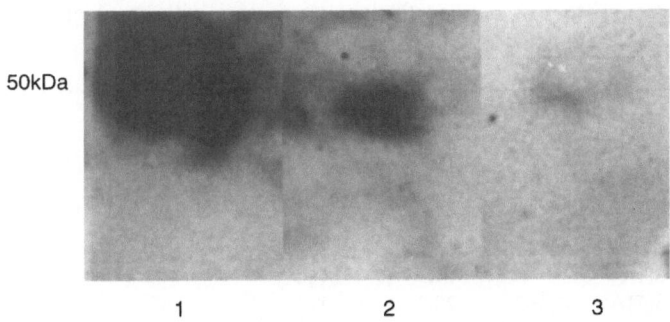

FIG. 5. Activity of PAI-1 in articular cartilage of the knee joint from patients with osteoarthritis and rheumatoid arthritis measured by electrophoretic reversed enzymography. *Lane 1*, PAI-1; *lane 2*, rheumatoid arthritis; *lane 3*, osteoarthritis

lage of the WS contained significantly decreased amounts of PAI-1 antigen ($P < .001$).

The activity of PA in extracts from OS, WS, RA, and control cases were measured using electrophoretic enzymography (Fig. 4). In all the extracts, bands of 55kDa and 33kDa appeared, and these coincided with bands for the u-PA marker. All the bands disappeared in the presence of the anti-u-PA antibody and thus were concluded to the u-PA. No band corresponding to the 72-kDa band of the t-PA marker was ever observed. The intensity of bands of u-PA in different samples was of the gradation RA > control > WS > OS.

Reverse fibrin autography was used to measure PAI-1 activity in extracts from articular cartilage with OA and RA (Fig. 5). Bands corresponding to

50 kDa were evident, and these coincided with the band for the PAI-1 marker. The intensity of the bands was of the order OS > RA > WS.

Effect of HA for Fibrinolytic Factors on Cartilage Exposed to Mechanical Stress

Mechanical stress of 5 kg/0.25 cm^2 was applied for 10 min at 37°C in cases of cartilage tissues of OS (64 years), WS (64 years), RA (61 years), and a normal case (63 years). The antigens of u-PA and PAI-1 were measured using ELISA kits before and after treatment with HA. The levels of u-PA and PAI-1 antigens increased in all specimens after mechanical stress. In contrast, the release of u-PA and PAI-1 antigens from specimens was suppressed in the case of HA (RA > WS > control > OS). In RA, 180 HA suppressed u-PA and PAI-1 antigens compared with the suppression rate of 80 HA treatment. HA cartilage was protected from mechanical stress (Table 2).

TABLE 2. Effect of HA on fibrinolytic factors with cartilage subjected to mechanical stress

Protocol	RA	WS	Control	OS
u-PA, no stress	100	100	100	100
u-PA, with stress	667	458	244	170
+80HA	243	83	127	142
+180HA	156	91	131	125
PAI-1, no stress	100	100	100	100
PAI-1, with stress	559	428	199	148
+80HA	298	156	145	116
+180HA	202	124	150	108

Mechanical stress of 5 kg/0.25 cm^2 was applied for 10 min to cartilage samples. The quantity of u-PA and PAI-1 released was measured using ELISA kits and is indicated as a percent of control.
HA, hyaluronic acid; RA, rheumatoid arthritis; WS, weight-bearing site in osteoarthritis; OS, osteophyte-formed site.

Measurement of TIMP-1 Antigens and Activities in Cartilage Tissue

The amount of TIMP-1 antigens in the control cartilage was 11.8 ± 4.6 ng/mg protein, while the cartilage with OA gave a value of 9.2 ± 4.1 ng/mg protein in the WS and 23.7 ± 2.0 ng/mg protein in the OS. In cartilage from RA patients, the amount was 33.8 ± 8.2 ng/mg protein. A significant increase in the amount of TIMP-1 occurred in cartilage from RA ($P < .001$) and OS subjects ($P < .01$).

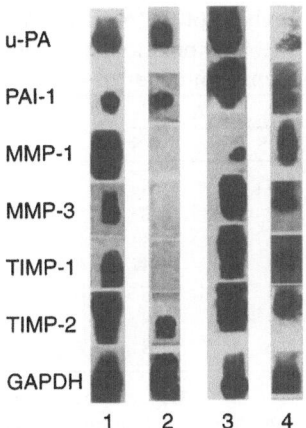

FIG. 6. Northern blot analysis of u-PA, PAI-1, matrix metalloproteinase (MMP-1), MMP-3, tissue inhibitor of MMP (TIMP-1), and TIMP-2 mRNA from articular cartilage from patients with osteoarthritis (OA) and rheumatoid arthritis and control. Total RNA was fractioned on a denaturated formamide agarose gel. After gel electrophoresis, RNA was blotted onto a nitrocellulose membrane and hybridized to cDNA probes for u-PA, PAI-1, MMP-1, MMP-3, TIMP-1, and TIMP-2. *Lane 1*, OA (osteophyte-forming site); *lane 2*, OA (weight-bearing site); *lane 3*, control; *lane 4*, rheumatoid arthritis. GAPDH, glyceraldehyde 3-phosphate dehydrogenase

MMP, TIMP, PA, and PAI mRNA Expression in Cartilage Tissue

The mRNA expression of u-PA, PAI-1, MMP-1, MMP-3 TIMP-1, TIMP-2, and GAPDH was investigated using Northern blot analysis of extracts from seven cases with OS (65 ± 8 years), all eight with WS (61 ± 7 years), five with RA (62 ± 5 years), and three normal cases (63 ± 16 years) (Fig. 6).

The expression of u-PA mRNA, PAI-1 mRNA, MMP-1 mRNA, MMP-3 mRNA, TIMP-1 mRNA, and TIMP-2 mRNA as determined for in each specimens was tabulated (Table 3). The amounts of mRNA expressed were corrected with the amount of expression of GAPDH after densitometric analysis. Thus, u-PA and MMP-1 mRNA were expressed at higher levels in the WS, while TIMP-1 and TIMP-2 mRNA expression was greater in cases of OS.

In 17 positive cases (10OA, 5RA, and 2 control) of mRNA expression for u-PA, 14 cases of mRNA expression for MMP-3 and 10 cases of mRNA expression for MMP-1 were positive. In 19 positive cases (12OA, 5RA, and 2 control) of mRNA expression for PAI-1, 16 cases of mRNA expression for TIMP-1 and 15 cases of mRNA expression for TIMP-2 were positive. In 6 cases of negative mRNA expression for u-PA, all cases of mRNA expression for TIMP-1 and TIMP-2 were positive.

248   H. Kikuchi et al.

TABLE 3. Positive numbers of mRNA (u-PA, PAI-1, MMP-1, MMP-3, TIMP-1, TIMP-2) expression in articular cartilage from OA patients, RA patients, and control

Protocol	OA		RA	Control
	OS	WS		
Total number	7	8	5	3
u-PA	2	8	5	2
PAI-1	6	8	5	2
MMP-1	3	3	5	1
MMP-3	4	8	5	1
TIMP-1	7	8	5	1
TIMP-2	6	8	5	3

MMP, matrix metalloproteinase; OA, osteoarthritis; RA, rheumatoid arthritis; TIMP, tissue inhibitor of metalloproteinase.

Discussion

Intraarticular administration of HA is used worldwide to treat subjects with OA. In Japan, 80HA is commonly used for the treatment of OA, and clinical trials of 180HA for the treatment of OA and RA are under way. The effects of HA on fibrinolytic factors, metalloproteinases, and mechanical stress require further study. There are reports that HA acts on chondrocytes or synovial fibroblasts [10–12]. The mechanism of action has remained obscure, and the effects of HA on the fibrinolytic system are unclear. We demonstrated that matrix metalloproteinases (MMPs), serine proteinases, and their inhibitors are related to the destruction of articular cartilage and that the production of u-PA induces destruction of articular cartilage. High fibrinolytic status induced activation of MMPs. In the weight-bearing site of OA cartilage, the levels of u-PA and MMP mRNA expression were high, and levels of PAI-1 and TIMP mRNA expression were low. The antigen of u-PA and PAI-1 in the synovial fluid showed a tendency to increase 3h after the administration of HA in both improved and unimproved patients, and compressive mechanical stress on the cartilage tissue of WS led to high fibrinolytic status, determined by the decrease in the PAI-1:u-PA ratio. Mechanical stress of the cartilage tissue of OS led to a low fibrinolytic status as a result of increase in the PAI-1:u-PA ratio. This increase may be a mechanical stress of the articular cartilage or the synovial tissue, which produce serine proteinase and their inhibitors by the administration of HA. HA decreased the attachment ability of interarticular cell sources (lymphocytes, neutrophils, macrophages, etc.) to the cartilage surface, the propagation of synovial membrane, and the permeability of synovial vessels resulting from stress [1].

However, u-PA activity gradually decreased from the second to the fourth week; furthermore, the PAI-1 antigen to u-PA antigen ratio also gradually decreased from the second to the fourth week after the initial administration of HA in improved cases. These results suggest that exogenous HA imparts increasing viscosity of synovial fluid in a concentration and has an important role in marginal lubrication for the inhibition of fibrinolysis. Administration of HA eventually led to an increase in PAI-1 levels and a decrease in PAI-2 levels. These reactions might be caused by either the reduction in u-PA levels and MMP levels in antigens and mRNAs, or the induction of PAI-1 levels and TIMP levels in antigens and mRNA. It therefore prevents mechanical damage of the synovium and cartilage tissues in the OA joint by treatment with HA. Activation of cytokines and other factors related to PAs acts destructively in aggravation of OA. HA inhibited the activation of the MMP system and also inhibited the secretion of gas mediators [13] and interleukins [8,9]. Many of the HA reactions mentioned here and inhibition of fibrinolysis, may cause a improvement for 9 of 12 patients. Therefore, this study suggests that the increase of PAI-1:u-PA on synovial fluids may be good parameters to use to determine improvement for the clinical status of patients with OA. In OA, intraarticular HA reduces fibrinolytic activity in the synovial fluid, and on the surface of cartilage tissues it is protective against joint destruction caused by the serine-metalloproteinase cascade.

References

1. Tanaka S, Hamanishi C, Kikuchi H, Fukuda K (1998) Factors related to degradation of articular cartilage in osteoarthritis. Semin Arthritis Rheum 27:392–399
2. Kikuchi H, Shimada W, Nonaka T, Ueshima S, Tanaka S (1996) Significance of serine protease and matrix metalloproteinase systems in the destruction of human articular cartilage. Clin Exp Pharmacol Physiol 23:885–889
3. Suzuki K, Enghild JJ, Morodomi T, Salvesen G, Nagase H (1990) Mechanism of activation of tissue procollagenase by matrix metalloproteinase-3 (stromelysin). Biochemistry 29:10261–10270
4. Okada Y, Nagase H, Harris ED Jr (1989) A metalloproteinase from human rheumatoid synovial fibroblasts that digests connective tissue matrix components: purification and characterization. J Biol Chem 264:14245–14255
5. Kikuchi H, Tanaka S, Matsuo O (1987) Plasminogen activator in synovial fluid from patients with rheumatoid arthritis. J Rheumatol 14:439–445
6. Nonaka T, Matsumoto H, Shimada W, Miyagi I, Okada K, Fukao H, Ueshima S, Kikuchi H, Tanaka S, Matsuo O (1995) Effect of cyclic AMP on urokinase-type plasminogen activator receptor and fibrinolytic factors in a human osteoblast-like cell line. Biochim Biophys Acta 1266:50–56
7. Estreicher A, Muhlhauser J, Carpentier JL, Orci L, Vassali JD (1990) The receptor type of plasminogen activator polarizes expression of the protease to leading edge of migrating monocytes and promotes degradation of enzyme inhibitor complex. J Cell Biol 111:783–792
8. Pelletier JP, Martel-Pelletier J (1989) Evidence for the involvement of interleukin-1 in human osteoarthritic cartilage degradation. Protective effect of NSAID. J Rheumatol 18:19–27
9. Fukuda K, Dan H, Takayama M, Kumano F, Saitoh M, Tanaka S (1996) Hyaluronic acid increases proteohlycan synthesis in bovine articular cartilage in the presence of interleukin-1. J Pharmacol Exp Med 277:1672–1675

10. Shimazu A, Jikko A, Iwamoto M (1993) Effects of hyaluronic acid on the release of proteoglycan from the cell matrix in rabbit chondrocyte cultures in the presence and absence of cytokines. Arthritis Rheum 36:247–253
11. Ghosh P (1994) The role of hyaluronic acid (hyaluronan) in health and disease. Interactions with cell, cartilage and components of synovial fluid. Clin Exp Rheumatol 12:75–82
12. Ghosh P, Holbert C, Read R, Armstrong S (1995) Hyaluronic acid (hyaluronan) in experimental osteoarthritis. J Rheumatol 22:155–157
13. Miyagi I, Kikuchi H, Hamanishi C, Tanaka S (1998) Auto-destruction of the articular cartilage and gas mediators. J Lab Clin Med 131:146–150

F. Problems Following Total Joint Replacement

Thigh Pain After Total Hip Arthroplasty

Robin J.E.D. Higgs[1] and William A.J. Higgs[2]

Summary. The main aim of, and the most significant benefit to be derived from, total hip arthroplasty (THA) is the relief of pain. In this regard THA continues to be an extremely successful procedure with ever-broadening indications, frequent improvements in materials of implant fabrication and design and methods of fixation, and constant improvement in surgical technique. The success or failure of the surgical procedure correlates directly with the presence or absence of pain. Pain is probably the only true measure of the quality of the surgical result, and the symptom stands alone as an index of "end point" or failure in any survivorship analysis. Only pain correlates positively with the patient's expectations, and furthermore it is only pain that can define disappointment or predict the decision if there is a need for a revision procedure.

Thigh pain after THA has attracted considerable debate but only since the mid-1980s. The introduction of and the increasing popularity of cementless implant fixation has provoked much of the discussion as to its cause. This chapter reviews the observed incidence of thigh pain and debates the many morphologic reasons implicated in the causation of the symptom. This chapter also discusses many of the causes, the effects, the diagnosis, and the management of thigh pain, and relates the discussion to a clinical experience of more than 1000 THA procedures.

Various mechanical causes of thigh pain are reviewed, and it remains clear that many of these remain an enigma. Specifically, a review of the concept of homoelasticity and the (as yet theoretical) potential benefit to be derived from the use, in implant fabrication, of novel materials and designs to modify section modulus and to optimize stress transfer are reviewed.

The correlation between radiographic and scintigraphic findings and the clinical presentation is reviewed. It is concluded that any positive correlation

[1] Centre for Advanced Materials Technology and Orthopaedic Engineering, Faculty of Engineering & Medicine, and [2] Faculty of Engineering, University of Sydney, P.O. Box 561, Milsons Point, NSW 2061, Australia

between these imaging techniques and the incidence of thigh pain is questionable and is more likely, in the majority of cases, to be coincidental. Furthermore, it has not been possible to positively correlate changes in bone morphology, implant fit and fill, and mode of implant stabilisation (bony vs fibrous) with the incidence of thigh pain. The only positive correlation identified between persisting thigh pain and a specific cause has been found to be associated with revision arthroplasty and with the use of femoral stem implants of greater than 17 mm diameter. A lower-than-usual incidence of thigh pain has been associated with fully sintered femoral stems of the Mittelmeier Autophor design and with femoral implants proximally coated with hydroxyapatite.

The authors conclude that, at this time, thigh pain is an inevitable complication of total hip arthroplasty. The morphologic reasons for the symptom remain unclear. Fortunately, the symptom is not always a clinical problem and in a great many cases the symptom is observed to improve with time. Unfortunately, persistent thigh pain can be a significant clinical problem and a cause for failure of the expectation of both the patient and the surgeon. A program of management is recommended and the "Higgs" surgical stress by-pass procedure for relief of intractable thigh pain of mechanical origin is described.

Key Words. Thigh, Pain, Hip, Arthroplasty, Homoelasticity

Introduction

The major aim of, and the most significant benefit to be derived from, total hip arthroplasty (THA) is relief of pain. In this regard, THA continues to be an extremely successful procedure with ever broadening indications, frequent improvements in materials of fabrication, design, and methods of fixation, and constant improvement in surgical technique. The success or failure of the surgical procedure correlates directly with the presence or absence of pain. Pain is, probably, the only true measure of the quality of the surgical result, and this symptom stands alone as an index of "endpoint" or of failure in a survivorship analysis. Pain correlates positively with the expectations of the patient, and this symptom alone is able to define disappointment or to predict the decision that a revision procedure may be needed.

Thigh pain after THA has attracted considerable debate, but only since the mid-1980s. The association of this debate with the introduction and increasing popularity of cementless implant fixation has provoked much of the discussion as to the cause. There are a great many causes for thigh pain after THA; some are rare, some are common. Much is known about a few of the causes, but for many the pathogenesis remains little more than speculative. Major causes of thigh pain following THA include prosthetic loosening, infection, osteolysis, and fracture of the bone or of the implant (Fig. 1). The diagnosis of these

FIG. 1. The "failed" total hip arthroplasty (THA)

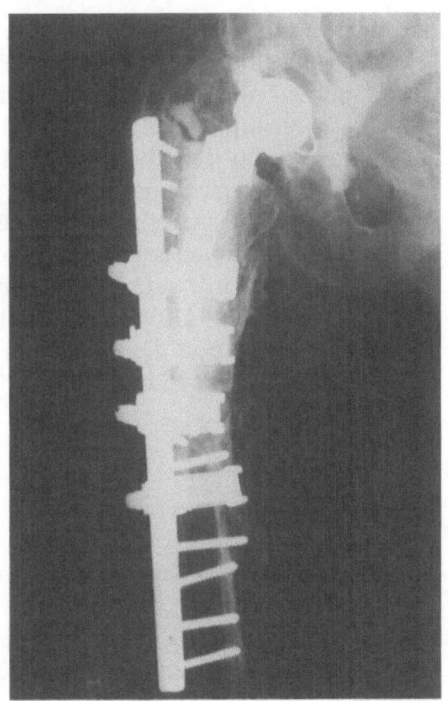

conditions should not be difficult. Each is generally accompanied by character-istic historical and clinical findings, and in almost every case there is no diagnostic dilemma. Thus, these four major causes for thigh pain after THA are not discussed further in this chapter.

It is important to establish that there is a considerable and significant differ-ence between groin pain and thigh pain after THA. Groin pain is a far more sinister symptom and may reflect either an acetabular or a femoral complica-tion or both, and for discussion groin pain stands alone as a subject on its own. This discussion is concerned with that pain which is truly thigh in distribution. It is a pain that the patient often describes as being "like a muscle ache" and which is generally indicated, often with the pointing finger, to be experienced in the midlateral and anterior thigh regions. The severity of the symptom varies greatly. Fortunately, in most cases, it is a discomfort that can be toler-ated and one that, in our experience, has been observed to lessen with time. Unfortunately, the symptom more rarely is intolerable and bears the respon-sibility for further surgical intervention.

A view can be taken, in the Western World, that regards Peter Ring as the "father" of the uncemented arthroplasty. In 1971, Ring was recorded as stating that "aching" in the thigh is an occasional complaint after THA. Ring thought that the symptom indicated that there was "some fault within the articulation" [1]. Although this observation is relevant, it is a generalization, and one that is now known not to be entirely valid. There are now known to be a great many factors implicated in a causal sense for thigh pain after THA. The causes have so far defied useful classification. The cause may be local, that is, related to the surgical implantation, and may be intrinsic or extrinsic to the implant. Intrinsic causes may be biological or mechanical in origin or, as is most likely, a combination of the two. Extrinsic causes generally relate to the consequences of the surgical procedure, for example, broken trochanteric wires or vastus lateralis hernia [2]. The latter is, in our experience, a more common complication than has been dislocation. Other more general causes are rarer but most commonly are of pain referred from some neurological cause [3].

Incidence

There is considerable variance in regard to the incidence of thigh pain following THA, as has been reported in the literature [4,5]. The reported incidence has been as low as 0.7% [6] and as great as 40.0% [7]. Generally, most authors have tended to agree that the incidence of thigh pain decreases with time [8,9], and this has certainly been our experience. During the period January 1980 to December 1995, 1000 total hip arthroplasties were performed by the senior author. The minimum review period is 2 years, and the maximum review period is now in its 18th year. During the course of this surgical experience, five different designs of uncemented femoral component and one single type of cemented femoral component have been used. The incidence of thigh pain at 3 years has been identified as 5%. Furthermore, in agreement with the internationally reported experience, a decrease in the incidence of thigh pain has been observed to occur with each year (up to the 3rd year) after surgery. Persisting thigh pain has been observed as 12% at 1 year, 6% at 2 years, and to have stabilized at 5% at year 3.

A comparison of the experience identified with the use of the five different uncemented femoral prosthetic systems has permitted the identification of the "best" and the "worst" scenarios. To date, the most gratifying results have been derived from the use of the fully sintered Mittelmeier Autophor Femoral Prosthesis [10]. The fully sintered Mittelmeier implant has been used in 250 cases. The incidence of thigh pain persisting at 5 years after surgery remains at only 4%. Not 1 case of loosening has been identified, and there has been no requirement for revision arthroplasty. The worst case scenario has been associated with use of the "Isoelastique" uncemented femoral device [11]. The incidence of persisting thigh pain at 5 years following the surgical implantation of this device remains at 9%. Of 117 Isoelastique femoral stems implanted, 30 (25.6%) have required revision within the first 3 years for loosening or material failure.

Cement Versus Cementless Fixation

There is a general consensus that cementless THA is more often associated with thigh pain (in the long term) than is cemented arthroplasty. If this consensus was without doubt true, then the fact could be explained by the more normal strain patterns identifiable in the femur following cemented arthroplasty [12]. There is good evidence that the femoral strain patterns are more physiological after cemented THA than are the strain patterns identified following uncemented femoral stem fixation. The literature reflects a difference of opinion with regard to the incidence of thigh pain following cemented and uncemented hip arthroplasty. A Mayo Clinic review of cemented Charnley total hip arthroplasties reported there to be no pain in 80% of cases at 5 years [13]. It is permissible to conclude that pain was a feature in 20% of cases. In fairness to the authors, however, the site of the pain was not stated, but it certainly appears that cemented THA is not necessarily an insurance for freedom from some long-term pain and discomfort. Professor D. Howie (Adelaide, South Australia 1997) has addressed this contentious issue for a number of years. A recent communication concluded that a prospective study did identify thigh pain following cemented THA and that the early 2-year results did not show any major difference in respect of the incidence of thigh pain when comparing cemented against uncemented implants. Furthermore, the patient-reported incidence was similar in both the cemented and the uncemented cohorts. There is some evidence that the "consensus" in the literature may be more apparent than real. Most reports review experience gained from the uncemented use of porous-coated anatomical devices fabricated from cobalt metal alloy. If it is permissible to review the literature with the exclusion of these reports, then it is seen that the incidence of thigh pain after the use of cemented and uncemented devices is not significantly different. This also has been our experience.

Implant Fit, Fill, and Size

Associated with most new experiences in life there is a period (or process) of learning. New surgical experiences are no different from other new experiences, and the use of the term learning curve in defining any new surgical experience is not uncommon in the literature. In regard to both cemented and uncemented femoral prosthetic implantation, it may be that results in general, and the incidence of thigh pain in particular, improved with experience. It has been our experience that the so-called learning curve does not have a statistical relationship with the incidence of persisting thigh pain after THA. Any incident of a less than optimal femoral component fit and fill was not necessarily associated with persisting thigh pain. However, a less than optimal fit and fill has certainly been associated with an increased incidence of loosening. Between 1980 and 1987, a prospective analysis of the fit and fill of 337 uncemented femoral components was undertaken by the senior author. A less than optimal fit and fill was not, in the long term, associated with persisting thigh pain, but when an imperfect fit and fill was identified, there was a causal relationship with the incidence of component loosening. During this period of time 17 femoral stems were revised for loosening; 11 (64.7%) of those femoral stems revised were classified as being undersized, that is, too small. It was observed that many undersized femoral implants "migrated" by angulation into a varus position, thereby to achieve three-point fixation. The incidence of thigh pain in this group of patients was not observed to be different from that of the general group.

This was also the experience reported by Smith et al. [14], in which a 30% incidence of varus shift was observed to be associated with an incidence of only 6% persisting thigh pain. There can be no disagreement that good fit and fill is desirable, particularly at the proximal (metaphyseal) region of the implant. We believe there will be no disagreement in stating that femoral implant undersizing should be avoided. However, in endeavoring to achieve perfection with regard to fit and fill, there is an impetus to implant the largest size of femoral component that can safely be inserted and accommodated within the medullary canal of the femur. It has been our experience that the use of femoral stems of diameter greater than 17 mm is associated with a slightly higher incidence of persisting thigh pain. The association between the "over-sized" implant (diameter more than 17 mm) and the incidence of thigh pain has been reported elsewhere [15,16]. We agree with Dujovne et al. [17] that the cause of the persisting thigh pain is a consequence of the significant modulus (stiffness) mismatch that can occur between these large stems and the bone. We have no doubt that implant undersizing is associated with loosening and that oversizing is likely to be associated with an increased incidence of persisting thigh pain. Implant oversizing (and revision arthroplasty) have been the only two factors that we have been able to correlate directly with a higher than expected incidence of persisting thigh pain. The more important implication of this experience is to permit a reminder of the importance and benefits to be derived from adequate and skillful preoperative planning and to acknowledge that bone cement may, and perhaps should, be used in those cases in which it has not been possible to achieve a proper fit and fill.

Femoral Stem Design

We have discussed the implications of femoral stem size and of the appropriateness of good fit and fill. The gross shape of the stem is no less important. Although somewhat of a generalization, femoral stem design can be categorized into one of two groups. Femoral stems may be straight or curved. The latter are (too) often described as "anatomic" in design. Curved stems may be further subdivided into those characterized by a single curve and those characterized by a double curve. Other curved femoral stems can be justifiably described as custom-made stems, being more exact in respect of their anthropometric design. The evidence is that the incidence of thigh pain is significant following the use of the so-called anatomic femoral stems [4]. We are not surprised by this finding. It is impossible to insert a double-curved device into a canal that has been perfectly reamed to the same double-curved dimensions. A double-curve design can only be inserted into the femoral medullary canal if the canal has either been overreamed or allowed to fracture, or if the implant chosen is a little undersized. A simple experiment can confirm this observation to be true. Take a double-curved stem. Fabricate a perfect methylmethacrylate mold of the stem. Split this mold into two halves after setting. Remove the stem and reconstruct the mold. It may now be observed that it is impossible to reinsert the femoral stem into its custom-made mold. The exercise is little different from attempting to put a banana back into its unbroken skin.

This is a contentious issue but our observations, more likely than not, hold true also for the custom-made anthropometric design philosophy. The clinical results reflect some disagreement, but overall the experience has generally been poor. Robinson et al. reported an incidence of thigh pain of 37% in association with a revision rate of 17% at 2.5 years after surgery [18]. The less than optimal results following the use of "anatomically" designed femoral stems provides no great optimism for any benefits from the introduction of mechatronic robotic reaming procedures. It is probable that the more ideal implant is one that can assume the anatomical shape on insertion. The prosthetic design and the material of fabrication necessarily must be flexible and elastic yet sufficiently strong to withstand the duration and magnitude of the anticipated load.

Homoelastic Femoral Stem Design

In discussion of the more elastic femoral stem philosophy, we have chosen to use the term homoelasticity rather than the more generally used terminology of isoelasticity. We believe that the use of the term isoelastic or isoelasticity is inappropriate to any discussion of the more elastic femoral stem design philosophy. Bone is anisotropic, and it does seem logical to conclude, at the outset, that the achievement of isoelasticity is not only impossible but is also inappropriate. The use of the terms homoelastic and homoelasticity is perceived as more appropriate in that this terminology describes a condition of "sameness" between the physical properties of the femoral implant on the one hand and of the femoral bone on the other. The argument as to the possible benefits of the more flexible implant as compared to the more rigid implant continues unresolved (Fig. 2). The question remains as to whether low stiffness is associated with a durable pain-free arthroplasty. The argument to date has largely concerned the differences of opinion about the use of titanium (and its alloys) and the use of cobalt chrome alloys for the fabrication of femoral

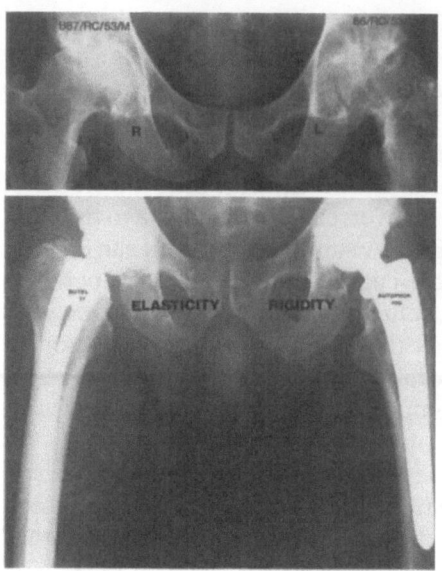

Fig. 2. Elasticity versus rigidity

stems. This argument debates the issue of the flexible metal versus the stiff metal. There is no doubt that the use of implants of titanium (and its alloys) is associated with a relatively lower incidence of thigh pain following THA [19,20]. This has also been our experience, if it is permissible to exclude the isoelastique cohort. This superiority has been achieved in spite of the fact that titanium and its alloys remain at least ten times stiffer than is bone. The modulus (stiffness) mismatch between the two materials is still considerable.

The perceived benefits to be derived from the concept of the homoelastic implant have escaped satisfactory development, probably because we have so far been unable to reproduce the femoral section modulus in the implant design. Section modulus refers to the stiffness and to the behavior of the femoral bone at each level, from proximal to distal, in the transverse or horizontal plane. The section modulus of an implant is as much influenced by its design as by its material properties. The concept of the section modulus is better understood by a consideration of the analogy with a spring. Steel is a very stiff material, and yet it is possible to fabricate great springs for trucks and trains and delicate springs for watches and chairs. The stiffness of the spring required for each very different application is greatly altered by change in design. The "clothespeg" split that characterizes the distal femoral stem design of some implants represents an endeavor to alter the section modulus so as to provide a more flexible implant. This mechanical concept was in part a characteristic of the so-called isoelastique femoral component [11]. In cross section this femoral stem was fabricated from a four-tyne configuration. Unfortunately, our experience with this stem design has not been satisfactory, as we previously mentioned.

It does seem logical and more nearly ideal for the implant and the bone to deform as one. The homoelastic environment should improve load transfer from the one to the other, reduce proximal stress shielding, and reduce the consequences of distal femoral strain and bone remodeling. However, even with the use of more flexible materials and designs there remains the potential for interface instability [21], especially when perfect fixation is not achieved. This potential for interface instability when there is imperfect fixation can be easily demonstrated by a simple experiment. Consider your right and your left hand. If they are both healthy then they are as homoelastic as any two structures can be. Place the palms of the hands together as if making a religious gesture. Bend the fingers in contact from one side and then to the other. A very slight interfacial movement will be perceived between the two hands in spite of both being in perfect apposition and in spite of both being perfectly homoelastic in respect of their design and their materials of fabrication. This interfacial movement may be prevented if perfect (osseo)integration of the implant to the bone can be achieved. The solution to interface instability may be to transfer the unstable interface from the implant–bone region to a region within the substance of the implant itself. The use of composite materials for femoral stem fabrication may permit this.

Femur Type and Bone Quality

We have identified a positive correlation between revision arthroplasty and the occurrence of persisting thigh pain. Thigh pain is more common following revision THA. Not infrequently a femoral window has been required to facilitate the removal of bone cement during the course of the revision procedure. In such cases we have observed a negative correlation with, and no increase in the incidence of, thigh pain. It is generally the case that the femoral bone identified at revision arthroplasty is, more often than not, of less than optimal quality. We have been unable to identify any other positive correlation between the incidence of thigh pain and the quality of, or type of, femoral bone identified at surgery. We have observed a low incidence of thigh pain following THA in those suffering from severe rheumatoid arthritis and from severe juvenile rheumatoid arthritis. We have, as have others [22], identified a negative correlation between thigh pain and these two conditions.

The normal process of skeletal aging is associated with a gradual deterioration in the quality of tubular bone. The significant changes include osteopenia and a progressive reduction of cortical thickness, which is initiated at the endosteal surface. The medullary canal of the aging tubular bone can be seen to gradually increase in diameter at the expense of the thinning cortex. We have been surprised to observe that this natural process is not associated with an increased incidence of thigh pain following THA. It has also been our experience that femoral stem loosening is only rarely associated with the morphological changes that occur with skeletal aging. Only one case of

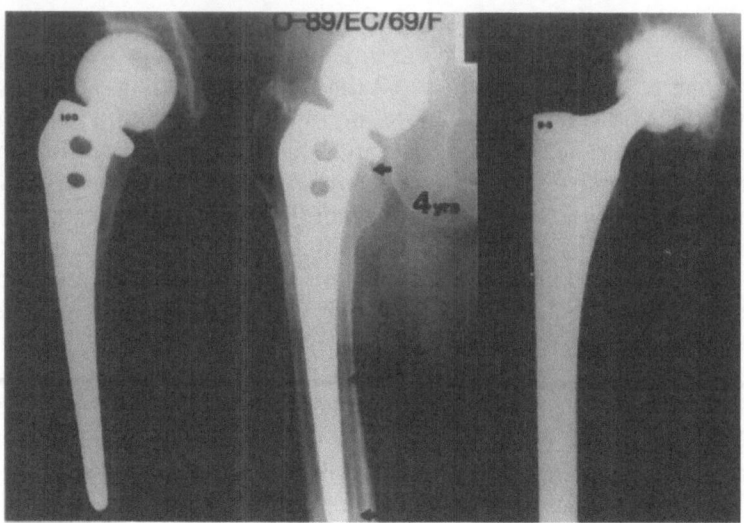

FIG. 3. Age-related changes and THA

femoral stem loosening was observed to have been associated with age-related medullary canal enlargement (Fig. 3). The X-ray of a 69-year-old woman demonstrates the enlargement of the medullary canal dimensions that are associated with aging. In this case the age changes were determined as being the cause for the femoral implant loosening. We have identified no correlation between the type of femur, whether classified according to the Dorr type [23] or by the Spotorno Romognoli Index [24], and the occurrence of thigh pain after THA.

Biology and Mechanics

Few, if any, would dispute that in life there is a constant interaction between biology and mechanics. The fabric of this philosophy is held together by Wolff's law. Put simply, Wolff's law can be interpreted as stating that what you put into life determines what you get out of it. This philosophy is fundamental to Wolff's law, and the philosophy is no less valid than when applied to the biological response of the musculoskeletal system to its mechanical environment. The mechanical stresses that are applied to a bone determine the nature of that bone's response. In Fig. 4, Wolff's law has been captured in action. The patient, a man of 66 years, has undergone a total hip replacement procedure. Eight months following surgery the patient complains of mild midregion anterior thigh pain. X-Rays taken at that time clearly reveal the presence of periosteal new bone formation. Further x-rays taken some few months later confirm that this periosteal new bone formation has progressed to

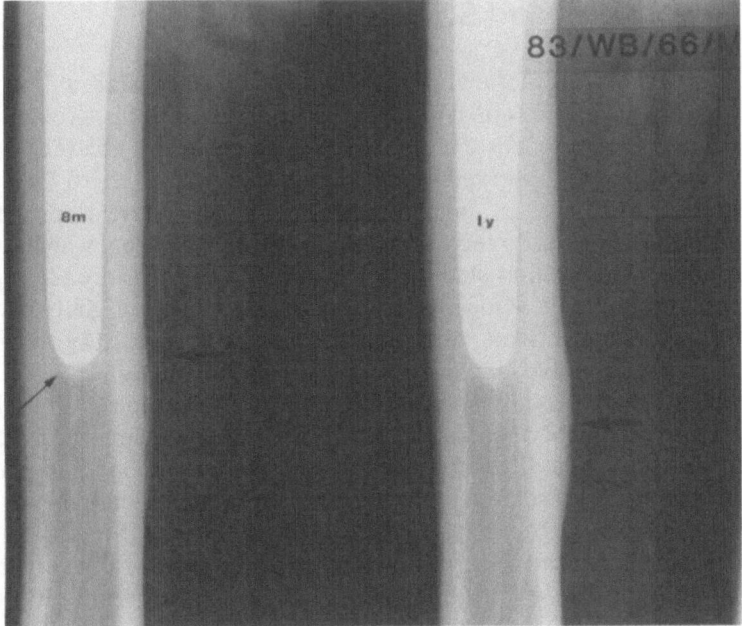

FIG. 4. Wolff's law in action

cancellization and to cortical densification. Subsequent months witnessed a progressive improvement in symptoms.

It is the authors' view that we are here, radiologically, visualizing Wolff's law in action: mechanical stress producing biomechanical strain, causing biological (bone) activity, resulting in a change to the structure to effect a biomechanical equilibrium by reducing the modulus mismatch in the new mechanical environment. These biological changes to the mechanical environment can be well seen both with plain X-rays and with bone scintigraphy. Two questions present themselves. First, why is the biological response to the mechanical environment symptomatic in some but asymptomatic in others? Second (and also relevant), why is persisting thigh pain associated with femoral prosthetic stem implantation in some, yet upper arm pain is seldom associated with humeral stem replacement? It is the authors' view that the answer to these two questions may be the same: there may be a threshold stress level below which there is no stimulation for a perception of pain. The loads on the proximal humerus, following shoulder arthroplasty, approach approximately 1.5 to 2 times body weight when the arm is elevated with a small weight in the hand. The loads on the proximal femur following THA are considerably greater (by an order of magnitude of 3- or 4 fold). It is permissible to suggest that there is a threshold to the stress level at which pain is experienced and at which there are bone reactions and identifiable bony morphological responses.

Roentgenological and Scintigraphic Findings

The radiological features following THA have received considerable attention in the literature. There remains some agreement and much disagreement as to the significance of these observed changes. It is generally accepted that implant loosening can be observed radiologically to be represented by a change in implant position, that is, angulation or migration. There is probably no doubt that these changes do represent an episode of loosening, which for some may fortunately be the first step toward fixation. We have already seen that varus angulation may be associated with three-point fixation. Similarly, distal migration may be associated with femoral stem impaction. In both cases the observed episode of loosening is just one step toward the process of fixation. Hosli believes that the only radiological feature of loosening after the first postoperative year is an observation of subsidence exceeding 4 mm [25].

The radiolucent zone often observed around the femoral stem implant may reflect an episode of loosening, but it is our view that this is only the case if the lucent zone, bordered by linear sclerosis, diverges from the surface of the implant. A radiolucent zone that is seen to be parallel to, or convergent with, the implant is consistent with satisfactory implant fixation, albeit including an intervening fibrous tissue zone. Observe the fixation of the human tooth (Fig. 5). Each healthy tooth demonstrates a parallel or convergent lucent zone around its root or stem. While the fixation of teeth remains unaccompanied by any evidence of osseointegration they can, in health, survive for three score and ten years and continue to permit (even) the cracking of nuts without pain. Healthy dentition is not associated with jaw pain.

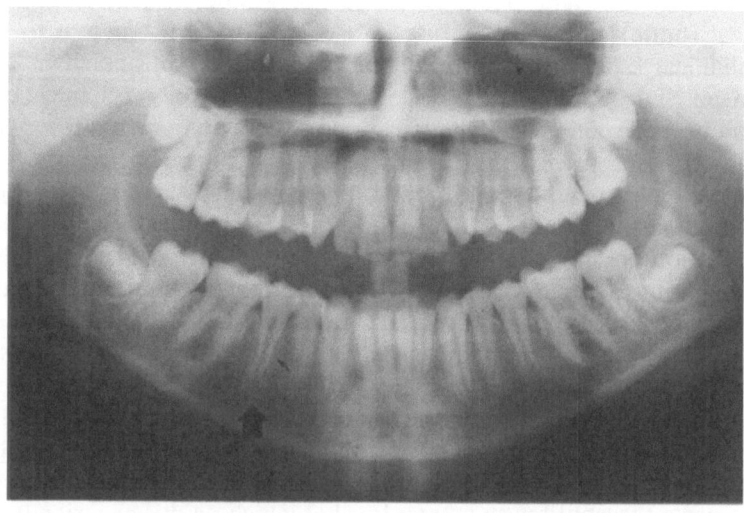

FIG. 5. Fixation of human tooth

Femoral skeletal changes are frequently observed after THA. The commonly observed skeletal manifestations are clearly seen on X-ray, and these are best described according to their Gruen zone [26] location. Distal and middle cortical hypertrophy may be seen in zones 3 and 5, and distal endosteal bone formation is frequently observed in zone 4. These skeletal changes reflect the biological response to mechanical stress, whether this stress transfer be over a discrete area or whether it be transferred over a more generalized area. In contradistinction, in zones where there is no stress transfer, that is, stress shielding, then the skeletal response is manifestly osteopenic. It is well known that distal femoral fixation may be frequently associated with significant osteopenia in Gruen zones 1 and 7. It has been the authors' experience that the skeletal changes associated with both stress transfer and stress shielding are common to both the cemented and to the cementless THA. We have been unable to correlate clinical findings with radiographic findings. We are in agreement with other reports that any association between the clinical and radiographic findings is purely incidental [27], that the radiological changes are secondary to changes in respect of stress transfer [28], and that there is no correlation between thigh pain after THA and the skeletal changes [29].

The scintigraphic findings observed following cementless THA are well known. The scintigraphic findings of increased Tc-99 m uptake, like the radiographic findings, are similarly an image of the biological response of bone activity responding to stress transfer (Fig. 6). It has been our experience that similar scintigraphic findings can be seen with both the cemented and with the uncemented THA and, interestingly, with both the successful and the unsuccessful arthroplasty. We have been unable to identify any correlation between the scintigraphic findings and the presence or absence of thigh pain, and

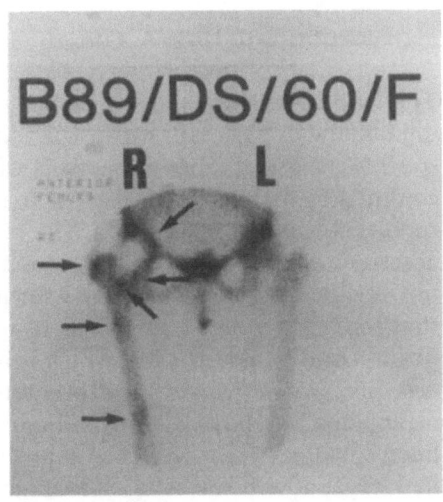

FIG. 6. Scintigraphic findings after cementless THA

furthermore we have not identified any correlation with femoral implant loosening. However a positive scintigraphic study utilizing Tc-99 m stannous colloid-labeled leukocytes in the evaluation of the painful THA is highly suggestive of infection and warrants appropriate further investigation and treatment [30].

Ingrowth Fixation

The debate continues unresolved as to whether or not fibrous tissue integration is associated, in a causal sense, with persisting thigh pain after THA. There is also some disagreement as to whether the incidence of thigh pain is less in the presence of a fully osseointegrated implant. It is again relevant and permissible to observe the fixation of the human tooth (see Fig. 5). The human tooth is not secured through osseointegration but is clearly in a state of secure and stable fixation within the fibrous tissue mantle of the periodontal membrane. The findings presented in the international literature reflect significant differences of experience. Moreland and Bernstein [31] observed a significantly higher incidence of thigh pain in the presence of fibrous tissue ingrowth than was the case in the presence of bone ingrowth, 18.5% and 4.2%, respectively. On the other hand, Shaw et al. [32] reported an extremely high incidence of thigh pain (34.0%) in a series of 178 THAs in which bone ingrowth was observed to have taken place in 92.3% of cases. It is significant that no loose femoral stems were identified in this series. Although we have not observed such a high incidence of thigh pain, we are in agreement that rigid fixation, whether it be with good bone ingrowth or whether it be associated with fibrous tissue fixation, does not necessarily guarantee the clinical presentation and the absence of thigh pain.

Enhanced Surface Coating (Hydroxyapatite)

The world literature reflects an optimistic view following the use of femoral implants with hydroxyapatite coatings in general, and in particular with respect to the use of those implants in which the hydroxyapatite coating has been confined to the proximal third of the implant. The incidence of thigh pain is reportedly extremely low [33]. The radiological and the clinical evidence does add some validity to the so far theoretical advantages exposed in regard to the use of enhanced hydroxyapatite surface coatings. It has been our experience that in Gruen zones 1 and 7 there is good radiological evidence of implant fixation and stress transfer, which is associated with new bone formation and osseointegrated "welds." Furthermore, cortical densification is the norm and osteopenia has been a rare finding. However, although our experience has been small, we have observed that the femoral stem that is fully coated with hydroxyapatite behaves in a similar manner to the uncoated femoral stem and the incidence of thigh pain following the use of these fully coated stems is no different from that following the use of the uncoated stem.

Prevention and Treatment

Experience has caused us to conclude that some measures for prevention may be undertaken. We make no apology for emphasizing the importance of meticulous pre-operative planning and attention to surgical technique. We recommend the use of low-modulus, straight-stem femoral implant design with hydroxyapatite surface coating in the proximal one-third metaphyseal region. We believe that it is vital to achieve a primary stable endosteal interference (friction) fit of the femoral implant at the metaphyseal region. If perfect proximal fit and fill is not achievable, for whatever reason, then the use of polymethylmethacrylate bone cement must be considered.

The fundamental consideration in respect of the treatment of persisting thigh pain following THA is to accept that the symptom is a normal consequence of total hip replacement in a percentage of cases. If this can be accepted then a necessary part of treatment should be to warn, and to reassure, patients as to the nature, pathophysiology, and natural history of the symptom. Treatment should also include advice as to the benefit to be derived from reducing the load on the femoral implant by the simple measures of moderating activity, the use of walking aids, and the preservation of an acceptable body mass index through attention to diet and acceptable exercise. We have found that the use of nonsteroidal antiinflammatory agents in general, and the use of Feldene in particular, has been beneficial. The beneficial effects of antiinflammatory agents has been reported in the literature. Campbell et al. reported in 1992 the achievement of partial to complete relief from thigh pain in two-thirds of those patients thus treated [4]. The therapeutic dilemma remains the treatment of the patient suffering from severe, persisting, intolerable, and disabling thigh pain after THA. We have endeavored to revise one such case without success because the femoral implant was so securely fixed as to deny its removal. Three further cases have been surgically treated by a procedure that we have described as a stress bypass procedure (Fig. 7). The aim of this procedure is to unload the femur at a region of discrete overload and, in so doing, also to stiffen the femur so as to reduce the modulus mismatch between the implant and the bone. This is achieved by plating the convex surface of the femur, at the region of discrete overload, using the Dall-Miles plate and cerclage cable technique. This procedure has been performed in three patients with a successful outcome in two cases. The case of a 69-year-old man who had experienced disabling thigh pain for 5 years is shown in Fig. 7. Careful observation of the X-ray permits visualization of a femur that has been stiffened and straightened so as to bypass the effects of a region of discrete implant overloading. The success of this procedure depends on the viscoelastic nature of bone and on the ability of living bone to creep.

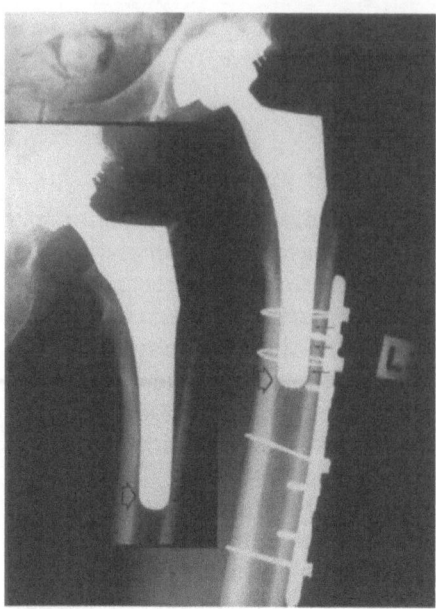

FIG. 7. The "Higgs" stress bypass procedure

Conclusion

In this chapter, we have discussed those factors implicated in the causation of persisting thigh pain after THA that have interested us most. There are obviously a great many other factors that may be considered as causative which we have neglected to discuss. Our experience has permitted us to conclude three things without any doubt. The first is that persisting thigh pain is a normal consequence of total hip arthroplasty in a percentage of cases. Second, the incidence of thigh pain following THA improves with time. Third, we believe that persisting thigh pain is only rarely caused by loosening.

We have identified only two factors that we have been able to positively correlate with the incidence of persisting thigh pain: the use of oversized implants of diameter 17 mm or more and the procedure of revision arthroplasty. In respect of all other factors reviewed, we have failed to identify any statistically secure positive correlation. The pathophysiology of the symptom of thigh pain remains debatable, but there is sufficient evidence to permit a view that the cause, and the solution, reflect both a surgical and a biomechanical etiology.

The authors, an orthopaedic surgeon and an aeronautical engineer, predict that the solution to the achievement of optimal femoral implant fixation, without persisting thigh pain, rests in the successful development of the concept of homoelasticity and in the control of the zone of interfacial instability.

References

1. Ring PA (1971) Ring total hip replacement. In: Jayson M (ed) Total hip replacement. Sector, London, pp 26–46
2. Higgs JE, Chong A, Haertsch P, et al (1995) An unusual cause of thigh pain after total hip arthroplasty, J Arthroplasty 10(2):203–204
3. Austin RT (1990) Spinal lesions simulating hip joint disorders. Clin Rheumatol 9(3):414–420
4. Campbell ACL, Rorabeck CH, Bourne RB, et al (1992) Thigh pain after cementless hip arthroplasty—annoyance or ill omen? J Bone Joint Surg 74B:63–66
5. Callaghan JJ, Dysart SH, Savory CG (1988) The uncemented porous-coated anatomic total hip prosthesis. Two year results of a prospective consecutive series. J Bone Joint Surg 70A:337–346
6. Bulow JU, Scheller G, Arnold P, et al (1996) Uncemented total hip replacement and thigh pain. Int Orthop 20(2):65–69
7. Haddad RJ Jr, Skalley TC, Cook SD, et al (1990) Clinical and roentgenographic evaluation of noncemented porous-coated anatomic medullary locking (AML) and porous-coated anatomic (PCA) total hip arthroplasties. Clin Orthop 258:176–182
8. Amstutz HC, Nasser S, Kabo JM (1989) Preliminary results of an off-the-shelf press fit stem. The anthropometric total hip femoral component using exact fit principles. Clin Orthop 249:60–72
9. Engh CA, Bobyn JD, Glassman AH (1987) Porous coated hip replacement. The factors govening bone ingrowth, stress shielding, and clinical results. J Bone Joint Surg 69B:45–55
10. Mittelmeier H (1984) Eight years of clinical experience with self-locking ceramic hip prosthesis "Autophor." J Bone Joint Surg 66B:300
11. Butel J, Robb JE (1988) The isoelastic hip prosthesis followed for 5 years. Acta Orthop Scand 59(3):258–262
12. Djerf K, Gillquist J (1987) The effects of different stem designs on femur loading in total hip replacement. Medical dissertation, no 252, Linkoping University, pp 89–107
13. Kavanagh BF, DeWitz MA, Ilstrup DM, et al (1989) Fifteen year results of cemented Charnley total hip arthroplasty. J Bone Joint Surg 71A:1496
14. Smith SE, Garvin KL, Jardon OM, et al (1991) Uncemented total hip athroplasty. Prospective analysis of the tri-lock femoral component. Clin Orthop Relat Res 269:43–50
15. Chandler HP, Ayres DK, Tan RC, et al (1995) Revision total hip replacement using the S-Rom femoral component. Clin Orthop 319:130–140
16. Vresilovic EJ, Hozack WJ, Rothman RH (1996) Incidence of thigh pain after uncemented total hip arthroplasty as a function of femoral stem size. J Arthroplasty 11(3):304–311
17. Dujovne AR, Bobyn JD, Krygier JJ, et al (1993) Mechanical compatibility of noncemented hip prostheses with the human femur. J Arthroplasty 8(1):7–22
18. Robinson RP, Clark JE (1996) Uncemented press-fit total hip arthroplasty using the Identifit custom-molding technique. A prospective minimum 2-year follow-up study. J Arthroplasty 11(3):247–254
19. Mulliken BD, Bourne RB, Rorabeck CH, et al (1996) A tapered titanium femoral stem inserted without cement in a total hip arthroplasty. Radiographic evaluation and stability. J Bone Joint Surg 78A:1214–1225

20. Robinson RP, Deysine GR, Green TM (1996) Uncemented total hip arthroplasty using the CLS stem: a titanium alloy implant with a corundum blast finish. Results at a mean 6 years in a prospective study. J Arthroplasty 11(3):286–292
21. Huiskes R, Weinans H, Dalstra M (1989) Adaptive bone remodeling and biomechanical design considerations for noncemented total hip arthroplasty. Orthopedics 12(9):1225–1267
22. Lachiewicz PF (1994) Porous coated total hip arthroplasty in rheumatoid arthritis. J Arthroplasty 9(1):9–15
23. Dorr LD (1986) Total hip replacement using the APR system. Tech Orthop 1:22–29
24. Spotorno L, Romagnoli S: Indications for the CLS stem. Product monograph—CLS prosthesis. Protek, Bern, Switzerland
25. Hosli P (1993) Cement-free hip endoprosthesis: PCA shaft prosthesis, 5–7 year results. Z Orthop Grenzgeb 131(6):518–523
26. Gruen TA, McNeice GM, Amstutz HC (1979) "Modes of failure" of cemented stem-type femoral components. A radiographic analysis of loosening. Clin Orthop 141:17–27
27. Fumero S, Dettoni A, Gallinaro M, et al (1992) Thigh pain in cementless hip replacement. Clinical and radiographic correlations. Ital J Orthop Traumatol 18(2):167–172
28. Bands R, Pelker RR, Shine J, et al (1991) The noncemented porous-coated hip prosthesis. A three-year clinical follow up study and roentgenographic analysis. Clin Orthop Relat Res 269:209–219
29. Kutsuna T, Kasahara T, Tsutsumi Y, et al (1992) Radiological changes in the femoral side after cementless total hip arthroplasty. Nippon Seikeigeka Gakkai Zasshi (J Jpn Orthop Assoc) 66(10):985–995
30. Chik KK, Magee MA, Bruce WJ, et al (1996) Tc-99 m stannous colloid-labeled leukocyte scintigraphy in the evaluation of the painful arthroplasty. Clin Nuclear Med 21(11):838–843
31. Moreland JR, Bernstein ML (1995) Femoral revision hip arthroplasty with uncemented, porous coated stems. Clin Orthop 319:141–150
32. Shaw JA, Bruno A, Paul EM (1992) The influence of age, sex and initial fit on bony ingrowth stabilization with the AML femoral component in primary THA. Orthopedics 15(6):687–692
33. D'Antonio JA, Capello WN, Jaffe WL (1992) Hydroxylapatite-coated implants. Multicenter three-year clinical and roentgenographic results. Clin Orthop 285:102–115

Polyethylene Properties and Their Role in Osteolysis After Total Joint Arthroplasty

Bassam A. Masri[1], Eduardo A. Salvati[2], and Clive P. Duncan[1]

Summary. Polyethylene continues to be the weak link in total joint arthroplasty. Wear particles, regardless of their source, are capable of inducing osteolysis by the induction of cytokines, which stimulate osteoclastic bone resorption. This, ultimately, leads to failure, and if allowed to continue for a long time, potentially very difficult reconstructions. Although materials other than polyethylene generate wear debris, polyethylene wear continues to be the most important source of these particles. Oxidation after gamma irradiation leads to worsening of the wear characteristics of polyethylene. Techniques to minimize oxidative degradation are therefore of great importance. Unconsolidated polyethylene particles, also known as fusion defects, may also be responsible for increased polyethylene wear. Strict quality control for the prevention of these defects is also important.

Key Words. Polyethylene, Osteolysis, Wear, Total hip arthroplasty, Total knee arthroplasty

Introduction

The introduction of low-friction arthroplasty by Sir John Charnley has revolutionized the treatment of osteoarthritis of the hip. This operation, with its high success rate, has improved the quality of life for millions of people worldwide. Currently, about 200000 such procedures are performed annually in the United States alone. Rorabeck et al. [1] have shown that total hip arthroplasty is not only highly effective, but also improves the quality of life of patients at

[1] Department of Orthopaedics, University of British Columbia, 930-943 West Broadway, Vancouver, B.C., Canada V5Z 4E1.
[2] Hip and Knee Services, The Hospital for Special Surgery and New York Hospital, 535 E. 70th Street, Cornell University College of Medicine, New York, NY 10021, U.S.A.

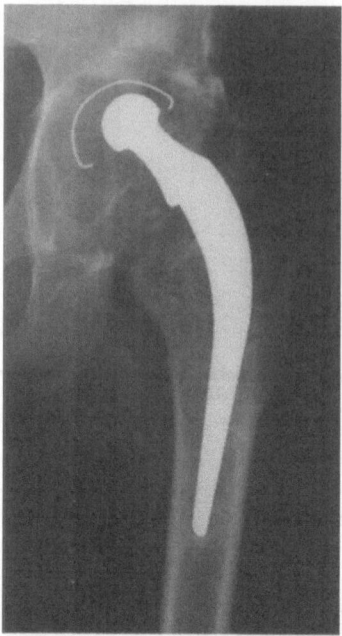

a

FIG. 1. Osteolysis secondary to excessive poly-ethylene wear is seen with (**a**) cemented implants, (**b**) solidly fixed cementless implants, and (**c**) loose cementless implants. The status of fixation of the hip replacements shown in this figure was confirmed at the time of surgery

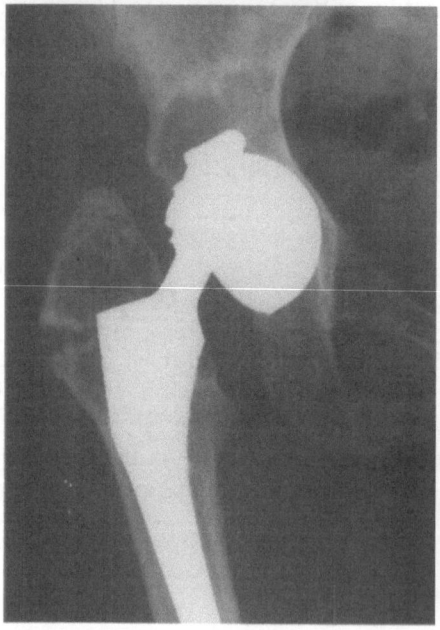

b

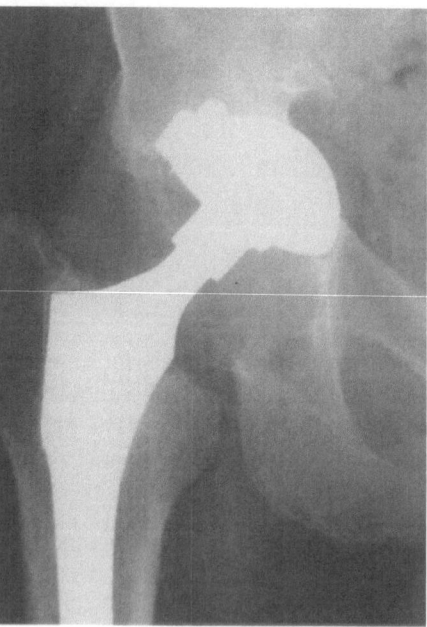

c

a relatively low cost. In fact, when compared to a variety of common medical and surgical treatments, total hip arthroplasty was only second to the insertion of a pacemaker in terms of cost-effectiveness.

Regardless of the excellent result of total hip arthroplasty, the implants ultimately fail, requiring revision, particularly in the young patient. Thirty percent of all hip replacements performed in the United States are revision procedures. The prevalence of these revision procedures is certainly increasing, as the population ages, and also as the indications for this operation are relaxed, allowing many young, otherwise healthy patients to undergo hip replacement. Because of the difficulty in component fixation and bone loss, revision procedures have a worse outcome than primary procedures; therefore, prevention of failure is of much more importance than improving revision techniques. It is therefore important to understand the mechanisms of failure so that the longevity of hip and knee replacements may be improved.

Cement was thought to be a cause of failure in cemented implants. Cementless fixation was introduced for hip and knee replacements as a means of improving fixation and increasing the longevity of these reconstructions. In 1987, Jones and Hungerford [2] coined the term cement disease, and postulated that the elimination of cement, particularly for the young patient, will prolong the longevity of hip replacements in such patients. Since then, however, the use of cementless implants has not been shown to prevent osteolysis. In fact, osteolysis has been noted around loose as well as solidly fixed cementless implants (Fig. 1) [3–6]. At the present time, it is clear that cement is not the main culprit in failure of total joint replacement. Instead, it is now apparent that wear particles play a major role in bone resorption, leading to osteolysis and implant failure [7–11].

Since the introduction of total hip arthroplasty, few bearing surfaces have been used. In addition to metal and ceramic, ultrahigh molecular weight polyethylene continues to be the most common acetabular bearing surface in hip replacements and the tibial and patellar bearing surface in knee replacements. Polyethylene wear, however, has been the weak link in total joint arthroplasty, and it is now believed that minimizing wear should improve the longevity of total hip and knee replacements.

In this chapter, the various material properties of polyethylene that may influence wear are discussed.

The Relationship Between Wear and Loosening

In a study of the wear rate of Charnley total hip arthroplasties, Charnley and Halley [12] measured the wear rates of polyethylene cups in low-friction arthroplasties. The wear rate during the first 5 years was 0.18 mm/year; in the last 4 years of a 9- to 10-year period it was 0.1 mm/year. In a subgroup of these patients, the wear rate was on average 0.35 mm/year. There was no correlation between age, activity level, and excessive polyethylene wear. The authors could not account for the unusually high wear rate in these patients. This perhaps was related to polyethylene properties; however, this is only a speculation. The authors' concern was not that wear could lead to osteolysis and loosening, but that wear will remove the bearing surface and lead to failure of the reconstruction.

In 1977, Willert [9] published the first reference of which we are aware to the relationship between wear particles and possible loosening. The authors retrieved tissue from the capsule surrounding hip replacements as well as the membranes at the cement–bone junction. The authors noted a histiocytic response, with multinucleated giant cells, with small phagocytosed particles within the histiocytes. These cells are capable of inducing bone resorption if sufficient wear particles are present. The authors also described a process of equilibrium between the body's ability to remove these wear particles and the resulting bone resorption when the body's ability to remove these cells is overwhelmed. The authors concluded that polyethylene, compared to Teflon and polyester, was more capable of achieving that equilibrium, leading to fibrosis rather than bone resorption. On the other hand, Mirra et al. [13] found a correlation between excessive polyethylene wear debris and loosening. Finally, Revell et al. [14] confirmed that polyethylene wear particles are capable of producing clinically significant osteolysis. With osteolysis, the bond between the cement or implant and bone is weakened, allowing loosening of the implant. At present, there is no doubt that osteolysis resulting from excessive polyethylene wear is the initiating event in aseptic loosening.

Causes of Excessive Polyethylene Wear

Although polyethylene wear cannot be eliminated, certain factors can increase polyethylene wear to alarmingly high rates. These factors can be classified as patient related, prosthetic related, and polyethylene related.

Although Charnley and Halley [12] were not able to correlate excessive polyethylene wear with patient weight, the median weight in that series was 140 lb, and the heaviest patient weighed just over 180 lb. By today's standards, even the heavy patients in that series are considered relatively light. It is therefore understandable that no correlation was noted. García-Cimbrello and Manuera [15] found a greater wear rate in patients less than 50 years of age or weighing more than 80 kg. Feller et al. [16] found a higher rate of wear in patients with higher levels of activity.

Prosthetic design and implantation techniques also influence polyethylene wear rates. Excessive lateral opening of the acetabular component causes excessive polyethylene wear. Figure 1b shows a solidly fixed porous coated anatomic (PCA; Howmedica, Rutherford, NJ, USA) acetabular component that was placed in excessive lateral opening, with catastrophic failure of the polyethylene liner from excessive wear. Furthermore, thin polyethylene, as the result of a very small socket with a large internal diameter or excessive metal backing, also increases the wear rate. Finally, the characteristics of the femoral head also affect polyethylene wear properties.

Livermore et al. [17] showed that femoral head size influences the degree of polyethylene wear; 32-mm heads cause the largest amount of volumetric wear, whereas 22-mm heads cause the largest amount of linear wear. Neither is ideal, and the middle ground is probably best. In North America, the most commonly used head sizes at present are 28 mm or 26 mm, provided that the socket allows enough polyethylene thickness. Otherwise, a smaller head diameter such as 22 mm is recommended. The surface finish of the femoral head is also important; the rougher the femoral head, the higher the rate of polyethylene wear in the acetabulum [18,19]. The material of the femoral head also influences the rate of polyethylene wear. It has been clearly shown that titanium is an inferior bearing surface [20], compared to cobalt-chromium alloys and stainless steel. While it is common for the tibial tray in total knee replacements to be made of a titanium alloy, the femoral components, for the most part, are made of cobalt-chromium alloys. In an effort to reduce polyethylene wear even further, ceramics have been used. There is no definite evidence, however, that a ceramic femoral head is better than a highly polished cobalt-chromium head.

In addition to polyethylene wear from the articulating surface, it is important to also consider polyethylene wear on the backside of an acetabular component [21]. Excessive micromotion can be a cause of excessive backside wear. The presence of screwholes may allow wear particles access to the underlying bone and potentially accelerate osteolysis. Furthermore, the presence of screws may increase wear if the screw heads are not well seated within their holes, and screws may also act as conduits for polyethylene debris; however, this is more common in the knee than in the hip. At the present time, the current trend is to use acetabular components without screwholes and without screws if at all possible. In total knee arthroplasty, although cementless tibial trays with screw fixation have been popular in the past decade, the trend is to return to cemented fixation and to avoid screw fixation altogether.

Certain steps in the manufacturing and sterilization process of polyethylene can results in various properties that may result in excessive polyethylene wear. Inclusion defects within the polyethylene, commonly known as fusion defects, have been implicated as causes of excessive wear. Furthermore, a white band that is seen within sectioned polyethylene in retrieved implants has also been suspected as a cause of excessive polyethylene wear. These properties, particularly as they relate to polyethylene wear, are discussed next.

Polyethylene Manufacturing

Polyethylene is a generic term for a plastic polymer of ethylene molecules. There has been some confusion about the proper terminology for the polyethylene used in joint replacement prostheses. The term high-density polyethylene, albeit used interchangeably [22,23] with ultrahigh molecular weight polyethylene, refers to a form of polyethylene that has a lower molecular weight and a higher density than the commonly used ultrahigh molecular weight polyethylene [24]. This difference is not simply semantics. High-density polyethylene tends to have a lower molecular weight, has lower impact strength, and has a poorer wear profile than ultrahigh molecular weight polyethylene. It also has a higher density (0.953 mg/ml to 0.965 mg/ml) than ultrahigh molecular weight polyethylene (0.925–0.935 mg/ml). Oxidation of ultrahigh molecular weight polyethylene renders its properties more like high-density polyethylene, with its poorer wear profile.

Ultrahigh molecular weight polyethylene is synthesized from ethylene gas, which is bubbled through a generator with a catalyst in the form of titanium chloride and aluminum alkyl compound [24]. The powder particles are then filtered and then processed to generate the familiar polyethylene components. The three processes that are generally used [24] include compression molding, in which the powder is directly molded in the form of an implant; other methods include ram extrusion and sheet molding. In ram extrusion, a cylindrical bar stock ranging from 2 to 6 in. in diameter is generated and the implants are then machined from this rod. In machine molding, sheets up to 8 in. thick are generated and, as in ram extrusion, components are then manufactured. These processes require varying conditions of high temperature and pressure. At any time during this complex manufacturing process, impurities or defects may interfere with the final product. These are discussed later in this chapter under ultrahigh molecular weight polyethylene quality.

Polyethylene Sterilization

The most common method by which polyethylene is sterilized is gamma irradiation, in a dose between 2.5 and 4.0 megarads. Ultrahigh molecular weight polyethylene oxidizes after gamma irradiation in an oxygen-containing environment [25]. There is also some evidence that this is a dynamic process that continues for some time after sterilization [25–27]. Irradiation causes chemical changes that adversely alter the physical properties of polyethylene. The hydrocarbon chains in polyethylene are fragmented by radiation, and free radicals are formed at the broken ends. If oxygen is present, free oxygen radicals are also formed. Carbonyl groups as well as carbon–carbon cross-links can then form. This process, also knows as chain scission and oxidative degradation, leads to a decrease in molecular weight and an increase in polyethylene density. This reaction, therefore, converts the polyethylene into a material that is more similar to high-density polyethylene than ultrahigh molecular weight polyethylene.

Although increase of polyethylene density is highly suggestive of oxidative degradation, Fourier transform infrared spectroscopy allows the detection and quantification of the carbonyl groups, therefore confirming that oxidation is the cause of this density increase. Using both techniques, Rimnac et al. [25]

showed that these changes continue for at least 1 year after sterilization. These changes can occur to at least 3 mm from the surface of the implant. Therefore, for a 6-mm-thick implant, it would be expected that changes throughout its thickness are present 1 year after sterilization.

The chemical changes within polyethylene are accompanied by physical changes as well. The modulus of elasticity of polyethylene rises by about 35%. This increase of elastic modulus is accompanied by mechanical changes on the surface of the implant, which lead to altered stresses within the articular surface and thus to higher degrees of wear [28]. To minimize the degree of damage, it is therefore important to decrease the shelf life of the implants before their use.

Ultrahigh Molecular Weight Polyethylene Quality

As previously mentioned, because of the complexity of the process of polyethylene manufacturing, and because of the high degree of temperature and pressure required, it in not inconceivable that defects may occur in the manufacturing process. Indeed, defects within the polyethylene have been observed [24,29]. These defects can often be seen by the naked eye (Fig. 2). There has been some speculation that these are impurities within the polyethylene containing calcium, titanium, aluminum, and silica, all of which are part of the catalysis system or a known additive. These defects, however, are too numerous to represent such impurities, and have since been demonstrated to be unconsolidated polyethylene particles, as demonstrated by electronic spectroscopy for chemical analysis (ESCA), scanning electron microscopy, and x-ray fluorescence, which failed to detect any significant levels of metal or

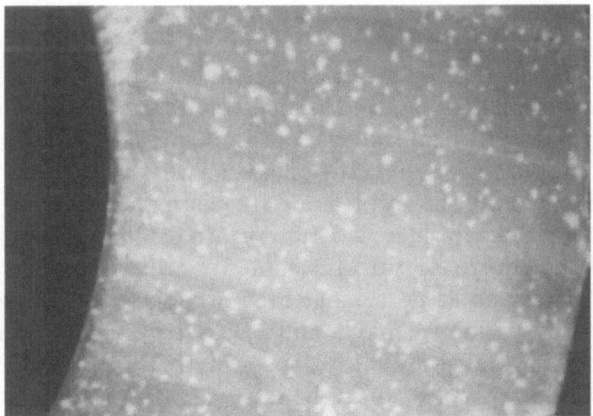

FIG. 2. This 200-μm slice of polyethylene shows the so-called fusion defects, also known as unconsolidated polyethylene particles

mineral. Furthermore, the melting point of these defects corresponded to that of polyethylene, suggesting that these are polyethylene particles. Finally, on cooling, these particles coalesced with the other particles [30]. For these reasons, these are now known as fusion defects, or as unconsolidated polyethylene particles.

Interaction Between Clinical Features and Material Properties in Polyethylene Wear in Total Hip Arthroplasty

The influence of unconsolidated polyethylene particles on polyethylene wear in total joint arthroplasty is difficult to study because of the multitude of factors that influence wear. Such factors include clinical factors, such as obesity, age, and activity level, as well as surgical technique and material properties of the polyethylene. We studied retrospectively a series of 98 cases of failed Charnley total hip replacements [31], retrieved at the Hospital for Special Surgery. Average follow-up was 124.8 months after the index operation. To avoid problems with different designs, we chose a single design, namely, the Charnley low-friction arthroplasty.

The patients' clinical characteristics, including age at implantation, activity level, and underlying diagnosis, were recorded; these data were available in the hospital chart. Acetabular component wear was measured using the uniradiographic method as well as direct wear measurement from the retrieved implants. The material characteristics of the polyethylene were examined by sectioning the cups along the plane of major wear. Sections between 100 and 200 μm in thickness were then obtained and inspected under light microscopy. Images from the worn areas as well as the less worn areas were correlated. Morphometric analysis of these sections was then performed using digital photography. The unconsolidated polyethylene particles were carefully noted, and the percentage area of the polyethylene that was occupied by these defects was recorded; this was used as an estimate of the polyethylene quality. Using appropriate statistical models, the influences of clinical variables and polyethylene properties on polyethylene wear were studied.

Radiographic wear in the whole series measured, on average, 1.93 mm, for an annual average wear rate of 0.2 mm/year. On direct measurement, the average thickness decrease was 1.34 mm for an average decrease rate of 0.13 mm/year. The average percentage area occupied by unconsolidated polyethylene particles was between 3% and 3.9%, depending on the depth away from the articular surface and also depending on whether the polyethylene was sampled in the worn area or in the less worn area. In each cup, there was a statistically significant difference between the distribution of unconsolidated polyethylene particles within the worn or less worn areas of the acetabular components, with the more worn area showing a higher percentage. This difference may reflect the fact that the measured wear is a combination of true wear and creep.

It is conceivable that the difference in distribution of these fusion defects is caused by creep-related compacting of the polyethylene in the more worn regions of the cups. All polyethylene cups wear in a superolateral direction because of the mechanical forces applied to the cup. Therefore, we cannot postulate that the difference in distribution of unconsolidated particles is related to this wear phenomenon. The interesting finding, however, is that head penetration within the polyethylene strongly correlated with the percentage distribution of unconsolidated particles, even when the polyethylene in the less worn area of the cup was examined. This suggests that larger numbers of unconsolidated polyethylene particles correlate with a higher degree of head penetration and therefore with wear.

Clinical factors, such as the length of time between implantation and revision, correlated well with polyethylene wear, which is not surprising because wear is a time-dependent phenomenon. Controlling for this factor, there was a strong correlation between activity level, younger age at implantation and weight, and polyethylene wear. These factors were all independent predictors of higher degrees of polyethylene wear. In conclusion, this study confirms our suspicion, through a rather indirect correlation, that fusion defects may have an adverse influence on polyethylene wear in total joint arthroplasty.

Subsurface Polyethylene Defects: The "White Band"

Analysis of retrieved polyethylene components revealed, in addition to unconsolidated polyethylene particles, a white band in the subsurface region of some polyethylene acetabular and tibial components [29,32–34]. This has been interpreted differently by different authors. Landy et al. [35] interpreted this region as that of cracking secondary to stress application. Li and Burstein [33] considered it as a region of high concentration of unconsolidated polyethylene particles. Sun et al. [34] was the first to refer to this region as the so-called white band, and thought that it was related to compression molding of components. Finally, Wrona et al. [29] related this to the polyethylene machining process. Regardless of the cause of this white band, there was agreement that it most likely represented an adverse characteristic that potentially resulted in worsening of the wear characteristics of the polyethylene.

In an effort to further define the nature of this white band and to further correlate its presence with that of unconsolidated polyethylene particles, we investigated two groups of retrieved Charnley acetabular components [32]. Each group consisted of eight cups that were matched not only to their duration of implantation, but also to the duration between retrieval and analysis, because of concerns that degradative oxidation of polyethylene may continue long after gamma irradiation. All cups were sterilized by gamma

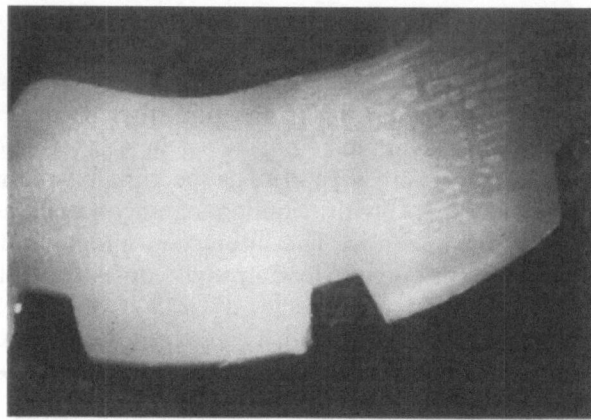

FIG. 3. The direction of the microtome blade was changed halfway through the cut of this 200-μm section of polyethylene. The orientation of the white lines within the so-called white band turns as the microtome blade is rotated, always remaining perpendicular to the direction of the cut. This confirms that this white band is an artifact of sectioning, caused by the brittle nature of the highly oxidized polyethylene

irradiation in air. The difference between the groups is that one group contained cups with a white band while the cups in the other group did not.

The white band was inspected under light microscopy, which consistently revealed a series of parallel lines that made up the white band. In an effort to determine whether these lines were cracks within the polyethylene, each cup was sectioned, and 100- to 200-μm slices were obtained using a microtome. Using each same cup with a white band, the orientation of the parallel lines within the white band rotated by 90° when the direction of the microtome cut was rotated by 90°. Furthermore, the lines within the white band were always perpendicular to the direction of the cut. This is characteristic of polyethylene cracking, because the crack lines are always perpendicular to the line of force application. Figure 3 shows a polyethylene slice that was cut at two different microtome orientations, with reversal of the orientation of the lines within the white band.

In an effort to rule out the contribution of unconsolidated polyethylene defects to the white band, the percentage distribution of the unconsolidated polyethylene particles was measured in the two groups. There was no statistically significant difference in the distribution of these particles within the two groups. This supported our hypothesis that the white band was not related to unconsolidated polyethylene particles.

Finally, we hypothesized that the white band was simply a region of degraded polyethylene, with a higher density caused by marked oxidation. The polyethylene density profiles were measured in the two groups. The typical density profile within the polyethylene is shown in Fig. 4. There is a subsurface

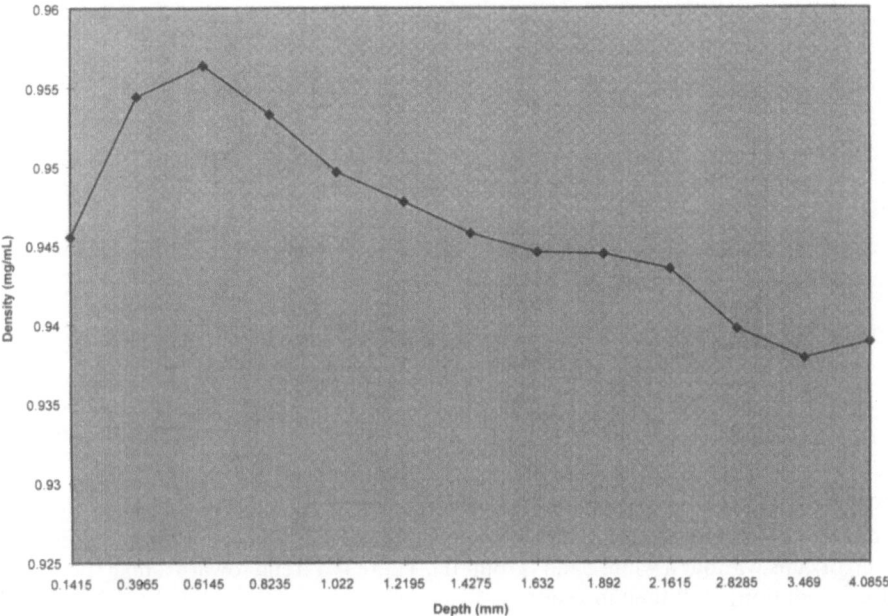

F<small>IG</small>. 4. Density profile within polyethylene. In the subsurface region of the poly-ethylene, the density is highest (peak density). This gradually plateaus to a steady-state level deep within the polyethylene (core density)

density peak, with rapid decline to a steady-state core polyethylene density, deep within the polyethylene. The maximum density was referred to as the peak density, and the plateau density was referred to as the core density. The peak density in the group with the white band was significantly higher than that in the group without the white band (Fig. 5). This confirmed our hypoth-esis that the white band is simply an indication of significant polyethylene oxidative degradation, causing marked brittleness within the polyethylene.

The Effect of Time on Oxidative Degradation After Gamma Irradiation of Polyethylene

Sutula et al. [36] as well as Rimnac et al. [25] have shown that oxidative degradation of polyethylene continues long after the gamma irradiation ceases, when polyethylene is sterilized by gamma irradiation. It therefore stands to reason that polyethylene components should be implanted shortly after sterilization. To study the influence of implantation on this continued oxidative degradation, we compared the oxidative degradation in a group of 16 retrieved Charnley acetabular components with a group of 9 stored, but

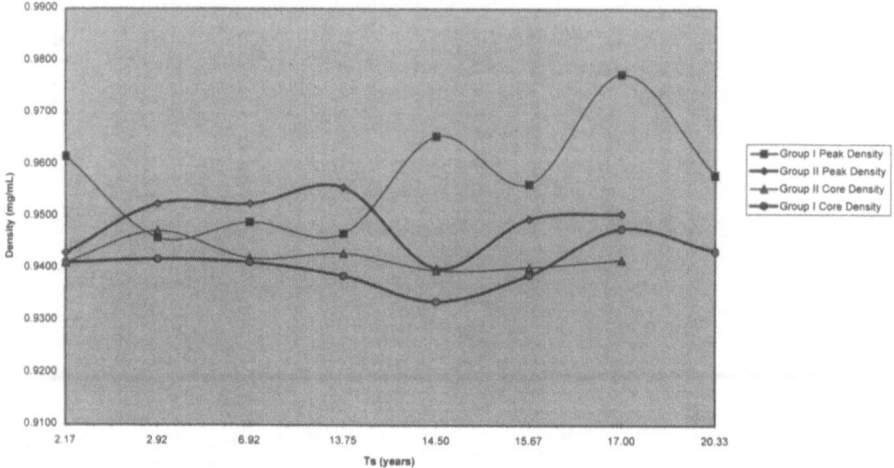

FIG. 5. Polyethylene density versus time in service (T_s). The peak polyethylene density in the group of Charnley cups with a white band (group I) is higher than that in the group of cups without a white band (group II). There is a trend toward a higher density (more oxidation) with time in group I

never used, similar acetabular components [37]. Despite finding that the implants that were never used were newer than the implanted prostheses, the degree of oxidation in the cups that were never implanted was significantly higher. More importantly, there was no significant trend toward worsening oxidation with time within the core polyethylene in the implanted cups. There was a statistically significant trend, however, in the never implanted group, toward worsening oxidation with time. This suggests that implantation of a polyethylene cup tends to delay the progression of oxidative degradation and confirms the need for implanting polyethylene prostheses soon after irradiation.

Mechanisms by Which Oxidation Can Be Reduced

The dose of gamma rays currently used for sterilization of polyethylene is 2.5–4.0 megarads. In a study of the killing potential of gamma rays, we found that a dose of at most 400000 rads was sufficient to kill *Staphylococcus epidermidis*, *Staphylococcus aureus*, *Pseudomonas aerugenosa*, and *Bacillus stearothermophilus*, a spore-forming organism commonly used in sterility checks. In this study, however, the bacterial load was controlled to maintain a realistic bioburden based on bacterial counts done at a manufacturing facility affiliated with our hospital [38]. Sutula et al. [36] showed that a reduction in the gamma radiation dose from 2.5 to 1.25 megarads resulted in a significant reduction in oxidative degradation.

More recently, however, gamma radiation has been found to have beneficial effects, so long as oxygen is eliminated. When polyethylene implants are irradiated in an oxygen-free environment, chain scission continues; however, oxidation cannot occur because of the lack of oxygen free radicals. When irradiation stops, the broken chains coalesce in a manner that causes cross-linking of the polyethylene chains, leading to strengthening of the polyethylene rather than weakening as is seen with oxidation. Many manufacturers have now switched to an oxygen-free environment for irradiating their implants. Whether this makes a clinically significant difference remains to be seen. In the meantime, however, every effort to minimize oxidative degradation should be practiced.

References

1. Rorabeck CH, Bourne RB, Laupacis A, et al (1994) A double-blind study of 250 cases comparing cemented with cementless total hip arthroplasty. Cost-effectiveness and its impact on health-related quality of life. Clin Orthop 298:156–164
2. Jones LC, Hungerford DS (1987) Cement disease. Clin Orthop 225:192–206
3. Brown IW, Ring PA (1985) Osteolytic changes in the upper femoral shaft following porous-coated hip replacement. J Bone Joint Surg [Br] 67:218–221
4. Jasty MJ, Floyd WE III, Schiller AL, et al (1986) Localized osteolysis in stable, non-septic total hip replacement. J Bone Joint Surg [Am] 68:912–919
5. Santavirta S, Hoikka V, Eskola A, et al (1990) Aggressive granulomatous lesions in cementless total hip arthroplasty. J Bone Joint Surg [Br] 72:980–984
6. Smith E, Harris WH (1995) Increasing prevalence of femoral lysis in cementless total hip arthroplasty. J Arthroplasty 10:407–412
7. Howie DW, Vernon RB, Oakeshott R, Manthey B (1988) A rat model of resorption of bone at the cement-bone interface in the presence of polyethylene wear particles. J Bone Joint Surg [Am] 70:257–263
8. Dannenmaier WC, Haynes DW, Nelson CL (1985) Granulomatous reaction and cystic bony destruction associated with high wear rate in a total knee prosthesis. Clin Orthop 198:224–230
9. Willert H-G (1977) Reactions of the articular capsule to wear products of artificial joint prostheses. J Biomed Mater Res 11:157–164
10. Maguire JK Jr, Coscia MF, Lynch MH (1987) Foreign body reaction to polymeric debris following total hip arthroplasty. Clin Orthop 216:213–223
11. Howie DW (1990) Tissue response in relation to type of wear particles around failed hip arthroplasties. J Arthroplasty 5:337–348
12. Charnley J, Halley DK (1975) Rate of wear in total hip replacement. Clin Orthop 112:170–179
13. Mirra JM, Marder RA, Amstutz HC (1982) The pathology of failed total joint arthroplasties. Clin Orthop 170:175–183
14. Revell PA, Weightman B, Freeman MAR, Vernon-Roberts B (1978) The production and biology of polyethylene wear debris. Arch Orthop Trauma Surg 91:167–181
15. García-Cimbrello E, Munuera L (1992) Early and late loosening of the acetabular cup after low-friction arthroplasty. J Bone Joint Surg [Am] 74:1119–1129

16. Feller JA, Kay PR, Hodgkinson JP, et al (1994) Activity and socket wear in Charnley low-friction arthroplasty. J Arthroplasty 9:341–345
17. Livermore J, Ilstrup D, Morrey B (1990) Effect of femoral head size on wear of the polyethylene acetabular component. J Bone Joint Surg [Am] 72:518–528
18. Isaac GH, Wroblewski BM, Atkinson JR, et al (1992) A tribological study of retrieved hip prostheses. Clin Orthop 276:115–125
19. Weightman B, Light D (1986) The effect of the surface finish of alumina and stainless steel on the wear rate of UHMWPE. Biomaterials 7:20–24
20. Buly RL, Huo MH, Salvati EA, et al (1992) Titanium wear debris in failed, cemented, total hip arthroplasty: an analysis of seventy-one cases. J Arthroplasty 7:313–323
21. Huk OL, Bansal M, Betts F, et al (1994) Polyethylene and metal debris generated by non-articulating surfaces of modular acetabular components. J Bone Joint Surg [Br] 76:568–574
22. Wroblewski BM (1993) Charnley low-friction arthroplasty of the hip. Clin Orthop 292:191–201
23. Harris WH, Sledge CB (1990) Total hip and total knee replacement. N Engl J Med 323:725–731
24. Li S, Burstein AH (1994) Ultra high molecular weight polyethylene. J Bone Joint Surg [Am] 76:1080–1090
25. Rimnac CM, Klein RW, Betts F, et al (1994) Post irradiation aging of ultra high molecular weight polyethylene. J Bone Joint Surg [Am] 76:1052–1056
26. Eyerer P, Ke YC (1987) Property changes of UHMW polyethylene hip endoprostheses during implantation. J Biomed Mater Res 21:275–291
27. Streicher RM (1988) Influence of ionizing radiation in air and nitrogen for sterilization of surgical grade polyethylene implants. Radiat Phys Chem 31:693–698
28. Bartel DL, Bicknell VL, Wright TM (1986) The effect of conformity, thickness, and material on stresses in ultra-high molecular weight components for total joint replacement. J Bone Joint Surg [Am] 68:1041–1051
29. Wrona M, Mayor ME, Collier JP, et al (1994) The correlation between fusion defects and damage in tibial polyethylene bearings. Clin Orthop 299:92–103
30. Gomez-Barrena E, Chang J-D, Li S, Rimnac CM, Salvati EA (1996) The role of polyethylene properties in osteolysis in total hip replacement. Instrum Course Lect 45:171–197
31. Goméz-Barrena E, Masri BA, Furman BD, et al (1996) Polyethylene wear in Charnley acetabular components: the interaction between clinical factors and material properties. Presented at the 63rd annual meeting of the American Academy of Orthopaedic Surgeons, Atlanta, GA
32. Masri BA, Goméz-Barrena E, Furman BD, et al (1996) The nature of subsurface defects in retrieved Charnley acetabular components. Presented at the 63rd annual meeting of the American Academy of Orthopaedic Surgeons, Atlanta, GA
33. Li S, Burstein AH (1997) Current concepts review: ultra-high molecular weight polyethylene. The material and its use in total joint implants. J Bone Joint Surg [Am] 76:1080–1090
34. Sun DC, Stark C, Dumbelton JH (1994) Characterization and comparison of compression molded and machined UHMWPE components. Trans Orthop Res Soc 19:173
35. Landy M, Walker PS (1985) Wear in condylar replacement knees. A 10 year follow-up. Trans Orthop Res Soc 10:96

36. Sutula LC, Collier JP, Saum KA, Currier BH, Currier JH, Sanford WM, Mayor MB, Wooding RE, Sperling DK, Williams IR, et al (1995) The Otto Aufranc Award. Impact of gamma sterilization on clinical performance of polyethylene in the hip. Clin Orthop 319:28–40
37. Masri BA, Goméz-Barrena E, Furman BD, et al (1996) A comparison of in vivo and in vitro oxidation of Charnley acetabular components. Presented at the 63rd annual meeting of the American Academy of Orthopaedic Surgeons, Atlanta, GA
38. Duus LC, Masri BA, Salvati EA, et al (1996) Optimal dosage of gamma irradiation for the sterilization of UHMWPE used in total joint replacements. Presented at the 1996 Orthopaedic Research Society annual meeting, Atlanta, GA

Responses in the Underlying Bone During Migration of Hydroxyapatite Grafts in the Growing Rabbit

TOSHITAKA NAKAMURA[1] and AKIHIRO YANAGISAWA[2]

Summary. To clarify whether local bone turnover underneath hydroxyapatite grafts differs in nasal and mandibular bones, a single porous hydroxyapatite block was implanted on the respective surface of the right nasal bone and the mandibular ramus in 40 rabbits at the age of 4 weeks. The undecalcified sections of the bone specimens underneath the graft were histomorphometrically measured under a light microscope. In all grafted specimens, the hydroxyapatite graft was united, but sinking of the grafts proceeded during 16 weeks. In the nasal bone, bone area density beneath the graft was significantly decreased within 3 weeks and continued to be diminished thereafter. In the mandibular ramus, however, bone area density was maintained at a similar level to that of the sham-operated side. In the nasal bone, the parameters of mineralizing surface and bone formation rates obtained by fluorescence labels were significantly reduced. In the mandibular bone, however, these parameters of bone formation were significantly increased. Mineral apposition rates were reduced in either bone. The parameters of osteoclasts obtained by tartrate-resistant acid phosphatase (TRAP) staining were significantly increased in both the nasal and mandibular bones. These data clearly demonstrated that bone density and local turnover underneath the osteoblast recruitment in the face of increased bone resorption by the grafts depend on the intrinsic factors of individual bones. Osteoblast functions at a cellular level, however, appeared to be commonly disturbed in the neighboring bone of the hydroxyapatite grafts.

Key Words. Hydroxyapatite, Bone density, Osteoblast, Osteoclast, Histomorphometry

---

[1] Department of Orthopedics, University of Occupational and Environmental Health, 1-1, Iseigaoka, Yahatanishi-ku, Kitakyushu 807, Japan.
[2] Department of Plastic and Reconstructive Surgery, Nagaski University School of Medicine, Nagasaki, Japan.

Introduction

Loosening or migration of implants is always associated with reduction in bone mass in the periimplant region. Because the reduction in bone mass is the sequel of bone turnover and the negative balance of the amounts of bone formed and resorbed at the bone surfaces [1], data on local bone formation and resorption in the juxtaprosthetic bone tissue may provide useful information for preventing loosening and migration of the implants.

Hydroxyapatite implant has been used as a substitute for autologous bone graft to fill bone defects and contour deformities for plastic and orthopedic surgeries in adults [2,3]. However, there is a potential risk for the implant onlays to sink into the underlying bone [4]. Information is scant on bone metabolism in underlying bone when the implants migrate into the bone. We have established an animal model of implant migration by using rabbits that received hydroxyapatite grafts on their nasal bone [5]. In this model, when the microporous hydroxyapatite-tricalcium phosphate composite was placed subperiosteally on the nasal bone, the implants did sink into the bone tissue. Then, we performed experiments of histomorphometric analysis on bone density and turnover in the underlying bone tissues for nasal and mandibular bones that received the hydroxyapatite onlay grafts [6].

Because the use of porous hydroxyapatite bone graft causes induction of osteoclasts [7], it is expected that the intrinsic factors for the individual bone and bone marrow cells may be related to bone density and turnover in underlying bone tissues during migration of the hydroxyapatite grafts. The purpose of this chapter is to review the effects of hydroxyapatite onlays on bone density and turnover in the underlying bone tissues in the nasal and mandibular bone.

Different Modeling and Turnover Activities in the Nasal Bone and the Mandibular Ramus

The nasal bone is known to resorb materials deposited onto its periosteal surface and endosteal region. No muscle attaches to the nasal bone. Also, mechanical stimuli seem to be minimal on the nasal bone. The mandibular ramus, on the other hand, is resorptive onto its outer surface [8,9]. The mandibular bone has strong masseter muscles that receive a compressive force in daily movements of chewing.

Initially, we investigated the basal histomorphometrical conditions of the spongiosae for the nasal bone and the mandibular ramus in growing rabbits at the age of 4 weeks. Undecalcified bone specimens were embedded in methacrylate resin, and sections were studied. Osteoclasts were identified by tartrate-resistant acid phosphatase (TRAP) staining, and osteoblasts were observed by counterstaining with Meyer's hematoxylin. The trabecular osteo-

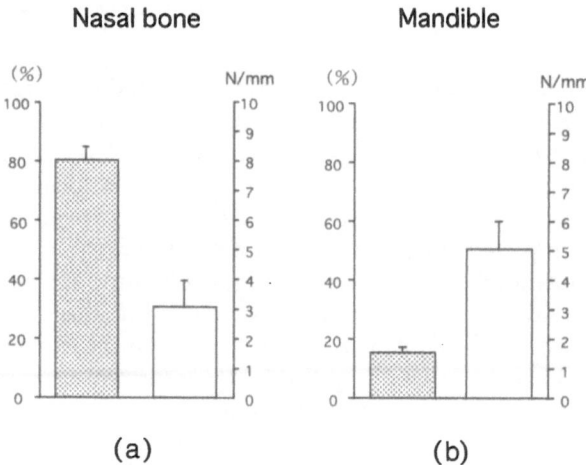

FIG. 1a,b. Parameters of osteoblast surface (*dotted bars*) and osteoclast number (*white bars*) in the nasal bone (**a**) and the mandibular ramus (**b**) in rabbits at the age of 4 weeks (means ± SD)

clast number values per bone perimeter (Oc.N/mm) in the mandibular bone were significantly larger than the values in the nasal bone, but trabecular osteoblast surface values (Ob.S/BS) in the nasal bone were significantly larger than the values in the mandibular bone (Fig. 1). The mean value of trabecular bone formation rate (BFR/BS) obtained by fluorescence labeling was 2.5 ± 0.1 in the nasal bone, whereas the value was $0.4 \pm 0.1 \mu m \cdot \%/day$ in the mandibular bone. Thus, it is expected that local bone turnover is higher in the nasal bone than in the mandibular bone.

Implants and Surgeries

Hydroxyapatite blocks 8 mm long, 4 mm wide, and 3 mm high with a porosity of 55%, sintered at 1200°C (Asahi Optical, Tokyo, Japan), were used. The blocks contained a pore structure of 100–500 μm with an interconnected microporous matrix.

A single porous hydroxyapatite onlay was implanted surgically on the respective surface of the right nasal bone and the mandibular ramus in 40 rabbits. The nasal bone was exposed through a midline incision and the hydroxyapatite implant was laid on the center of right bone after elevation of the periosteum. The longest side of the hydroxyapatite block was placed parallel with the internasal suture, and the height of the implant was set 2 mm from the bone surface. For the mandibular ramus, the periosteum was reflected from the edge of the mandibular angle after cutting the skin over the submandibular region. The hydroxyapatite block was placed on the outer surface of the mandibular ramus with its lateral side parallel with the mandibular plane (Fig. 2). The periosteum was redraped over the implant, and the wound was closed with sutures. Sham surgery including only the reflection of the periosteum was performed on the contralateral sides of the bone, respectively.

Assessments

The rabbits were killed at 3, 6, 9, 12, or 16 weeks postoperatively after respective bone labeling with tetracycline and alizarin complexone 9 and 4 days before sacrifice. The specimens were removed and embedded in methacrylate resin. Undecalcified ground sections, $40\,\mu$m in thickness, were prepared and used for contact microradiography. Serial 5-μm-thick unstained sections were used for fluoroscopic observation. Some sections were stained for TRAP activity and counterstained with hematoxylin [10]. In these sections, bone–bone marrow interfaces in the entire area within $200\,\mu$m below the base of the hydroxyapatite graft were measured. The interfaces in the counter area on the sham-operated contralateral side also were measured.

To obtain the parameter of bone density in the total bone tissue area, the bone area was measured within the area and the percentage of bone area was calculated. Mineral apposition rate (MAR, μm/day) and mineralizing surface (MS/BS, %) were obtained, and the bone formation rate (BFR/BS, μm·%/day) was calculated. Osteoblast surface (Ob.S/BS, %) and osteoclast number (Oc.N/BS, /mm) were measured on TRAP-stained sections. These parameters were determined according to the report of the ASBMR Histomorphometry Nomenclature Committee [11].

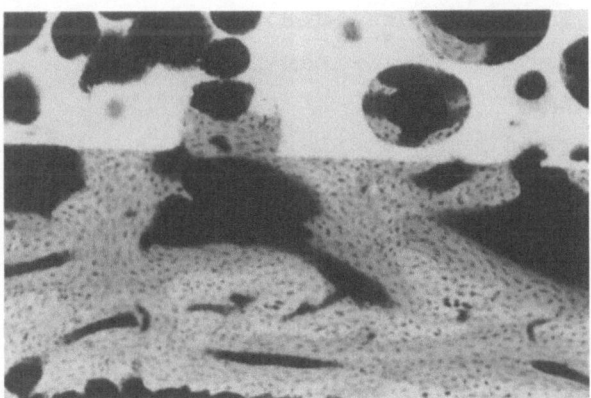

Fig. 2. Contact microradiographs of the mandibular ramus. The *upper region* represents the hydroxyapatite grafts. The graft was united directly with the underlying bone tissue 6 weeks after surgery

Sinking of Hydroxyapatite Grafts

In all grafted specimens, the hydroxyapatite matrix was united directly with the underlying bone tissue, and no intervening fibrous layer was observed (see Fig. 2). In the nasal bone, sinking of the graft was observed from 3 weeks after surgery, with further progressive increases in the area of migration occurring throughout the experimental period (Fig. 3a). Sinking of the graft in the mandibular ramus became apparent at 6 weeks after surgery, and the area of migration increased thereafter (Fig. 3b).

Local Bone Density and Turnover Beneath the Hydroxyapatite

In the nasal bone, bone density beneath the graft was significantly decreased within 3 weeks and continued to diminish thereafter (Fig. 4a). In the mandibular ramus, however, bone area density was maintained at a similar level to that of the sham-operated side at 16 weeks (Fig. 4b).

In the nasal bone, hydroxyapatite grafts caused significant reductions in osteoblast surface (Ob.S/BS) (Fig. 5a). Mineral apposition rate was significantly decreased in 3 weeks on the grafted surface and continued to decrease

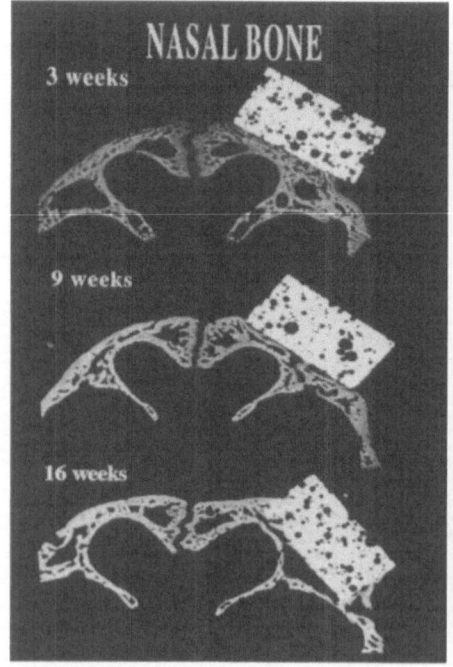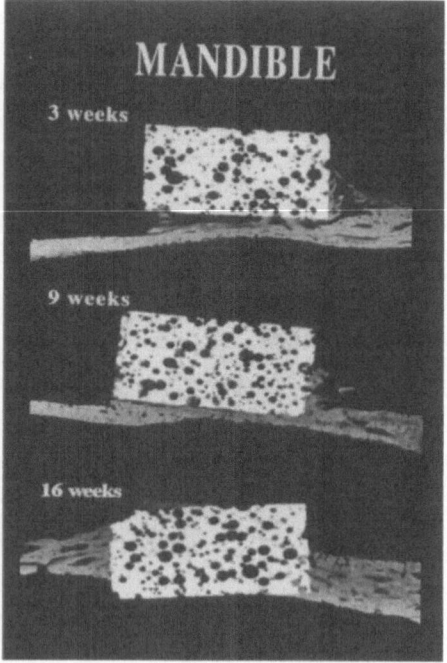

a   b

FIG. 3a,b. Contact microradiographs show the migration of hydroxyapatite grafts into the underlying bone. **a** Nasal bone; **b** mandibular ramus

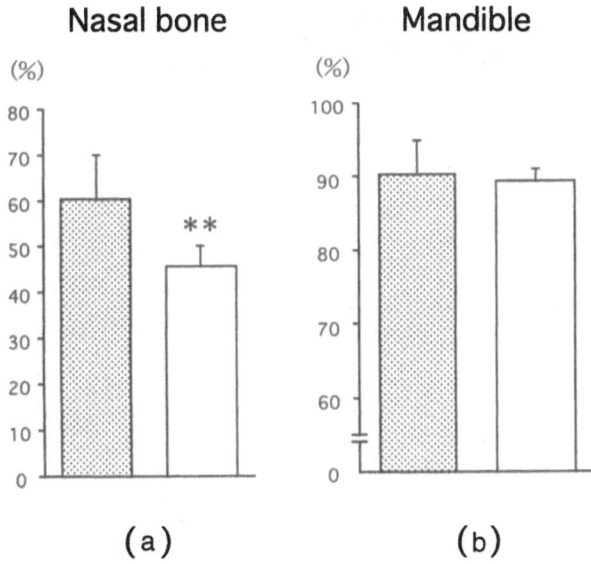

FIG. 4a,b. Bone density (trabecular bone volume) values at 16 weeks post surgery in the bone underlying hydroxyapatite grafts in the nasal bone (**a**) and the mandibular ramus (**b**). *Dotted bars*, sham-operated; *white bars*, grafted; **, $P < .01$ (means $\pm$ SD)

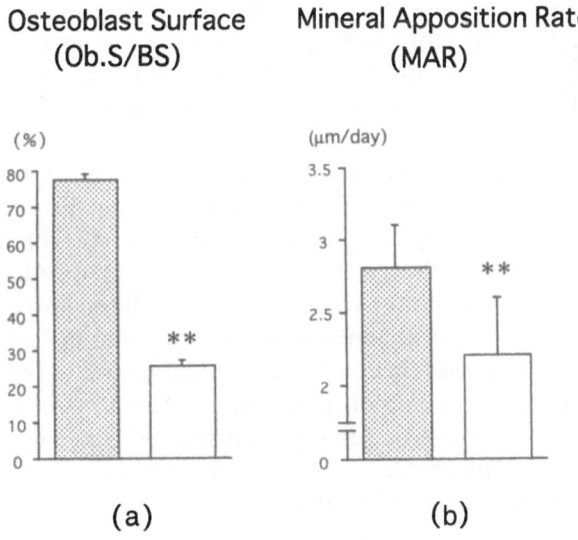

FIG. 5a,b. Parameters of trabecular osteoblasts (**a**) and mineral apposition rates (**b**) in bone tissue underneath hydroxyapatite grafts in the nasal bone. *Dotted bars*, sham-operated; *white bars*, grafted; **, $P < .01$ (means $\pm$ SD)

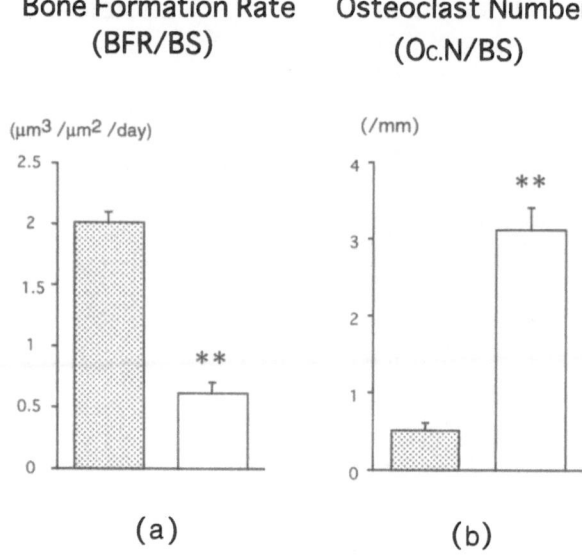

FIG. 6a,b. Parameters of trabecular bone formation rates (**a**) and osteoclast number (**b**) in bone tissue underneath hydroxyapatite grafts in the nasal bone, *Dotted bars*, sham-operated; *white bars*, grafted; **, $P < .01$ (means ± SD)

until 9 weeks after surgery (Fig. 5b). The bone formation rate (BFR/BS) values were also significantly reduced throughout the experimental period (Fig. 6a). The osteoclast number (Oc.N/BS) values were significantly increased 3 weeks postopertatively (Fig. 6b). The increases were maintained until the end of the experiment.

In the mandibular ramus, osteoblast surface (Ob.S/BS) values were significantly increased postoperatively. The parameter of bone formation remained elevated thereafter (Fig. 7a). Mineral apposition rate was diminished significantly within 6 weeks on the grafted side and remained reduced thereafter (Fig. 7b). The bone formation rate (BFR/BS) values, however, increased significantly and were larger than the values of the sham-operated side in 3, 6, and 9 weeks (Fig. 8a). Differences in bone formation rates between the grafted and sham-operated sides were not significant at 12 or 16 weeks. The values of osteoclast number (Oc.N/BS) on the grafted side were significantly increased at 3 weeks (Fig. 8b). The elevated values for the parameters of the osteoclasts remained elevated until the end of the experiment.

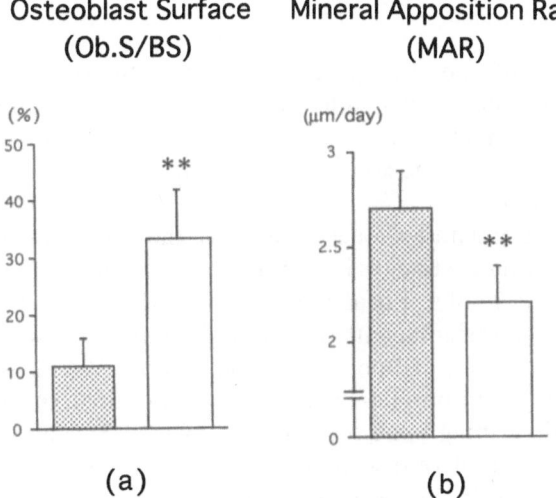

FIG. 7a,b. Parameters of trabecular osteoblast (**a**) and mineral apposition rates (**b**) in bone tissue underneath hydroxyapatite grafts in the mandibular ramus. *Dotted bars*, sham-operated; *white bars*, grafted; **, $P < .01$ (means ± SD)

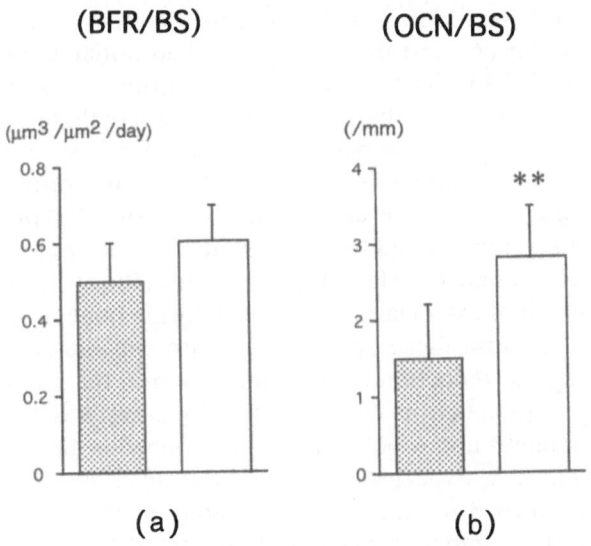

FIG. 8a,b. Parameters of trabecular bone formation (**a**) and osteoclast number (**b**) in bone underneath hydroxyapatite grafts in the mandibular ramus. *Dotted bars*, sham-operated; *white bars*, grafted; **, $P < .01$ (means ± SD)

Discussion

The current data confirmed that porous hydroxyapatite onlay grafts sink into the underlying nasal bone and mandibular ramus in growing rabbits. However, while bone density beneath the hydroxyapatite onlays was reduced in the nasal bone, it was maintained at the level of the contralateral sham-operated side in the mandibular ramus.

Histomorphometric data for local turnover of the underlying bones seemed to be compatible with the changes in their bone density for both the nasal bone and the mandibular ramus. Local bone resorption beneath the grafted hydroxyapatite block was significantly increased in both the nasal and mandibular bone. The uncoupling of bone formation to bone resorption apparently induced the reduction in bone density of underlying bone in the nasal bone. The parameters describing bone formation such as trabecular osteoblast surface and bone formation rate were significantly reduced in the face of the increases in osteoclasts in the nasal bone. However, it seems that bone density in the mandibular ramus was maintained by a concomitant increase in bone formation. The values of osteoblast surface indicated the extent of the area where osteoblasts are engaging in bone formation at bone and bone marrow interface. Thus, the number of osteoblasts underneath the hydroxyapatite graft is decreased in the nasal bone but increased in the mandibular ramus. Because the changes in surface parameters of resorption and formation were observed 3 weeks postoperatively, the recruitment of osteoblasts and osteoclasts from bone marrow cells would be modified within the early postimplantation period.

It has been well observed that the hydroxyapatite block induces direct bone formation on the surface and that resorption then initiates turnover on the osteoclastic bone [12,13]. The current data confirmed that the number of osteoclasts was increased 3 weeks after surgery underneath the hydroxyapatite onlays in the nasal bone and the mandibular ramus. Because osteoclastic bone resorption activates the bone surfaces, the hydroxyapatite grafts seem to stimulate the remodeling process in the underlying bone. Osteoclast production from bone marrow cells is now thought to be regulated by many cytokines, such as interleukins and tumor necrosis factors [14,15]. Thus, the hydroxyapatite grafts may cause induction of osteoclasts in the neighboring bone mediated through these cytokines. Because these cytokines are also capable of reducing bone formation [15,16], the reduction of bone formation in the nasal bone underneath the hydroxyapatite grafts may be caused by these cytokines.

Because the mineral apposition rates were reduced in the bone tissue beneath the implants, it is expected that osteoblast functions at a cellular level are commonly disturbed in either the nasal bone or the mandibular ramus. However, while the number of osteoblasts recruited onto the bone surface apparently was reduced in the nasal bone, it was increased in the mandibular ramus. The nasal bone is depository onto its periosteal surface, whereas the mandibular ramus is resorptive. The current data suggest that bone resorption is dominant in the local turnover of the mandibular ramus, while bone formation is dominant in the nasal bone. These differences in basal bone turnover may be one of the factors determining the changes in turnover and density of the neighboring bone tissues after transplanting the hydroxyapatite graft. Another explanation relates to mechanical stress. As the mandibular bone, used in eating, is the "biting bone" covered by the strong masseters, it is possible that compressive force on the grafted region facilitated osteoblast recruitment from the bone marrow cells.

By reviewing the data, it is obvious that direct bone fixation of the hydroxyapatite grafts does not eliminate possible migration in the growing animal. Because bone resorption initiates remodeling of the trabecular structure, migration of the implants would be initiated by increased bone resorption beneath the graft. However, because bone density in the neighboring bone appeared to depend on reduced bone formation, maintenance of bone formation would be important to prevent reduction in bone density around the grafts. The use of compressive force to the grafted bone may be helpful in preventing osteopenia in the neighboring bone of hydroxyapatite grafts.

References

1. Motoie PA, Nakamura T, O'uchi N, et al (1995) Effects of the bisphosphonate YM175 on bone mineral density, strength, structure and turnover in ovariectomized beagles on concomitant dietary calcium restriction. J Bone Miner Res 10:91–920
2. Salyer KE, Hall CD (1989) Porous hydroxyapatite as an onlay bone-graft substitute for maxillofacial surgery. Plast Reconstr Surg 84:236–244
3. Oonishi H, Yamamoto M, Ishimaru H, et al (1989) The effect of hydroxyapatite coating on bone growth into porous titanium alloy implants. J Bone Joint Surg 71:213–216
4. Fearon JA, Munro A (1995) Observations on the use of rigid fixation for craniofacial deformities in infants and young children. Plast Reconstr Surg 95:634–639
5. Arakaki M, Yamashita S, Mutaf M, et al (1995) Onlay silicone and hydroxyapatite-tricalciumphosphate composite (HAP-TCP) blocks interfere with nasal bone growth in rabbits. Cleft Palate-Craniofacial J 32:282–289
6. Yanagisawa A, Nakamura T, Arakaki M, et al (1997) Migration of hydroxyapatite onlays into the mandible and nasal bone and local bone turnover in growing rabbits. Plast Reconstr Surg 99:1972–1977
7. Basle MF, Chappard D, Grixon F, et al (1993) Osteoclastic resorption of Ca-P biomaterials implanted in rabbit bone. Calcif Tissue Int 53:348–342
8. Bang S, Enlow DH (1967) Postnatal growth of the rabbit mandible. Arch Oral Biol 12:993–996
9. Zins JE, Kusiak JF, Whitaker LA, et al (1984) The influence of the recipient site on bone grafts to the face. Plast Reconstr Surg 73:371–381
10. Murakami H, Nakamura T, Tsurukami H, et al (1994) Effects of tiludronate on bone mass, structure, and turnover at the epiphyseal, primary, and secondary spongiosa in the proximal tibia of growing rats after sciatic neurectomy. J Bone Miner Res 9:1355–1364

11. Parfitt AM, Drezner MK, Glorieux FH, et al (1987) Bone histomorphometry: standardization of nomenclature, symbols, and units. Report of the ASBMR Histomorphometry Nomenclature Committee. J Bone Miner Res 2:595–610
12. Holmes RE (1979) Bone regeneration within a coralline hydroxyapatite implant. Plast Reconstr Surg 63:626–633
13. Uchida A, Nade SML, McCartney ER, et al (1984) A comparative study of three different porous ceramics. J Bone Joint Surg 66B:269–278
14. Nguyen L, Dewhrist FE, Hauschka PV, et al (1991) Interleukin-1 beta stimulates bone resorption and inhibits bone formation in vivo. Lymphokine Cytokine Res 10:15–21
15. Bertolini DR, Nedwin GE, Bringman TS, et al (1986) Stimulation of bone resorption and inhibition of bone formation in vitro by human tumor necrosis factors. Nature (Lond) 319:516–518
16. Stashenko P, Dewhrist FE, Rooney ML, et al (1987) Interleukin-1 beta is a potent inhibitor of bone formation in vitro. J Bone Miner Res 2:559–565

Key Word Index